PATHOLOGY AND GENETICS

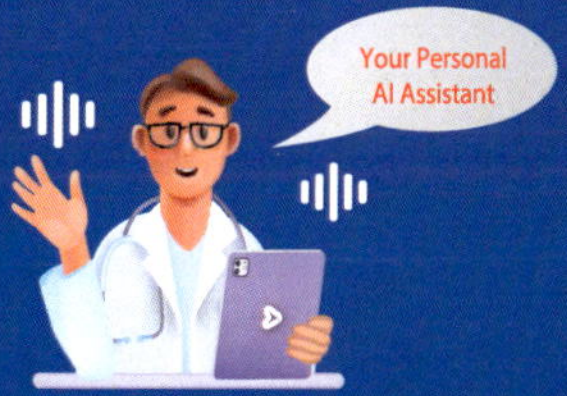

for Nurses

PATHOLOGY AND GENETICS
for Nurses

A Clinically Integrated Approach with Case Scenarios and Clinical Applications

Semester III and IV

As per the Revised INC Syllabus

FOURTH EDITION

K Swaminathan MD MPhil (HPE)
Professor and Head
Department of Pathology
Tirunelveli Medical College
Tirunelveli, Tamil Nadu, India

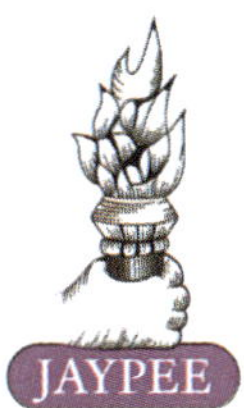

JAYPEE BROTHERS MEDICAL PUBLISHERS
The Health Sciences Publisher
New Delhi | London

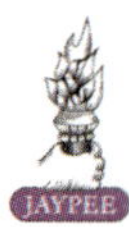

Jaypee Brothers Medical Publishers (P) Ltd

Headquarters
Jaypee Brothers Medical Publishers (P) Ltd
EMCA House, 23/23-B
Ansari Road, Daryaganj
New Delhi 110 002, India
Landline: +91-11-23272143, +91-11-23272703
+91-11-23282021, +91-11-23245672
Email: jaypee@jaypeebrothers.com

Corporate Office
Jaypee Brothers Medical Publishers (P) Ltd
4838/24, Ansari Road, Daryaganj
New Delhi 110 002, India
Phone: +91-11-43574357
Fax: +91-11-43574314
Email: jaypee@jaypeebrothers.com

Overseas Office
J.P. Medical Ltd
83 Victoria Street, London
SW1H 0HW (UK)
Phone: +44 20 3170 8910
Fax: +44 (0)20 3008 6180
Email: info@jpmedpub.com

Website: www.jaypeebrothers.com
Website: www.jaypeedigital.com

Inquiries for bulk sales may be solicited at: jaypee@jaypeebrothers.com

Pathology and Genetics for Nurses

First Edition: 2009

Second Edition: 2010

Third Edition: 2021

Fourth Edition: **2024** Reprint : **2025**

ISBN: 978-93-5696-856-1

Printed in India at Rajkamal Electric Press, Kundli, Haryana.

Preface to the Fourth Edition

In this edition, I have tried to explain the basic concepts of "General Pathology" with a few more illustrations. Another interesting feature of this book is that every chapter has a list of self-assessment questions which includes essay type questions, short answer questions, and multiple-choice questions. Yet another special feature of this edition is the case-based multiple choice questions at the end of all the major chapters. This will of immense help to the learner to correlate the pathology with relevant clinical features. This will make the reading more interesting and also paves a way for self-directed learning which may be profound help while preparing for the examination. Moreover, every chapter begins with a set of learning outcomes and ends with summary points to ponder which will make the learning experience holistic.

A lot of changes have been made in the text on genetics incorporating various advances in the field of genetics.

Have a happy reading.

K Swaminathan

Preface to the First Edition

Pathology is a medical science that deals with the scientific study of disease with special reference to the causative factors, development of the disease process, morphological alterations in the organs and clinical implications as a result of the disease.

The study of pathology provides an insight into the disease processes and their effects. Pathology is a very essential link between the basic medical sciences and the clinical disciplines. A proper understanding of pathology is mandatory to have a clear idea about the diseases.

This book is designed to provide a basic knowledge in pathology for the paramedical nursing students, who will be handling sick patients in the hospital wards.

For a logical understanding, this book is divided into five sections. Section 1 deals with General Pathology which provides a deep knowledge about the basic concepts of cellular pathology. Sections 2 deals with Systemic Pathology. It gives knowledge about the application of the concepts in General Pathology to specific organ systems.

Sections 3 and 4 deal with Clinical Hematology and Clinical Pathology and provide an overview on various methodologies of basic laboratory procedures, observation and interpretation of the laboratory investigations used in the diagnosis of various diseases. This section will be of immense help to the nursing students especially with regard to the bedside investigations.

Section 5 on genetics in nursing equips healthcare professionals with vital knowledge to assist patients in comprehending and managing genetic factors affecting their health

Have a happy reading!

K Swaminathan

Acknowledgments

I thank the Almighty for giving me enough courage and strength to take up this project.

I immensely thank all my teachers and seniors who have inspired me to take this specialty of pathology and their enduring guidance throughout this venture.

I express my gratitude with love to my dear wife, Dr Priya Swaminathan and my daughter Gigi Swaminathan for their consistent help and encouragement during the tenure as well as in preparing a few of the illustrations used in this book.

I profusely thank Ms Samina Khan (Executive Assistant to Director Publishing) for giving me this opportunity to be associated with them in improving the earlier version of this book.

I extend my heartfelt gratitude to Ms Jitika Royal (Content Strategist—Nursing) for her invaluable support, dedication, and insightful contributions throughout this book.

I am very grateful to Shri Jitendar P Vij (Group Chairman), Mr Ankit Vij (Managing Director), Mr MS Mani (Group President), Dr Madhu Choudhary (Director—Educational Publishing), Ms Pooja Bhandari [Director-Production (Books and Journals)], Ms Sunita Katla (Executive Assistant to Group Chairman and Publishing Manager), Mr Ajay Kumar Sharma [DGM (Books and Journals)], Mr Sabyasachi Hazra (Commissioning Editor, Kolkata Branch), Mr Rajesh Sharma (Production Coordinator), Ms Seema Dogra (Cover Visualizer), Mr Kulwant Singh (Typesetter), Mr Vakil Khan (Proofreader), Mr Radhe Shyam Singh (Graphic Designer), and team members of M/s Jaypee Brothers Medical Publishers (P) Ltd, New Delhi, India, for all their support to work in this project and make it a success.

Contents

Unit	Time (hours	Learning Outcomes	Content	Teaching/ Learning Activities	Assessment Methods
			• Wound healing • **Neoplasia:** Nomenclature, normal and cancer cell, benign and malignant tumors, carcinoma in situ, tumor metastasis: general mechanism, routes of spread and examples of each route • **Circulatory disturbances:** Thrombosis, embolism, shock • **Disturbance of body fluids and electrolytes:** Edema, transudates and exudates		
II	5 (T)	Explain pathological changes in disease conditions of various systems	**Special Pathology** **Pathological changes in disease conditions of selected systems:** **1. Respiratory system** » Pulmonary infections: pneumonia, lung abscess, pulmonary tuberculosis » Chronic obstructive pulmonary disease: Chronic bronchitis, emphysema, bronchial asthma, bronchiectasis » Tumors of lungs 2. Cardiovascular system » Atherosclerosis » Ischemia and infarction. » Rheumatic heart disease » Infective endocarditis **3. Gastrointestinal tract** » Peptic ulcer disease (gastric and Duodenal ulcer) » Gastritis—*H. pylori* infection » Oral mucosa: Oral leukoplakia, Squamous cell carcinoma » Esophageal cancer » Gastric cancer » Intestinal: Typhoid ulcer, Inflammatory bowel disease (Crohn's disease and ulcerative colitis), colorectal cancer **4. Liver, gallbladder and Pancreas** » Liver: Hepatitis, amoebic liver abscess, Cirrhosis of liver » Gallbladder: Cholecystitis. » Pancreas: Pancreatitis » Tumors of liver, gallbladder and pancreas	• Lecture • Discussion • Explain using slides, X-rays and scans • Visit to pathology lab, endoscopy unit and OT	• Short answer • Objective type

Syllabus

PATHOLOGY-I

PLACEMENT: III SEMESTER

THEORY: 1 Credit (20 hours) (includes lab hours also)

DESCRIPTION: This course is designed to enable students to acquire knowledge of pathology of various disease conditions, understanding of genetics, its role in causation and management of defects and diseases and to apply this knowledge in practice of nursing.

COMPETENCIES: On completion of the course, the students will be able to

1. Apply the knowledge of pathology in understanding the deviations from normal to abnormal pathology.
2. Rationalize the various laboratory investigations in diagnosing pathological disorders.
3. Demonstrate the understanding of the methods of collection of blood, body cavity fluids, urine and feces for various tests.
4. Apply the knowledge of genetics in understanding the various pathological disorders.
5. Appreciate the various manifestations in patients with diagnosed genetic abnormalities.
6. Rationalize the specific diagnostic tests in the detection of genetic abnormalities.
7. Demonstrate the understanding of various services related to genetics.

COURSE OUTLINE

T – Theory

Unit	*Time (hours*	*Learning Outcomes*	*Content*	*Teaching/ Learning Activities*	*Assessment Methods*
I	8 (T)	Define the common terms used in pathology Identify the deviations from normal to abnormal structure and functions of body system	**Introduction** • Importance of the study of pathology • Definition of terms in pathology • **Cell injury:** Etiology, pathogenesis of reversible and irreversible cell injury, Necrosis, Gangrene • **Cellular adaptations:** Atrophy, Hypertrophy, Hyperplasia, Metaplasia, Dysplasia, apoptosis • **Inflammation:** » Acute inflammation (Vascular and Cellular events, systemic effects of acute inflammation) » Chronic inflammation (Granulomatous inflammation, systemic effects of chronic inflammation)	• Lecture • Discussion • Explain using slides • Explain with clinical scenarios	• Short answer • Objective type

Unit	*Time (hours*	*Learning Outcomes*	*Content*	*Teaching/ Learning Activities*	*Assessment Methods*
			5. Skeletal system » Bone: Bone healing, osteoporosis, osteomyelitis, tumors » Joints: arthritis—rheumatoid arthritis and osteoarthritis **6. Endocrine system** » Diabetes mellitus » Goiter » Carcinoma thyroid		
III	7 (T)	Describe various laboratory tests in assessment and monitoring of disease conditions	**Hematological tests for the diagnosis of blood disorders** ◆ Blood tests: Hemoglobin, white cell and platelet counts, PCV, ESR ◆ Coagulation tests: Bleeding time (BT), prothrombin time (PT), activated partial prothrombin time (APTT) ◆ Blood chemistry ◆ Blood bank: » Blood grouping and cross matching » Blood components » Plasmapheresis » Transfusion reactions Note: Few lab hours can be planned for observation and visits (Less than 1 credit, lab hours are not specified separately)	◆ Lecture ◆ Discussion ◆ Visit to clinical lab, biochemistry lab and blood bank	◆ Short answer ◆ Objective type

PATHOLOGY - II AND GENETICS

PLACEMENT: IV SEMESTER

THEORY: 1 Credit (20 hours) (Includes lab hours also)

DESCRIPTION: This course is designed to enable students to acquire knowledge of pathology of various disease conditions, understanding of genetics, its role in causation and management of defects and diseases and to apply this knowledge in practice of nursing.

COMPETENCIES: On completion of the course, the students will be able to

1. Apply the knowledge of pathology in understanding the deviations from normal to abnormal pathology.
2. Rationalize the various laboratory investigations in diagnosing pathological disorders.
3. Demonstrate the understanding of the methods of collection of blood, body cavity fluids, urine and feces for various tests.
4. Apply the knowledge of genetics in understanding the various pathological disorders.
5. Appreciate the various manifestations in patients with diagnosed genetic abnormalities.
6. Rationalize the specific diagnostic tests in the detection of genetic abnormalities.
7. Demonstrate the understanding of various services related to genetics.

COURSE OUTLINE

T - Theory

Unit	*Time (hours*	*Learning Outcomes*	*Content*	*Teaching/ Learning Activities*	*Assessment Methods*
I	5 (T)	Explain pathological changes in disease conditions of various systems	**Special pathology: Pathological changes in disease conditions of selected systems** **1. Kidneys and urinary tract** » Glomerulonephritis » Pyelonephritis » Renal calculi » Cystitis » Renal cell carcinoma » Renal failure (acute and chronic) **2. Male genital systems** » Cryptorchidism » Testicular atrophy » Prostatic hyperplasia » Carcinoma penis and Prostate. **3. Female genital system** » Carcinoma cervix » Carcinoma of endometrium » Uterine fibroids » Vesicular mole and Choriocarcinoma » Ovarian cyst and tumors	• Lecture • Discussion • Explain using slides, X-rays and scans • Visit to pathology lab, endoscopy unit and OT	• Short answer • Objective type

Unit	Time (hours	Learning Outcomes	Content	Teaching/ Learning Activities	Assessment Methods
			4. Breast » Fibrocystic changes » Fibroadenoma » Carcinoma of the breast **5. Central nervous system** » Meningitis » Encephalitis » Stroke » Tumors of CNS		
II	5 (T)	Describe the laboratory tests for examination of body cavity fluids, urine and feces	**Clinical Pathology** ◆ Examination of body cavity fluids: » Methods of collection and examination of CSF and other body cavity fluids (sputum, wound discharge) specimen for various clinical pathology, biochemistry and microbiology tests ◆ Analysis of semen: » Sperm count, motility and morphology and their importance in infertility ◆ Urine: » Physical characteristics, analysis, culture and sensitivity ◆ Feces: » Characteristics » Stool examination: occult blood, ova, parasite and cyst, reducing substance, etc. » Methods and collection of urine and feces for various tests	◆ Lecture ◆ Discussion ◆ Visit to clinical lab and biochemistry lab	◆ Short answer ◆ Objective type

GENETICS COURSE OUTLINE

T - Theory

Unit	*Time (hours*	*Learning Outcomes*	*Content*	*Teaching/ Learning Activities*	*Assessment Methods*
I	2 (T)	Explain nature, principles and perspectives of heredity	**Introduction:** ◆ Practical application of genetics in nursing ◆ Impact of genetic condition on families ◆ Review of cellular division: Mitosis and meiosis ◆ Characteristics and structure of genes ◆ Chromosomes: Sex determination ◆ Chromosomal aberrations ◆ Patterns of inheritance ◆ Mendelian theory of inheritance ◆ Multiple allots and blood groups ◆ Sex linked inheritance ◆ Mechanism of inheritance ◆ Errors in transmission (mutation)	◆ Lecture ◆ Discussion ◆ Explain using slides	◆ Short answer ◆ Objective type
II	2 (T)	Explain maternal, prenatal and genetic influences on development of defects and diseases	**Maternal, prenatal and genetic influences on development of defects and diseases** ◆ Conditions affecting the mother: genetic and infections ◆ Consanguinity atopy ◆ Prenatal nutrition and food allergies ◆ Maternal age ◆ Maternal drug therapy ◆ Prenatal testing and diagnosis ◆ Effect of radiation, drugs and chemicals ◆ Infertility ◆ Spontaneous abortion ◆ Neural tube defects and the role of folic acid in lowering the risks ◆ Down syndrome (Trisomy 21)	◆ Lecture ◆ Discussion ◆ Explain using slides	◆ Short answer ◆ Objective type
III	2 (T)	Explain the screening methods for genetic defects and diseases in neonates and children	**Genetic testing in the neonates and children** ◆ Screening for » Congenital abnormalities » Developmental delay » Dysmorphism	◆ Lecture ◆ Discussion ◆ Explain using slides	◆ Short answer ◆ Objective type

Unit	*Time (hours*	*Learning Outcomes*	*Content*	*Teaching/ Learning Activities*	*Assessment Methods*
IV	2 (T)	Identify genetic disorders in adolescents and adults	**Genetic conditions of adolescents and adults** • Cancer genetics: Familial cancer • Inborn errors of metabolism • Blood group alleles and hematological disorder • Genetic hemochromatosis • Huntington's disease • Mental illness	• Lecture • Discussion • Explain using slides	• Short answer • Objective type
V	2 (T)	Describe the role of nurse in genetic services and counseling	**Services related to genetics** • Genetic testing • Gene therapy • Genetic counseling • Legal and ethical issues • Role of nurse	• Lecture • Discussion	• Short answer • Objective type

Overview

Pathology is a medical discipline that deals with the scientific study of the diseases with special reference to the causative factors, mechanism of the development of the disease, morphological alterations in the organs due to the disease and its clinical implications.

The study of pathology provides a deep insight into the disease process, and it serves as an essential link between the basic medical sciences and the clinical disciplines. A proper and methodical understanding of pathology has become mandatory for understanding the diseases.

Genetics, the science of heredity is now emerging as one the most dynamic specialties in medicine. It has been established that most of the diseases have an underlying genetic basis. Thereby, a knowledge of the basic concepts of genetics becomes very much essential.

This unique book provides the reader an excellent opportunity to understand the basic concepts in "Pathology" and "Genetics" together, especially for the paramedical nursing students, who will be handling sick patients in the hospital wards.

For a logical understanding, this book is divided into 5 sections which deals with" Pathology " and " Human Genetics". The section on pathology is further divided into Section I which deals with "General Pathology", which provides a deep knowledge about the basic concepts of cellular pathology. Section 2 deals with "Systemic Pathology" which is an application of the concepts of general pathology to organ systems.

Sections 3 and 4 deal with "Clinical Hematology and Clinical Pathology", which provides an overview on various methodologies of basic laboratory procedures, observation and interpretation of the investigations used in the diagnosis of various disease conditions. This will be of immense help for the nursing students, especially with regard to the bedside investigations.

Section 5 of the book is dedicated to basic concepts of "Human Genetics". Genetics itself is a vast specialty covering various topics, only the most essential concepts have been incorporated in this section. It deals with basic structure of the chromosome and the various anomalies associated.

The chapters on prenatal diagnosis, genetic counseling, and role of a paramedical personnel in diagnosis of genetic diseases have been dealt in a detailed manner as these will be areas of primary importance for a paramedical nursing student.

Have a happy learning.

UNIT

General Pathology

Section Outline

1. Introduction and Cell Injury Adaptation
2. Inflammation
3. Wound Healing and Repair
4. Fluid and Hemodynamic Disturbances
5. Neoplasia

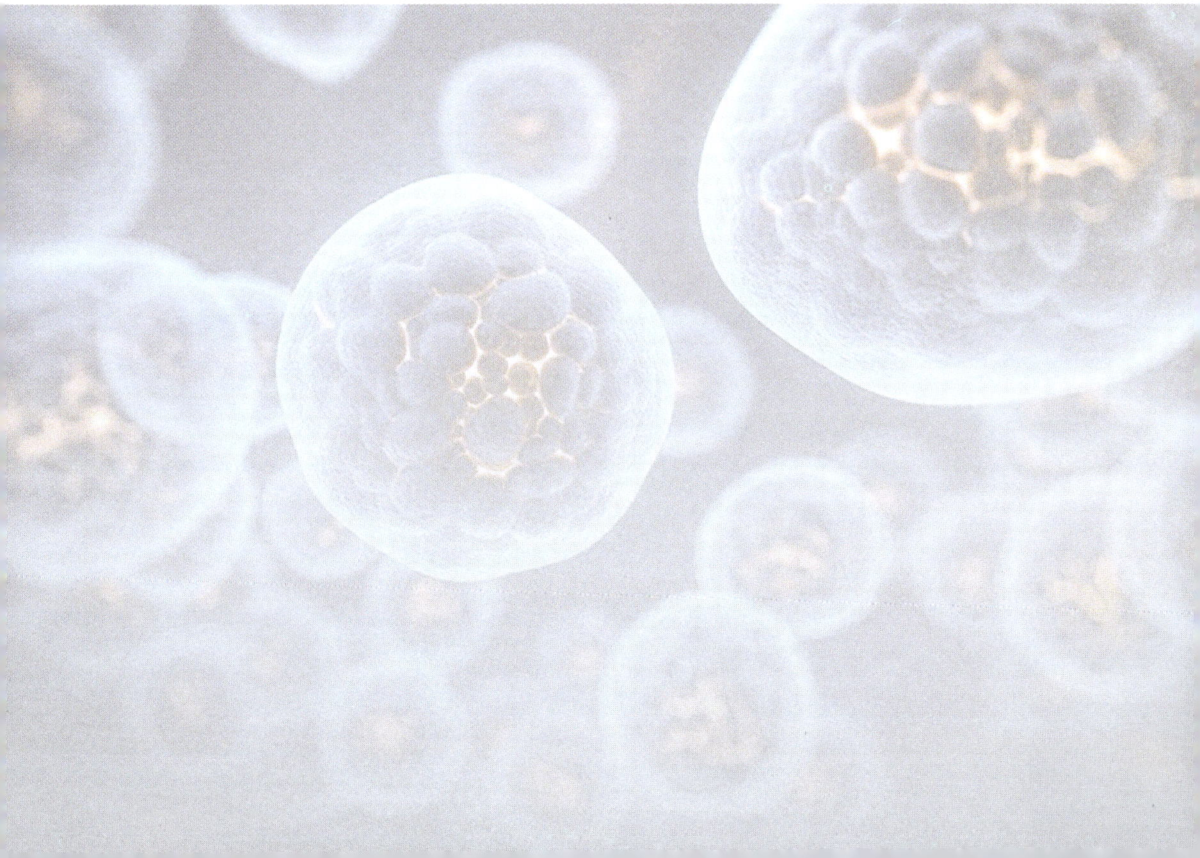

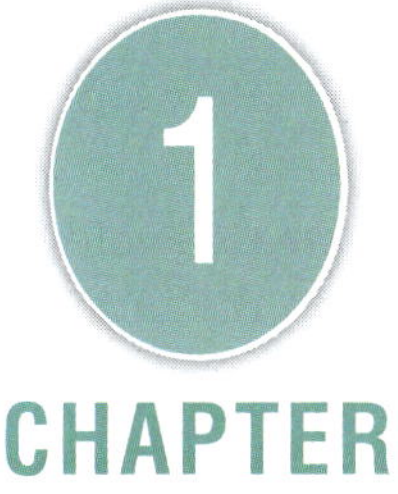

CHAPTER 1 Introduction and Cell Injury Adaptation

Learning Objectives

At the end of reading this chapter, the student shall be able to:

- Describe cellular adaptations and their significance.
- Enumerate the common causes for cell injury, mechanism of cell injury, distinguish between reversible and irreversible phase of cell injury and their clinical significance.
- Describe intracellular accumulation and fatty change.
- Describe the common types of cell death—types, mechanisms and morphology.
- Describe pathologic calcification with examples.

INTRODUCTION

The word *'Pathology'* is derived from two Greek words—*pathos* (meaning suffering) and *logos* (meaning study).

Pathology is the scientific study of diseases. It deals with the structural and functional changes in the cells and tissue that are expressed as diseases of organ systems.

It is categorized into general pathology, which involves the basic reactions of cell and tissues to injury and systemic pathology which involves the specific responses in specialized organ systems.

There are four main aspects which constitute the core of pathology. They are:

1.	Etiology	Cause of the disease
2.	Pathogenesis	Mechanism of the development of the disease
3.	Morphological changes	Alterations in the cells and tissues of the organ
4.	Clinical features	Functional consequences due to the disease process

Fundamental knowledge in pathology is very much essential for understanding the evolution of the disease process and to correlate the clinical features of the disease in the patient. It serves as a vital link between the basic sciences and clinical sciences.

KEYWORDS

- **Lesions** are pathological changes in cells and tissues, produced by the disease.
- **Etiology** is the cause/causal factor of disease.
- **Pathophysiology** is the study of deranged (patho) bodily functions (physiology), which occur as a consequence of the disease.
- **Pathogenesis** is the mechanism of disease evolution and progression.

CELLULAR RESPONSE TO INJURY

The cell is the basic structural and functional unit of a tissue/organ.

Rudolph Virchow, the father of modern pathology, proposed that injury to the cell forms the basis of all the disease process. So, it becomes very much essential to appreciate the changes that occur at the cellular level to understand the disease.

Every cell has a narrow range of structure and function. This is referred to as *homeostasis* **(Flowchart 1.1)**. When the cells are subjected to stress, they undergo certain structural and functional modifications which are called *adaptations*. When the stress is very severe then the cells are not able to adapt it gets injured and end up as *cell injury/death*.

CELLULAR ADAPTATIONS (FIG.1.1 AND FLOWCHART 1.1)

There are various methods by which a cell responds to stressful stimuli. They include:
- Hyperplasia
- Hypertrophy
- Atrophy
- Metaplasia

These cellular adaptations are reversible and the cells will return to normalcy when the stress is removed.

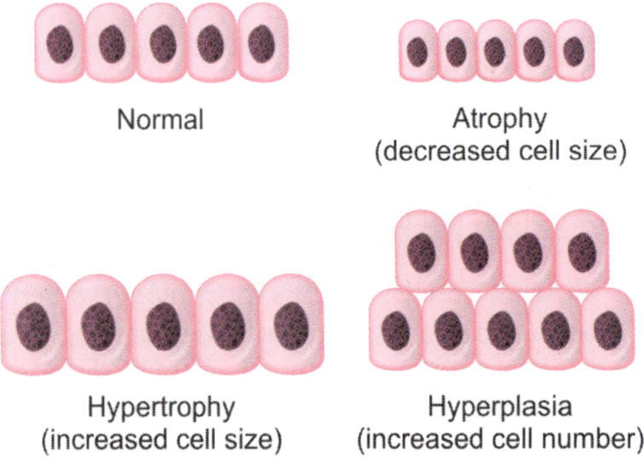

Fig. 1.1: Cellular adaptations.

Flowchart 1.1: Spectrum of cellular homeostasis.

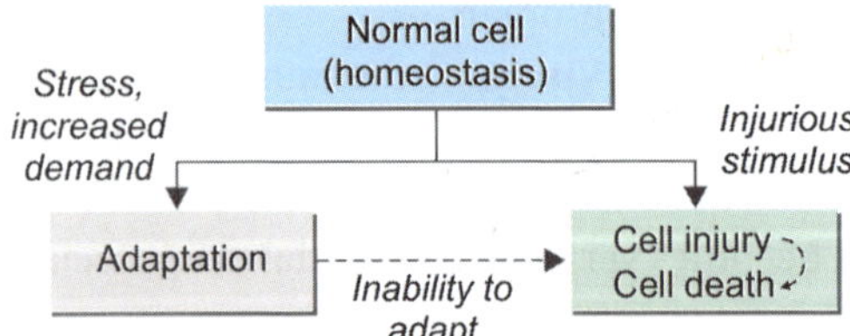

Hyperplasia

Definition: It is defined as increased volume of the organ due to increase in the number of cells in an organ/tissue. It occurs only in organs with dividing cells.

Types: There are two types of hyperplasia—physiological and pathological:
1. Physiologic hyperplasia may be induced by hormones, e.g., (1) increase in the size of female breast during puberty/ pregnancy, (2) increase in the size of uterus during pregnancy, or hyperplasia may also occur as a compensatory process, e.g., regeneration of liver following hepatectomy.
2. Pathologic hyperplasia usually occurs due to excessive hormonal stimulation, e.g., (i) estrogen-induced hyperplasia of the endometrial tissue, (ii) hormone-induced hyperplasia of prostate.

These hormone-induced pathologic hyperplasias constitute a fertile soil for cancerous growth **(Figs. 1.2 and 1.3)**.

Hyperplasia can also occur in the connective tissue. Example is the connective tissue hyperplasia that occurs in the process of wound healing. Hyperplasia of the surface epithelium usually produces warty lesions, e.g., viral warts caused by human papillomavirus.

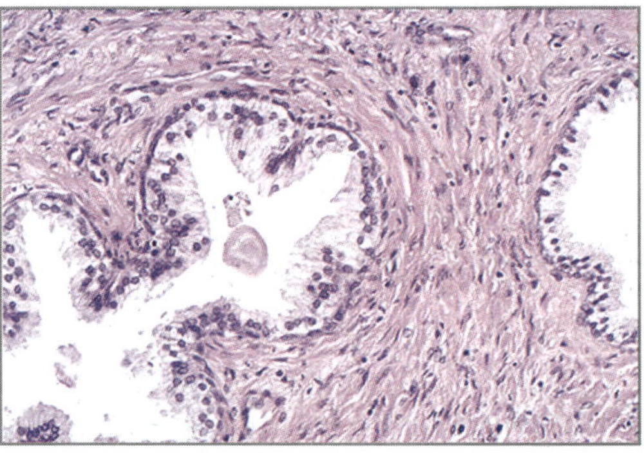

Fig. 1.2: Photomicrograph of normal prostatic glands.

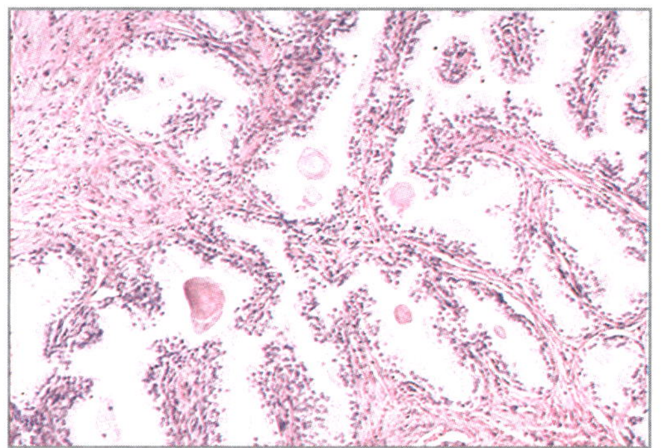

Fig. 1.3: Photomicrograph of prostatic hyperplasia.

Hypertrophy

Definition: It is defined as increase in the size of the organ due to increase in the size of the cells.

In contrast to hyperplasia, there are no new cells but the existing cells become larger.

Hypertrophy usually occurs in nondividing cells. There are two forms—physiologic and pathologic:

1. Physiologic hypertrophy, e.g., hypertrophy of the muscles due to exercise; hypertrophy of uterus in pregnancy **(Fig. 1.4)**.
2. Pathologic hypertrophy, e.g., hypertrophy of the cardiac chambers due to hemodynamic overload as in hypertension and valvular heart diseases **(Fig. 1.5)**.

The basic molecular mechanism for hypertrophy is due to the synthesis of newer cellular proteins or excessive secretion of growth factors.

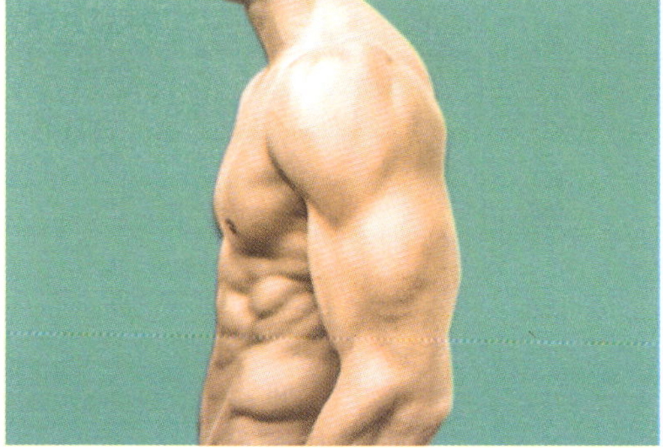

Fig. 1.4: Exercise-induced hypertrophy of muscle.

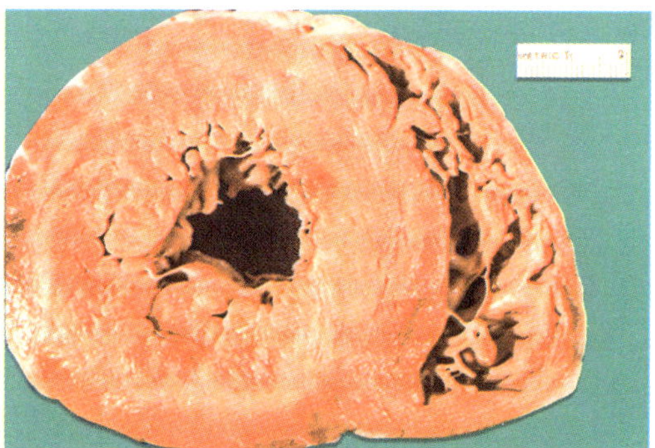

Fig. 1.5: Photomicrograph showing massive hypertrophy of the left ventricle.

Atrophy

Definition: It is defined as reduction in the size of the organ and due to decrease in the size of the cell. An atrophic cell has diminished function but it is not dead.

Atrophy can be physiological or pathological.

- Physiologic atrophy usually occurs during
  - Embryogenesis, e.g., atrophy of the thyroglossal duct or notochord
  - Adult life, e.g., atrophy of thymus, gonads, skin due to aging.
- Pathologic atrophy is due to
  - Decreased work load (disuse atrophy), e.g., limbs immobilized in plaster cast
  - Loss of nerve supply (denervation atrophy), e.g., muscle wasting
  - Loss of blood supply—changes in brain due to ischemia
  - Inadequate nutrition—protein energy malnutrition, cancer cachexia
  - Loss of endocrine stimuli—atrophy of uterus, ovaries
  - Aging (senile)
  - Pressure—tissue compressed for a longer duration.

The major molecular mechanism of atrophy is due to excessive degradation of structural proteins or an imbalance between the protein synthesis and degradation **(Fig. 1.6)**.

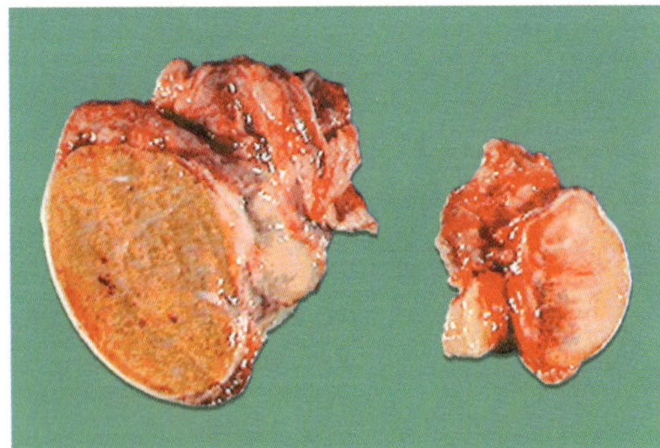

Fig. 1.6: Photomicrograph showing atrophic testis (right) and normal testis (left).

Metaplasia

It is defined as a reversible change of one adult type tissue into another. There are two forms of metaplasia—epithelial and mesenchymal.

Epithelial Metaplasia

- Change of columnar epithelium to squamous epithelium, e.g.,
  - Respiratory tract—chronic irritation, smoking
  - Ducts of salivary gland, pancreas—calculi
  - Urinary bladder—deficiency of vitamin A
- Change of squamous to columnar epithelium, e.g.,
  - Lower end of esophagus (Barrett's esophagus)—reflux of gastric acid **(Fig. 1.7)**.

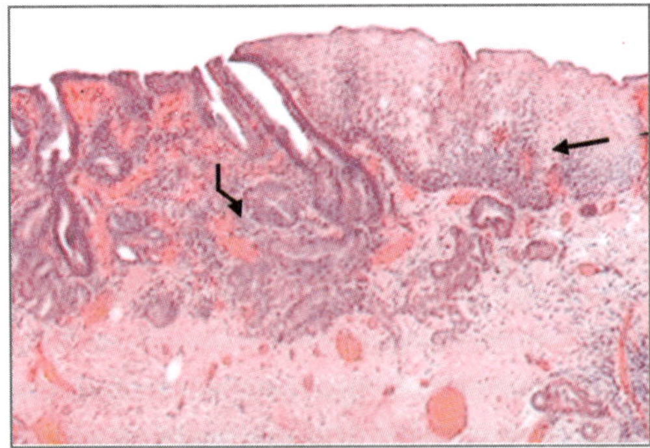

Fig. 1.7: Photomicrograph of Barrett's esophagus, squamous epithelium (straight arrow), columnar epithelium (bended arrow).

Mesenchymal Metaplasia

Myositis ossificans: It is condition of formation of bone within a muscle tissue induced by trauma.

The major underlying molecular mechanism of metaplasia is genetic reprogramming of the precursor stem cells. The metaplastic cell will be able to withstand the stress better than the original cell. Metaplastic tissue can also be a fertile soil of cancerous change.

CELL INJURY

It usually occurs when the cells are subjected to severe stress that they are no longer able to adapt.

There are two phases in cell injury—initial reversible phase and final irreversible phase (cell death) **(Flowchart 1.2)**.

Causes for Cell Injury

- Hypoxia—due to lack of oxygen—most common cause of cell injury
- Ischemia—decreased blood supply. It is the most common cause for hypoxia.
- Physical agents—trauma, pressure, radiation, shock, extremes of temperature
- Chemicals—drugs, insecticides, environmental pollutants
- Biological—viruses, bacteria, fungi, parasites

Flowchart 1.2: Reversible and irreversible phase of cell injury.

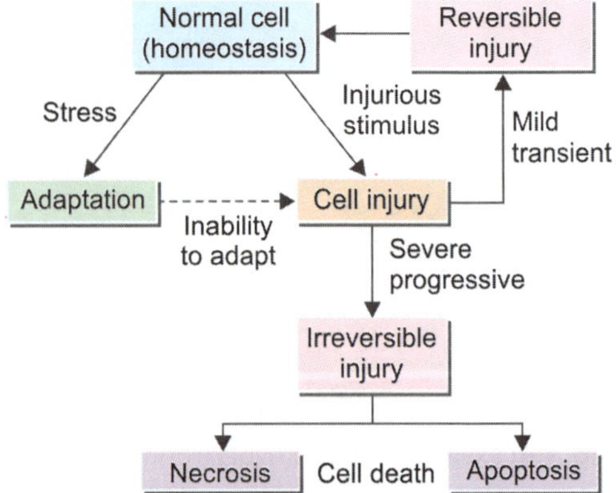

- Immunologic—derangements in the immune mechanisms
- Genetic derangements
- Nutritional imbalances—due to deficiency or excess of a particular nutrient

KEYWORDS

Cytopathology: It is a relatively new diagnostic discipline, which has branched out from surgical pathology. It deals with the study of cells collected from body organs/masses by fine-needle aspiration cytology (FNAC) or cells that are shed out from body surfaces (exfoliative cytology).

Mechanism of Cell Injury

The mechanism of cellular responses to various injurious stimuli depends on various factors, which include:

- Type of injurious stimuli
- Duration of injurious stimuli
- Severity of injurious stimuli
- Type of the cell
- Adaptability status of the cell

In any form of cell injury, there are few main cellular structures that are usually targeted, they include **(Fig. 1.8)**:

- Aerobic respiratory mechanism
- Integrity of the cell membrane
- Protein synthesis
- Cytoskeleton
- Genetic apparatus

The major biochemical mechanisms that are involved in cellular injury include **(Fig. 1.9)**:

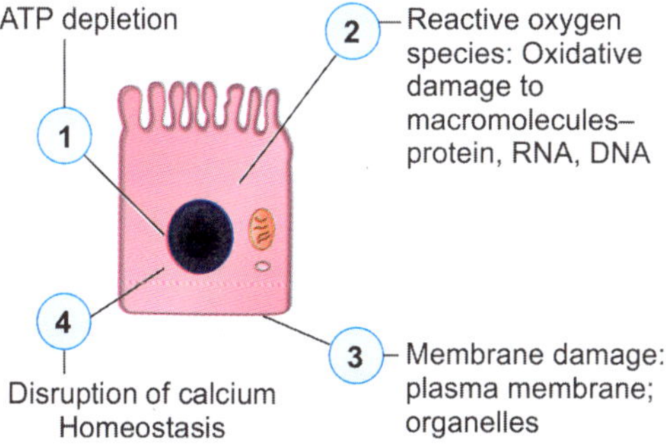

Fig. 1.8: Main targets of cell injury.

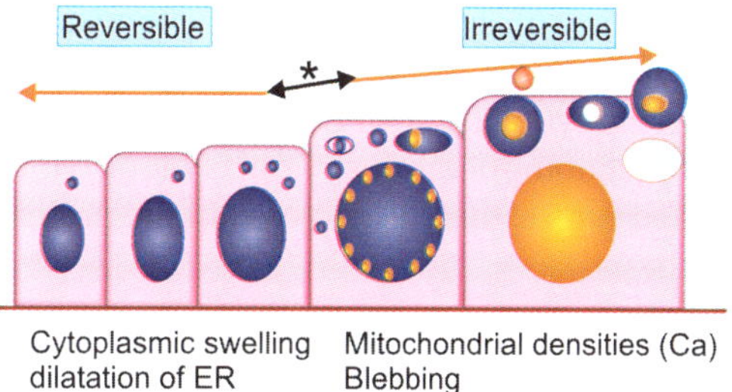

Fig. 1.9: Sequence of changes in reversible and irreversible cell injury.

- Depletion of adenosine triphosphate (ATP)
- Alterations in energy metabolism of cell
- Damage to cell membrane
- Failure of calcium homeostasis
- Mitochondrial damage

Depletion of Adenosine Triphosphate

It occurs in hypoxic and chemical injury. Normally, adenosine triphosphate (ATP) is required for the energy dependent functions, such as membrane transport, protein synthesis, and lipogenesis. Depletion of ATP leads to defective functioning of the Na/K dependent energy pump which causes excessive loss of potassium from the cell and high influx of sodium into the cell, whenever a molecule of sodium moves into the cell it carries a molecule of water. So, the net result there will be swelling of the cells and loss of the specialized structures like the microvilli and brush border.

Alterations in Energy Metabolism of Cell

As a result of the lack of energy molecules from the oxidative pathway, the cell tries to derive energy from other pathways. The most common pathway is glycolytic pathway. The glycogen breaks into lactic acid and pyruvic acid and in this process it liberates ATP which is used by the cell. This pathway is called anaerobic pathway. This leads to rapid depletion of glycogen stores producing moth eaten appearance of the cytoplasm with accumulation of lactic acid and pyruvic acid. Accumulation of the acids lead to fall in the cytoplasmic pH and as a result of this the functioning of various cytoplasmic enzymes is affected and there is decrease in the protein synthesis.

Damage to Cell Membrane

Damage to the cell membrane is a major event in the cellular injury. The damage is induced by various mediators of cell injury, such as free oxygen radicals, rise in the cytosolic calcium levels and others. Cell membrane damage leads to the following:

- Loss of osmotic balance of the cell
- Influx of water and ions into the cell
- Loss of proteins, enzymes, coenzymes, and metabolites
- Depletion of high energy phosphates
- Damage to the mitochondrial cell membrane leads to severe mitochondrial dysfunction
- Damage to the lysosomal membrane leads to leak of the lysosomal enzymes and activation which causes digestion of the cellular components.

Mitochondrial Damage

It is an important target for all types of injurious stimuli. Damage to the mitochondria occurs due to increased cytosolic calcium, oxidative stress, increased breakdown of phospholipids and breakdown of lipids. This leads to alteration in the mitochondrial membrane permeability and thereby defective oxidative phosphorylation. There is release of cytochrome C into the cytoplasm which triggers the death of the cell.

Failure of Calcium Homeostasis

Normally calcium is kept in a very low level within the cytoplasm within the endoplasmic reticulum and the mitochondria. Due to ischemia and certain toxins, the calcium is released from the organelles and intracellular calcium level is elevated. This leads to activation of various enzyme systems, such as ATPase, phospholipase, protease, and endonuclease. The elevated calcium levels also increases the membrane permeability of mitochondria.

Mediators of Cell Injury

The common mediators include the free oxygen radicals and cytosolic calcium. The role played by the cytosolic calcium is given above.

Free Oxygen Radicals

Definition: These are reactive oxygen molecules which have an unpaired electron in its outermost orbit. They are extremely reactive and capable of undergoing chain reactions with the generation of more free oxygen radicals. They are usually represented as O_2.

They mediate various forms of cell injury mostly due to radiation, chemical, and ischemia/reperfusion. They also play a vital role in mediating the cellular damage due to ageing and aid in microbial killing by the phagocytes.

The common free radicals include O_2, H_2O_2, OH, and NO.

The free radicals causes

- Lipid peroxidation of the cell membranes—cell membrane damage
- Oxidative modification of proteins—affects protein synthesis
- Damage to DNA

The action of the free oxygen radicals is usually balanced by substances which are normally present in our body called antioxidants. They inactivate the free radicals and terminate the damage induced by the radicals.

Common antioxidants include catalase, superoxide dismutase, glutathione peroxidase, transferrin, ferritin, lactoferrin, vitamins E, and A.

Usually, there is a well-maintained balance between the functioning of the free radicals and antioxidants.

When does the Cell Actually Die?

When the cell is unable to reverse the mitochondrial dysfunction as well as the cell membrane damage, the reversible phase of cellular damage transforms into an irreversible phase (cell death).

Morphological Patterns of Reversible Cell Injury

They include:
- Cellular swelling—hydropic/vacuolar degeneration
- Fatty change
- Hyaline and mucoid change

Cellular Swelling

It is the most common morphological form of cell injury. This occurs due to the loss of maintenance of the fluid and ionic balance as a result of the defective functioning of the Na/K-dependent pump.

This is manifested well in renal tissue and the change is called cloudy swelling of the renal tubules. The organ looks paler with increased turgor and weight. On light microscopy, the cells are swollen with small vacuoles within the cytoplasm and increased granularity of the cytoplasm. This leads to irregularity of the tubular lumina which is referred to as starry lumina **(Figs. 1.10A and B)**. Electron microscopy shows widespread alterations in the plasma membrane, mitochondria, endoplasmic reticulum, and nuclear chromatin.

Fatty Change

This is another form of reversible cell injury where the cell accumulates an intracellular substance in an excessive manner.

Lipid accumulation is the most common form and the cell accumulates triglycerides, cholesterol, phospholipids, and esters of cholesterol. Fatty change occurs in organs, such as liver, heart, muscle and kidneys. Most common site is liver as it is the seat of lipid metabolism.

Causes of Fatty Change Liver
- Chronic alcoholism (most common)
- Toxins—carbon tetrachloride
- Protein calorie malnutrition
- Diabetes mellitus
- Obesity
- Anoxia
- Infections—hepatitis C virus
- Late pregnancy
- Reye's syndrome
- Drugs—estrogen, corticosteroids, tetracycline

Gross: The liver is enlarged, yellowish, and greasy. The edges of the liver are blunt **(Fig. 1.11)**.

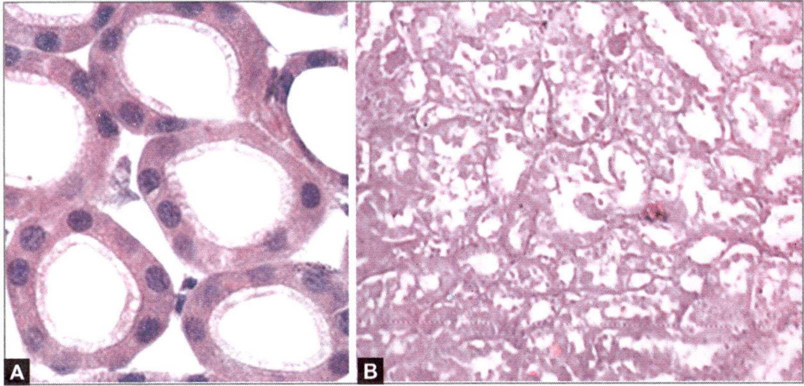

Figs. 1.10A and B: Cloudy swelling of kidney: (A) Normal proximal convoluted tubule; (B) Tubules with cloudy swelling.

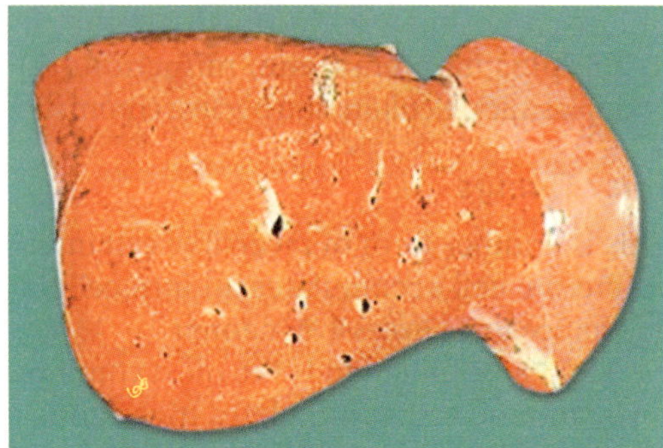

Fig. 1.11: Gross appearance of fatty liver.

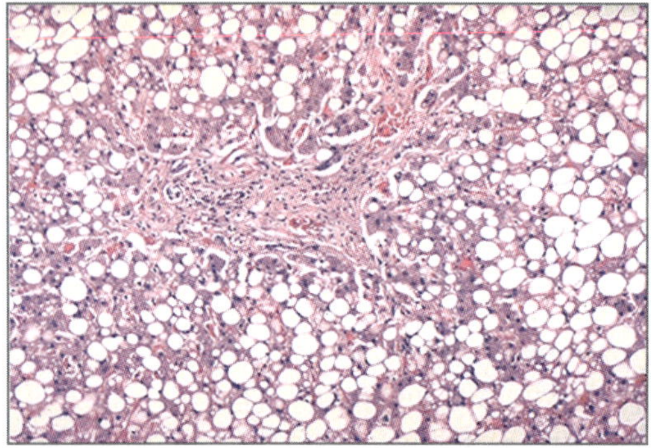

Fig. 1.12: Microscopic image with fat vacuoles within the hepatocytes.

Microscopy (Fig. 1.12): The hepatocytes are swollen with accumulation of microvesicles of fat which gradually fill the entire cell. The fat usually appears as clear spaces within the cytoplasm, because the fat is dissolved in the chemicals used for tissue processing in the laboratory. This pattern of staining is called **negative staining**. Fat can be demonstrated using special stains, such as Sudan Black B, Sudan III, Sudan IV, and Oil red O in a frozen section.

Fatty change of the heart is less common and it presents as two morphological forms depending on the cause. In cases of moderate hypoxia as in anemia, the change is called as **Tigered Effect**—fatty yellow myocardium alternates with normal brown myocardium and in cases of severe hypoxia as in diphtheria there is uniform fatty change within the myocardium.

MORPHOLOGY OF IRREVERSIBLE CELL INJURY (CELL DEATH)

The two major morphological forms of cell death include necrosis and apoptosis.

Necrosis

Definition: The spectrum of morphological changes that follow cell death in a living tissue. This is mostly induced by the proteolytic degradative action of the enzymes on the injured cell. The enzymes may be released from the same cell (autolysis) of from the adjacent cells and inflammatory cells (heterolysis).

The two major events that occur in necrosis are:

1. Denaturation of the cellular proteins
2. Enzymatic digestion of cells

Morphology of a necrotic cell:

- *Cytoplasmic changes:*
  - Increased eosinophilia of the cytoplasm due to denaturation of proteins
  - Glassy and moth eaten appearance of cytoplasm due to loss of glycogen
  - Presence of calcification
- *Nuclear changes* **(Fig. 1.13)**:
  - Small shrunken nuclei with condense chromatin—pyknosis

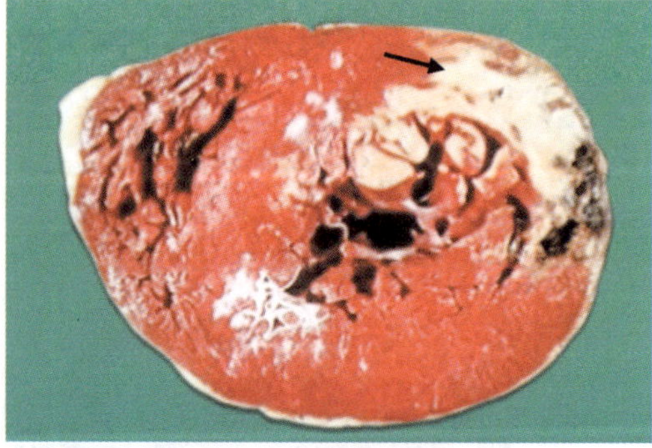

Fig. 1.13: Gross picture showing coagulative necrosis (arrow) of the wall of left ventricle.

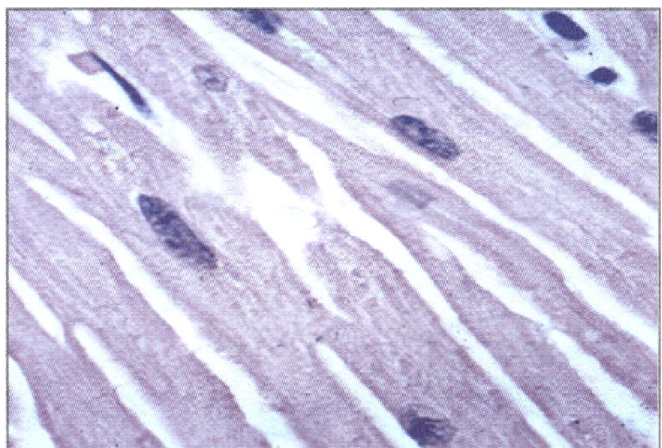

Fig. 1.14: Normal myocardial cells.

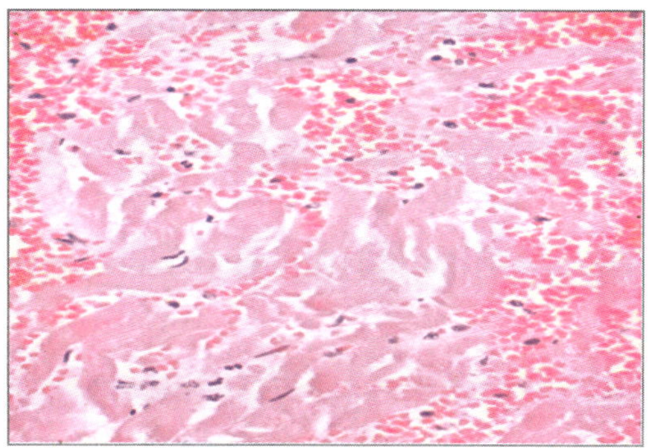

Fig. 1.15: Myocardium with coagulative necrosis.

   - Dissolution of the nuclei (due to activity of DNAse)—karyolysis
   - Fragmentation of the pyknotic nuclei—karyorrhexis
- *Ultrastructural changes* **(Fig. 1.14)**:
   - Cell membrane and plasma membrane damage
   - Mitochondrial alterations
   - Presence of amorphous densities in the mitochondria
   - Lysosomal membrane alterations
   - Aggregation of denatured proteins

Types of Necrosis (Table 1.1)

- Coagulative necrosis
- Liquefactive necrosis
- Caseation necrosis
- Fat necrosis
- Gangrenous necrosis
- Fibrinoid necrosis
- Osteonecrosis
- Zenker's degeneration

Coagulative Necrosis (Structured Necrosis) (Fig. 1.15)

- *Causes*: Ischemia and hypoxia.
- *Organs involved*: Heart, kidney, spleen (solid organs with end arterial blood supply).
- *Major event*: Denaturation of proteins.
- *Features*: The basic structure of the cell is retained, so the cell type can be recognized.

Liquefactive Necrosis (Fig. 1.16)

- *Causes*: Ischemia, bacterial infections (pyogenic)
- *Organs involved*: Brain (infarct brain), abscess
- *Major event*: Enzymatic digestion

TABLE 1.1: Summary of the major types of necrosis.

Type of necrosis	*Cause of necrosis*	*Organs involved*	*Major event*	*Features*
Coagulative	Ischemia, hypoxia	Heart, kidneys, spleen	Denaturation of proteins	Cellular structure retained
Liquefactive	Ischemia, toxins	Brain, other tissues	Enzymatic digestion	Cellular details lost
Caseation	Mycobacterial infection	Lung, lymph node	Immune mediated necrosis	Formation of dried cheese like material
Fat	Acute pancreatitis, trauma to breast	Omentum, breast	Enzymatic digestion	Formation of calcium soaps
Fibrinoid	Immune reaction	Blood vessel, glomeruli	Protein denaturation	Deposition of powdery fibrin like material

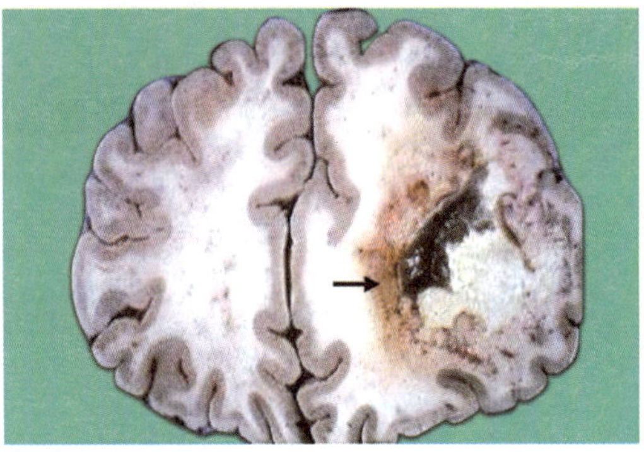
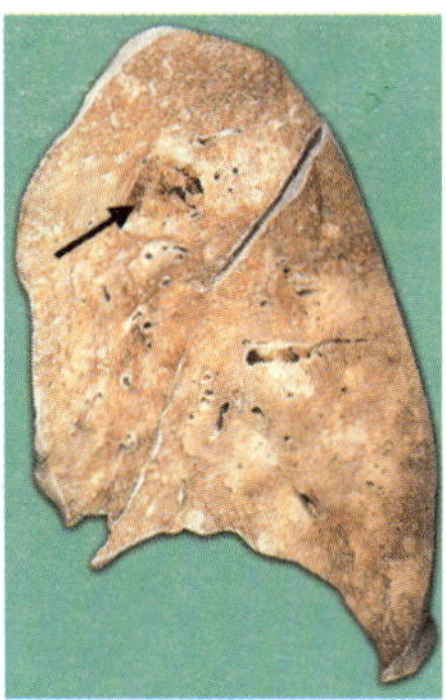

Fig. 1.16: Slice of brain with liquefactive necrosis (arrow) (left). Portion of lung with liquefactive necrosis (arrow) (right).

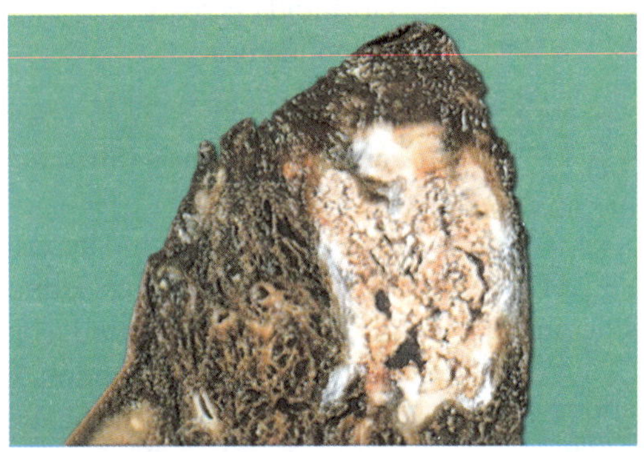
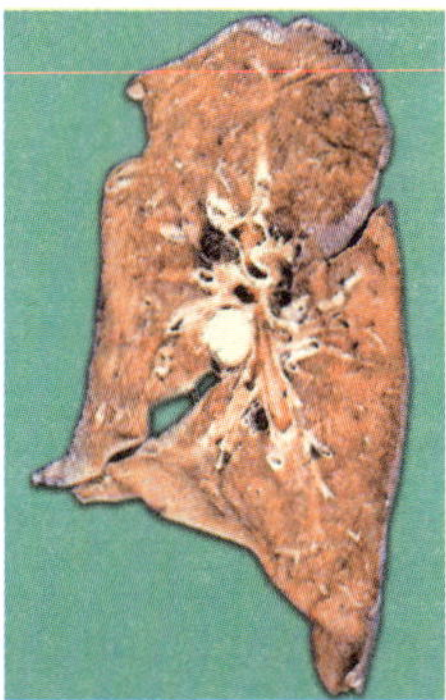

Fig. 1.17: Gross appearance of dry cheesy material indicative of coagulation necrosis in the lung.

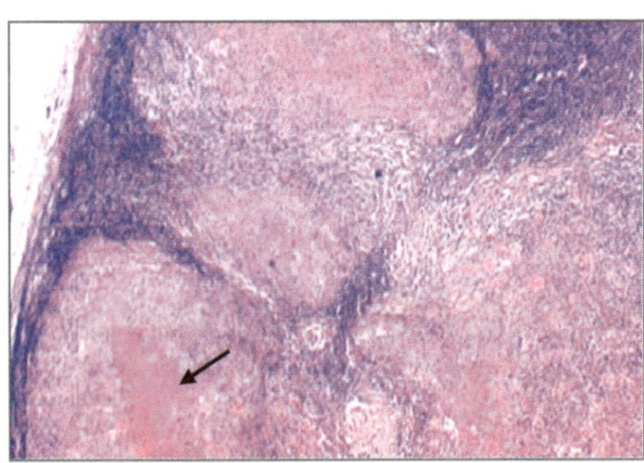

Fig. 1.18: Photomicrograph showing coagulative necrosis (arrow).

- *Features*: The necrotic area is converted into a liquid viscous mass which undergoes cystic change later.

Caseation Necrosis (Figs. 1.17 and 1.18)

- *Causes*: *Mycobacterium tuberculosis, Mycobacterium leprae.*
- *Organs involved*: Lung, lymph node, skin and other tissues.
- *Major event*: A combination denaturation of proteins and liquefaction necrosis—this is due to an immune mediated delayed hypersensitivity reaction to mycolic acid present in the cell membrane of the bacteria by the T lymphocytes.
- *Features*: The necrotic area appears firm, dry, and cheesy amorphous granular debris. The structure of the tissue is lost.

Fat Necrosis (Fig. 1.19)

- *Causes*: Acute pancreatitis, trauma (breast)
- *Organs*: Pancreas, abdominal fat, breast
- *Major event*: Enzymatic digestion with release of lipases
- *Features*: Formation of chalky white necrotic areas due to abnormal release of lipases and subsequent calcification.

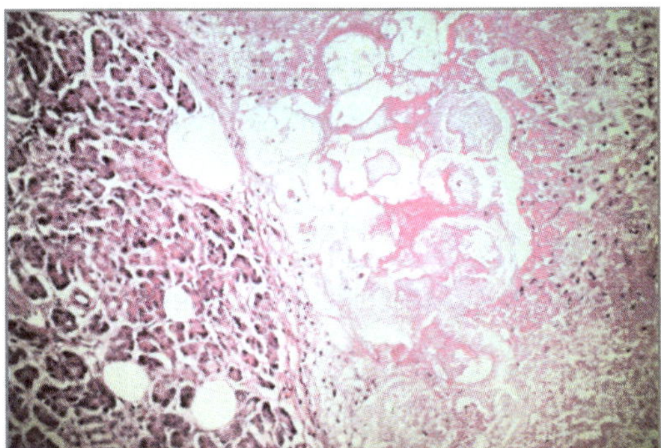

Fig. 1.19: Photomicrograph of fat necrosis in acute pancreatitis.

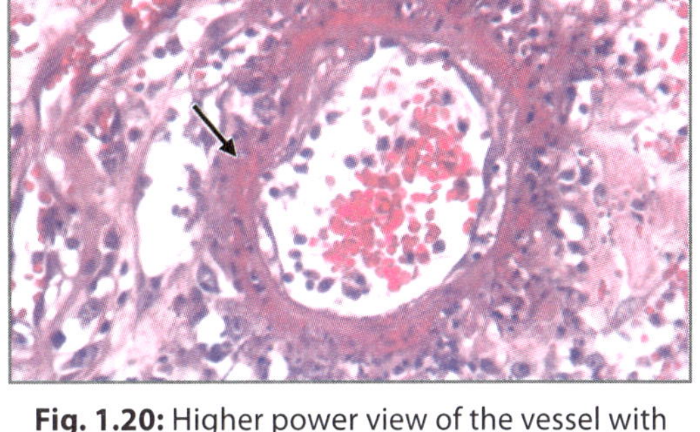

Fig. 1.20: Higher power view of the vessel with fibrinoid necrosis (arrow).

Fibrinoid Necrosis (Figs. 1.20 and 1.21)

- *Causes*: Immune mediated (antigen-antibody reaction).
- *Organs*: Blood capillaries, glomeruli.
- *Major event*: Immune-mediated protein denaturation.
- *Features*: Deposition of powdery pinkish amorphous granular substance in the blood vessels and capillaries.

Osteonecrosis

- *Causes*: Ischemia, radiation, traumatic
- *Organs*: Head of femur, navicular bone
- *Major event*: Protein denaturation

Zenker's Degeneration

- *Causes*: Enteric fever
- *Organ*: Rectus abdominus, diaphragm
- *Major event*: Protein denaturation
- *Features*: The muscle fibers loose the striations and appear as eosinophilic hyaline masses.

KEYWORDS

Molecular pathology: This is the detection and diagnosis of diseases at the nuclear level deoxyribonucleic acid (DNA) of cells. Molecular pathology emerged as a powerful research tool and is now being used widely for diagnostic purposes as well.

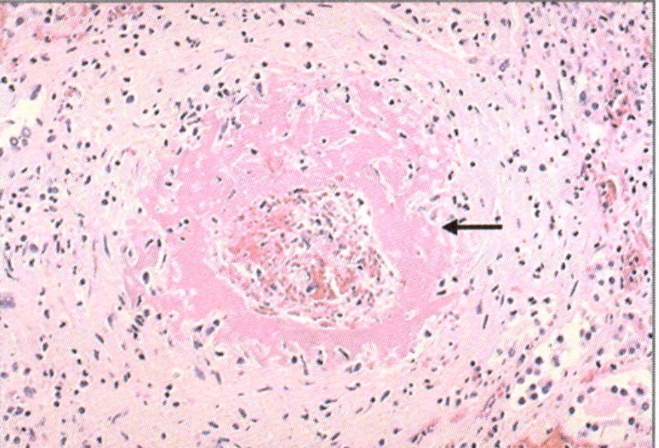

Fig. 1.21: Lower power view of fibrinoid necrosis (arrow).

GANGRENE

Definition: It is a type of coagulative necrosis with superadded putrefaction.

Cause: Due to ischemia with superadded severe bacterial infection.

Types

Three major types **(Figs. 1.22 and 1.23)**:

1. Dry gangrene
2. Wet gangrene
3. Gas gangrene

Dry gangrene: Usually occurs in the distal part of extremity mostly due to ischemia (arterial occlusion). Gradual in onset. The affected part appears dry, shrunken, and dark brown

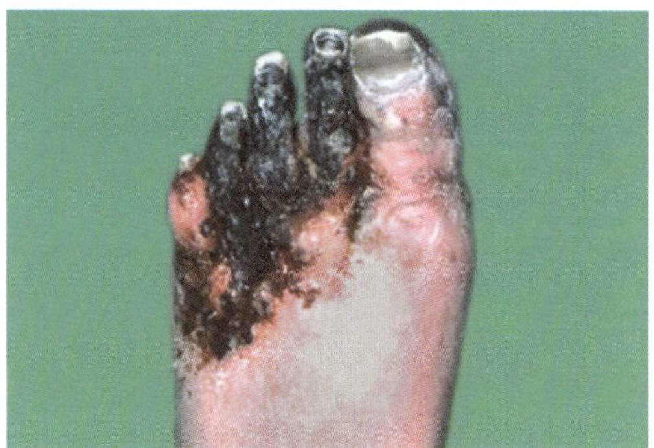

Fig. 1.22: Dry gangrene of the foot.

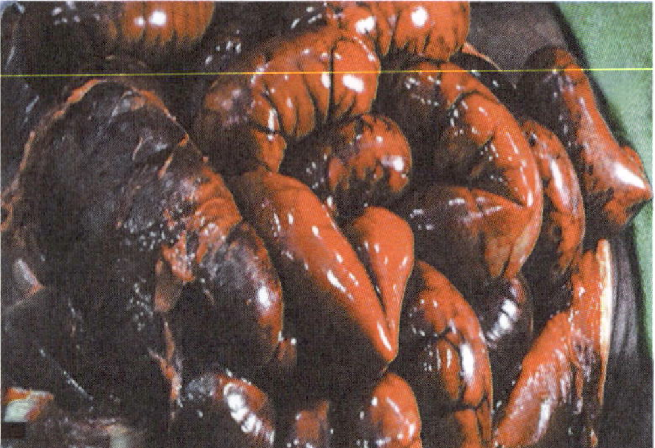

Fig. 1.23: Wet gangrene of a loop of small bowel.

to black in color. The color change is due to the oxidation of hemoglobin and myoglobin into ferric sulfide. The line of demarcation is very clearly made out.

Wet gangrene: Occurs in moist organs, such as small bowel, oral cavity, vulva, etc. The affected part appears swollen and dark. Mostly due to obstruction to the venous outflow. Rapid in onset. The line of demarcation is ill defined.

Contrasting features of dry and wet gangrene are summarized in **Table 1.2**.

Gas gangrene: Special type of wet gangrene due to infection with spore forming anaerobic bacteria of the *Clostridia* family—***Clostridium perfringens, Cl. novyi, Cl. septicum***.

The most common predisposing factor is lacerated wounds of the extremities as in road traffic accidents contaminated with spores of the bacteria in the soil. The bacteria grows well in the dead and devitalized tissues and secretes powerful exotoxins which causes myonecrosis. The muscle carbohydrate is fermented into lactic acid, hydrogen and carbon dioxide, which accumulate in the area of injury. The affected organ appears swollen, tense, greenish black, crepitant (due to gas accumulation) and foul smelling (due to formation of hydrogen sulfide).

This can be prevented by proper wound toileting, wound debridement, use of hyperbaric oxygen and Anti Gas Gangrene Serum (AGGS).

TABLE 1.2: Contrasting features of dry and wet gangrene.

Features	*Dry gangrene*	*Wet gangrene*
Cause	Arterial occlusion	Venous outflow obstruction
Sites	Extremities	Bowel loops, moist tissue
Onset	Gradual	Rapid
Macroscopy	Dry, shrunken and brownish black	Wet, congested, brownish black
Putrefaction	Moderate	Marked
Line of demarcation	Well defined	Ill defined

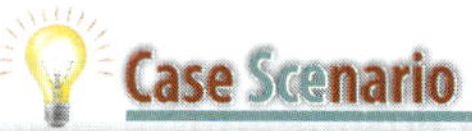

A female patient of 65 years admitted in hospital with a foot ulcer on her right foot. She reports localized pain, redness, and foul-smelling discharge. She is having history of type 2 diabetes, hypertension. During the initial assessment, the nurse address that the ulcer is located on the plantar aspect of the right foot, with signs of infection and has diminished sensation in her lower extremities. WBC are elevated.

Contd...

Contd...

Question:

Given the foot ulcer, diminished sensation, and elevated WBC count, what is the nurse's primary concern related to cell injury, and what nursing intervention is crucial?

A. **Risk of infection:** Initiate antibiotic therapy as prescribed and monitor wound care.
B. **Impaired circulation:** Administer pain medication and elevate the affected foot.
C. **Altered sensation:** Provide diabetic foot care education and assess neurovascular status regularly.
D. **Hyperglycemia:** Monitor blood glucose levels and administer insulin as needed.

Answer:

A. Risk of infection: Initiate antibiotic therapy as prescribed and monitor wound care.

Apoptosis

Definition: Type of coordinated and internally programmed cell death in which the cells destined to die, activate enzymes that degrade the cell's own DNA and cytoplasmic proteins.

Described in 1972, the term is derived from a Greek word of "Falling off" (as the leaves fall from the tree during autumn).

This is a process to eliminate the unwanted and potentially harmful cells.

Apoptosis can be physiological or pathological.

Physiological Apoptosis

- During embryogenesis—implantation, organogenesis, and developmental involution, e.g., disappearance of interdigital webs, involution of notochord, thyroglossal duct.
- Hormone-dependent involution, e.g., endometrial breakdown in menstruation, regression of lactating breast.
- Maintenance of cell balance, e.g., deletion of cells in intestinal crypts.
- Death of cells after they have served the function, e.g., neutrophils in acute inflammation, lymphocytes in immune reaction.
- Elimination of potential harmful self-reactive lymphocytes.
- Cell death by cytotoxic T-lymphocytes.

Pathological Apoptosis

- Cell death by various injurious stimuli—radiation, hypoxia, anticancer drugs
- Viral-induced cell injury—viral hepatitis (Councilman bodies)
- Cell death in tumors
- Induction of malignancy due to loss of apoptosis.

Morphological Features

- *Cell shrinkage:* The cell becomes small with dense cytoplasm and tightly packed cytoplasmic organelles. It becomes rounded and looses its specialized structures like the microvilli.
- *Condensation of chromatin:* It is the most characteristic feature with the aggregation of the chromatin under the nuclear membrane.
- *Formation of cytoplasmic blebs:* Extensive surface blebbing with fragmentation.
- Phagocytosis of the apoptotic bodies by the macrophages due to surface expression of vitronectin, beta 3 integrin, thrombospondin by the apoptotic cells.
- Absence of inflammatory response

The major biochemical events in apoptosis include cleavage of proteins, breakdown of DNA, and recognition by the phagocytes **(Figs. 1.24 and 1.25)**.

Mechanism: It occurs in two phases—initiation and execution.

1. *Initiation*: Initiation can occur by two pathways: (1) Intrinsic pathway, which is mediated by the mitochondria and (2) Extrinsic pathways mediated by the death receptors **(Flowchart 1.3)**.
   i. *Intrinsic pathway*: Due to the damage to the mitochondrial membrane, there will be release of proapoptotic

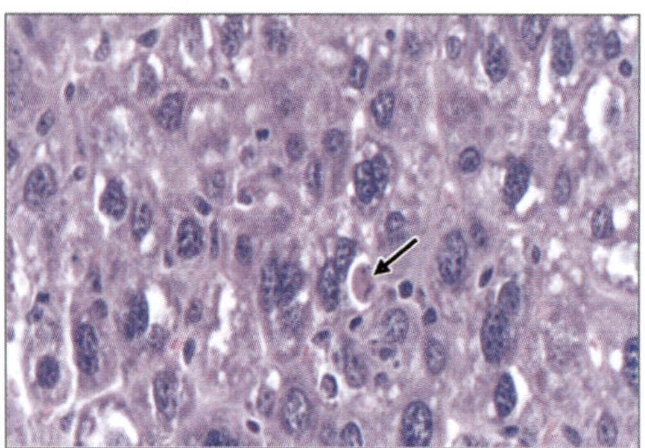

Fig. 1.24: Apoptotic body (arrow).

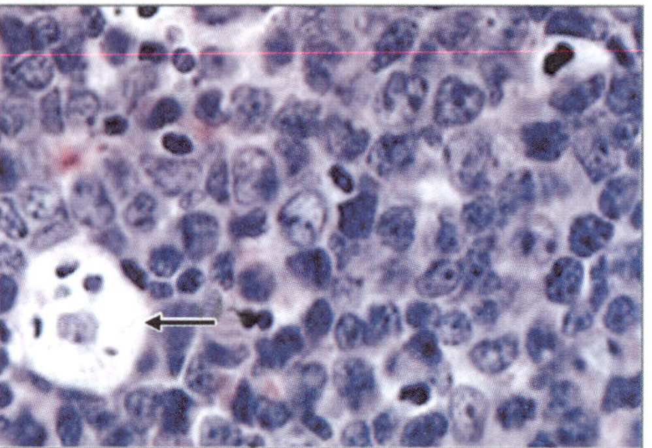

Fig. 1.25: Apoptotic body in a reactive lymph node (arrow).

signals from the mitochondria, e.g., BAK, BAX, BIM, and cytochrome C. The mitochondria also contains antiapoptotic molecules, such as bcl-2 and bcl-x. Due to stress, these molecules are lost and are replaced by the proapoptotic proteins which can also initiate the process of apoptosis.

ii. *Extrinsic pathway*: This pathway is mediated by extracellular signals. Many cells express death receptors on its surface. They belong to the tumor necrosis factor (TNF) family. When this receptor is activated by a related protein called **Fas (CD95)**, it leads to the activation of an adapter protein called **Fas associated death domain (FADD)** which in turn activates the enzymes of the execution phase and kills the cell.

2. *Execution*: It is mediated by enzymes of the caspase family, namely, transglutaminase and endonuclease. Transglutaminase causes cleavage of proteins and endonuclease causes chromatin condensation and DNA fragmentation.

Flowchart 1.3: Sequence of events in apoptosis.

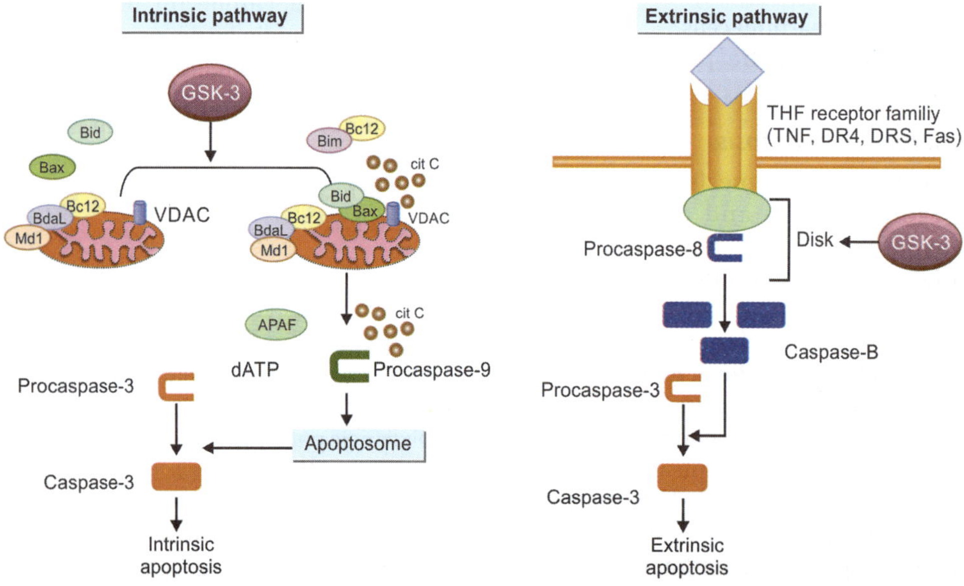

Disorders with dysregulated apoptosis are summarized below:

Disorders due to reduced apoptosis	♦ Autoimmune diseases ♦ Cancer
Disorders due to increased apoptosis	♦ Viral-induced cell injury ♦ Degenerative diseases ♦ Ischemia-induced cell injury

Contrasting features of necrosis and apoptosis are summarized in **Table 1.3**.

CALCIFICATION

Definition: Deposition of calcium salts in tissues other than teeth and enamel.

Types: Dystrophic and metastatic calcification

Morphology: Calcium is seen as granular deeply basophilic encrusted debris within the tissues. The special stains to demonstrate calcium are von Kossa and Alizarin red S.

Dystrophic: Calcification in dead and degenerate tissues. Plasma calcium levels are normal. Examples—calcification of:

TABLE 1.3: Contrasting features of necrosis and apoptosis.

S. no.	*Features in apoptosis*	*Features in necrosis*
1.	Involves single cells	Involves sheets of cell
2.	Intact tissue structure	Tissue structure lost
3.	Shrunken cell	Swollen cells
4.	Intact plasma membrane	Disrupted plasma membrane
5.	Compact organelles	Disorganized organelles
6.	Intact mitochondria	Amorphous densities in mitochondria
7.	Pyknotic nuclei	Pyknotic nuclei
8.	Active and Energy dependent	Passive process
9.	No inflammatory response	Inflammation present
10.	Physiological/ Pathological	Pathological

- Caseous necrotic material
- Dead parasites
- Fat necrosis
- Thrombi and infarct, hematoma
- Scar tissue
- Atherosclerosis
- *Monckeberg's sclerosis:* Deposition of calcium in the tunica media of the blood vessels, mostly uterine vessels seen in senility
- *Psammoma bodies:* Circumscribed spherules of calcium seen in tumors, such as papillary carcinoma of thyroid, meningioma, and serous papillary cystadenocarcinoma of ovary **(Figs. 1.26 and 1.27)**.
- *Metastatic*: Calcium deposition in normal tissues. Plasma calcium levels are elevated. Examples for metastatic calcification it must come in the next line.
- In the renal tubules—nephrocalcinosis or renal calculi formation **(Fig. 1.28)**.

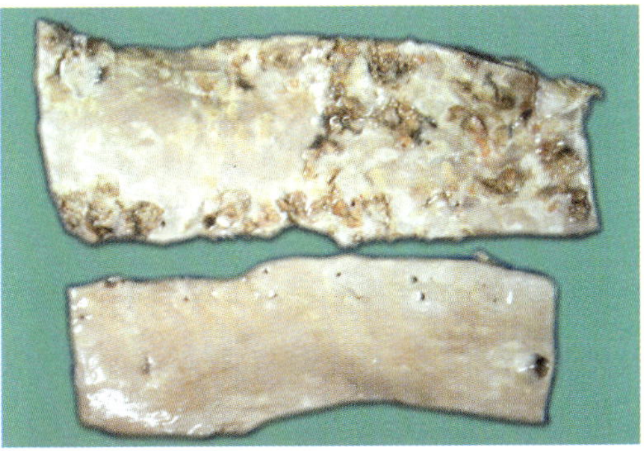

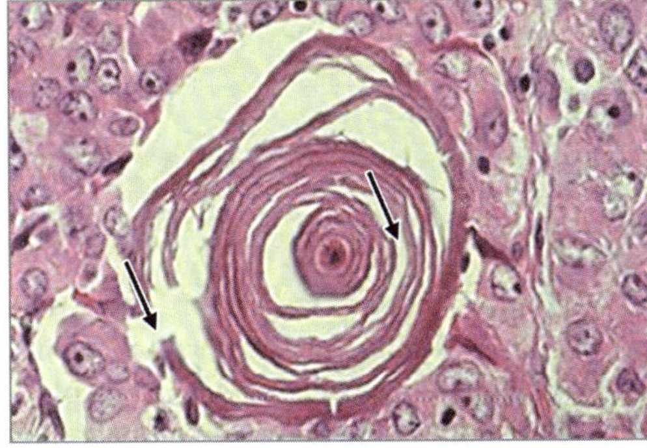

Fig. 1.26: Psammoma bodies (shown by arrows) in papillary carcinoma thyroid.

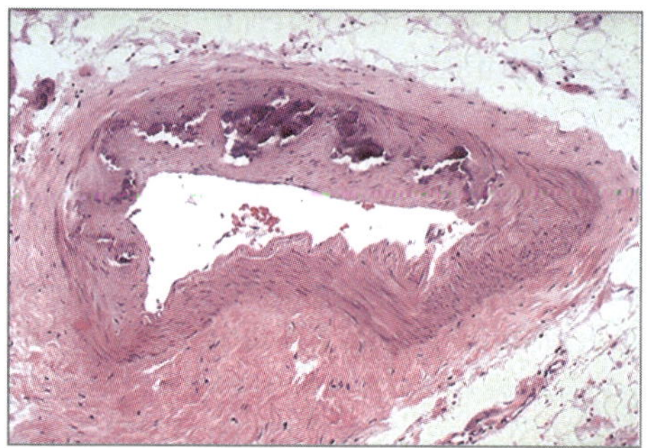

Fig. 1.27: Photomicrograph showing dystrophic calcification (reddish brown) areas in the tunica media of the blood vessel (Monckeberg's sclerosis).

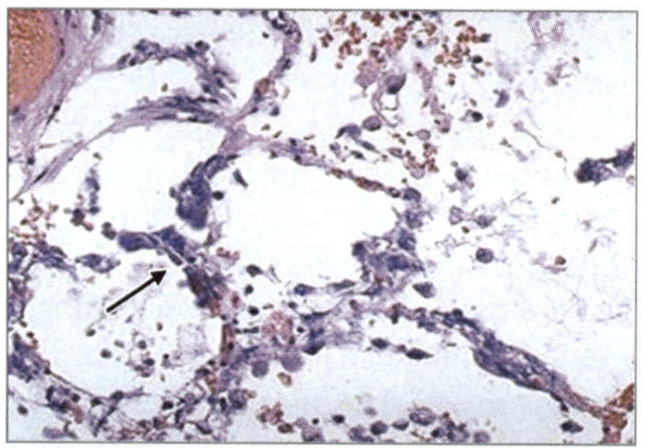

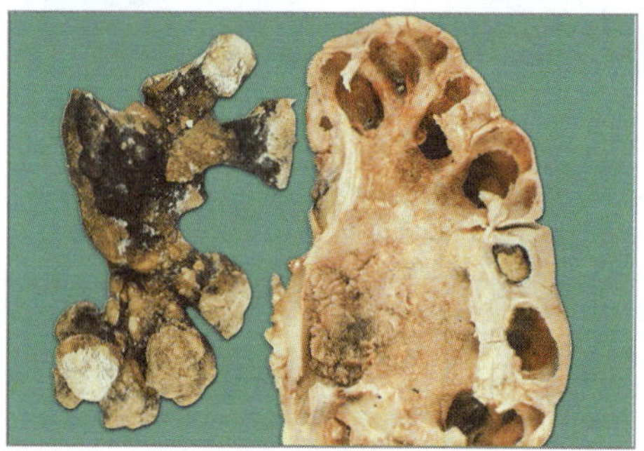

Fig. 1.28: Pulmonary alveolar microlithiasis, arrow points to the calcium deposits.

- In the alveolar walls of the lung, this condition is termed as pulmonary alveolar microlithiasis **(Fig. 1.28)**.

Wall of the blood vessels and cornea.

Common predisposing factors for hypercalcemia includes:

- Hyperparathyroidism
- Hypervitaminosis D
- Milk-Alkali syndrome
- Hypophosphatemia
- Destructive bone lesions

Points to Ponder

- There are four core areas in pathology—etiology, pathogenesis, pathological features and clinical features.
- There are four common cellular adaptations—hyperplasia, hypertrophy, atrophy and metaplasia.
- Cellular injury is mainly caused by physical, chemical, biological agents. The most common cause is hypoxia.
- The two phases of cell injury are reversible and irreversible phases. The death of mitochondria is the tell-tale sign of cellular death.
- The two common forms of cell death are apoptosis and necrosis.
- There are various types of necrosis which varies in their pathologic behavior.
- The two forms of pathologic calcification are dystrophic calcification and metastatic calcification.

ASSESSMENT QUESTIONS

Essay Type Questions

1. **Define necrosis. Describe the morphology of a necrotic cell. Describe in detail the various types of necrosis with suitable clinical examples.**
2. **Define apoptosis. Discuss the morphological features of apoptosis. Enumerate the salient differences between necrosis and apoptosis.**
3. **What is fatty change of liver? Enlist the common causes. Discuss in detail the morphology, microscopy and complications of fatty liver.**

Short Answer Questions

1. **What are the four main aspects that constitute the core of pathology?**
2. **Define hyperplasia. Give two examples.**
3. **What is metaplasia? Give examples.**
4. **What are the main cellular structures targeted in cell injury?**
5. **Enumerate the most common biochemical derangements in a cell injury.**
6. **Define free oxygen radicals. Give examples.**
7. **Enlist the causes for fatty change of liver.**
8. **Name the two most common morphological forms of irreversible cell injury.**
9. **What are the major types of necrosis?**
10. **Enlist the cause and common organs involved in osteonecrosis.**
11. **Define apoptosis.**
12. **Compare and contrast apoptosis and necrosis.**
13. **What are psammoma bodies?**
14. **Name the special stains for demonstration of fat.**
15. **What are the common organs affected in metastatic calcification?**

MULTIPLE CHOICE QUESTIONS

1. **One of the following is *NOT* an adaptation:**
   A. Hyperplasia
   B. Hypertrophy
   C. Dysplasia
   D. Metaplasia
2. **Antioxidants include all, *except*:**
   A. Cysteine
   B. Haptoglobin
   C. Transferrin
   D. Glutathione
3. **Free radicals cause all, *except*:**
   A. Lipid peroxidation
   B. Protein-protein crosslinking
   C. Protein strand scission
   D. Hydroxylation of amino acids
4. **Necrosis in brain is:**
   A. Liquefactive
   B. Coagulative
   C. Caseous
   D. Fibrinoid
5. **The most common cause of fatty liver is:**
   A. CCl4
   B. Starvation
   C. Alcoholism
   D. Steroids
6. **One of the following organelle is very critical in all cell injuries:**
   A. Ribosomes
   B. Golgi zone
   C. Lysosome
   D. Mitochondria
7. **Metastatic calcification occurs in all, *except*:**
   A. Hypoparathyroidism
   B. Addison's disease
   C. Vitamin D intoxication
   D. Systemic sarcoidosis
8. **The most common cause for cell injury is:**
   A. Genetic derangement
   B. Hypoxia
   C. Chemicals
   D. Biological

9. The enzyme that plays key role in protein denaturation of apoptosis is:

A. Ribonuclease
B. Endonuclease
C. Caspase
D. DNAase

10. The most common pattern of necrosis seen in immune mediated cell injury is:

A. Fibrinoid necrosis
B. Coagulative necrosis
C. Fat necrosis
D. Gangrenous necrosis

11. Which of the following is a characteristic feature of reversible cell injury?

A. Cellular swelling
B. Loss of membrane integrity
C. Irreversible DNA damage
D. Mitochondrial dysfunction

12. Father of modern pathology is _______

A. Rudolf Virchow
B. Gregor Mendel
C. Antonie van Leeuwenhoek
D. Herophilus

13. Which type of necrosis is often associated with tuberculosis?

A. Coagulative necrosis
B. Liquefactive necrosis
C. Caseous necrosis
D. Fat necrosis

14. Which of the following is a common consequence of ischemia in cell injury?

A. Increased ATP production
B. Acidosis
C. Enhanced cell function
D. Reduced oxidative stress

15. What is a hallmark of necrotic cell death?

A. Inflammation
B. Cell shrinkage
C. Preservation of cell structure
D. Controlled process

Answer Key for MCQs

1	2	3	4	5	6	7	8	9	10
C	B	D	A	C	D	A	B	C	A
11	**12**	**13**	**14**	**15**					
A	A	C	B	A					

2 CHAPTER

Inflammation

Learning Objectives

At the end of reading this chapter, the student shall be able to:

- Define inflammation. Describe the general features of acute and chronic inflammation. Discuss the vascular and cellular events in inflammation.
- Enumerate the chemical mediators and discuss its role in inflammation.
- Describe the various morphological patterns of acute inflammation.
- Describe the various morphological patterns of chronic inflammation.

INTRODUCTION

Definition: It is defined as the reaction of vascularized connective tissue to a sublethal injury. It is fundamentally a protective response to get rid of the offending injurious agents and if this goes unchecked it may be harmful.

Components: It includes the following **(Fig. 2.1)**:

1. Blood vessels
2. Plasma
3. Circulating cells—neutrophils, eosinophils, monocytes, lymphocytes, basophils, platelets and mast cells
4. Extracellular matrix proteins—collagen, fibronectin, laminin and others

Types: Inflammation is generally categorized as acute and chronic **(Table 2.1)**.

Cardinal signs of inflammation: There are four cardinal signs of an inflammatory response. This was described by Aulus Celsus in 1st Century AD. He was a Roman encyclopedist.

1. **Calor—heat**
2. **Rubor—redness**
3. **Dolor—pain**
4. **Tumor—swelling**

Rudolph Virchow added **loss of function**, as one more sign to the list of cardinal signs of inflammation.

ACUTE INFLAMMATION

The two most important events in acute inflammation includes

1. *Vascular events:*
   The main purpose of vascular events is to deliver circulating cells and plasma proteins to the site of injury. This is generally achieved by the following:
   a. Alteration in caliber of blood vessels
   b. Structural changes in the blood vessels
2. *Cellular events:* Emigration of leukocytes and their accumulation.

Vascular Events

The following are the vascular events that occur in acute inflammation. It includes:

1. *Transient vasoconstriction*—occurs immediately after the injury
2. Vasodilatation of the arterioles with increased blood flow (this is the factor which produces heat and redness in the site of inflammation)

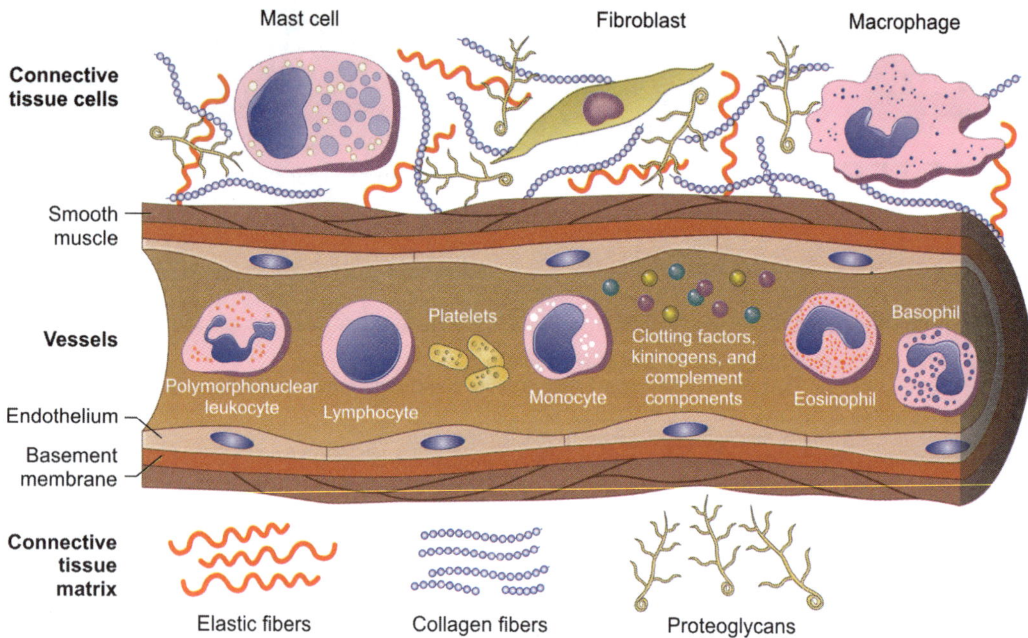

Fig. 2.1: Shows a blood vessel with its components and extravascular tissue components.

TABLE 2.1: Comparison of acute and chronic inflammation.

	Acute inflammation	*Chronic inflammation*
Duration	Short	Longer
Onset	Rapid (minutes to hours)	Slow and gradual
Predominant cell	Neutrophils	Lymphocytes/Macrophages
Cardinal event	Exudation	Tissue damage with proliferation of blood vessels and fibroblasts
Nature of tissue damage	Mild	Moderate to severe

3. *Increased vascular permeability:* It is the hallmark of acute inflammation. The endothelial lining becomes leaky and protein rich plasma escapes into the interstitial. This fluid is called **exudate**.
   Characteristics of an exudate:
   - Rich in protein
   - The specific gravity is more than 1.018
   - Rich in cells, mostly neutrophils **(Fig. 2.2)**.
   - High levels of lactate dehydrogenase [LDH]

     This can be distinguished from *transudate*—which is an ultrafiltrate of plasma that comes out of the vessel due to imbalances in the hydrostatic pressure. It has a very low protein content, specific gravity (< 1.018) and lactate dehydrogenase levels.

Causes for increase vascular permeability: The increase in vascular permeability is due to
- Formation of gaps between the endothelial cells
- Contraction and retraction of endothelial cells
- Direct injury to the endothelial cells
- Increased transcytosis

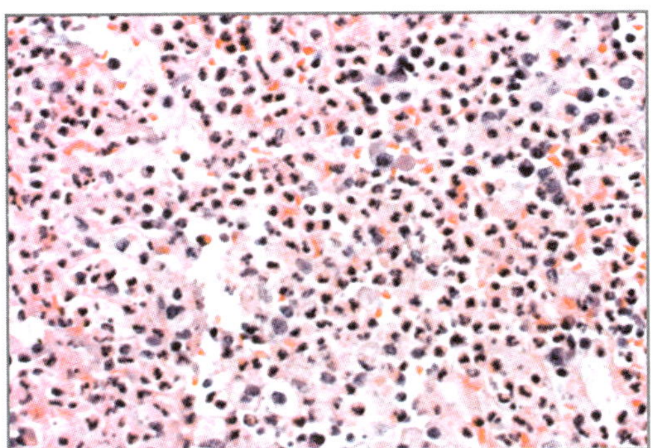

Fig. 2.2: Photomicrograph showing an inflammatory exudate with plenty of neutrophils.

4. *Slowing of circulation (stasis):* As the protein rich plasma escapes out of the vessels, there will be accumulation of red cells, white cells and platelets within the vessel.

Cellular Events

They play a critical role in inflammation and deliver the appropriate leukocytes to the site of injury. This can be grouped as intravascular and extravascular events.

Intravascular Events

It includes:

- *Margination:* During normal blood flow the leukocytes occupy the central column of flow rimmed by the red cells and platelets in the periphery. This is called the **axial flow**.
  During acute inflammation as a result of stasis, the leukocytes from the central column move to the periphery and this is referred to as margination.
- *Rolling and pavementing:* The leukocytes on reaching the periphery roll on the endothelium and arrange themselves on the endothelium which appears like the stones placed on the pavement. This event is called as **pavementing**.
- *Adhesion:* The leukocytes are tightly bound to the endothelial cells by a group of proteins called the adhesion molecules. They act as cellular glue and bridges leukocytes and endothelium.
  Adhesion molecules belong to three major families—selectins, immunoglobulin super family and integrins.
  Examples—E-selectin, P-selectin, L-selectin. ICAM-1 (intercellular adhesion molecule), VCAM-1 (vascular cell adhesion molecule), alpha and beta integrins.

Extravascular Events

It includes:

- Transmigration and diapedesis
- Chemotaxis
- Phagocytosis

Transmigration: Once the cell is adhered well to the endothelium, it slowly put forth long foot processes called the pseudopods which extend to the endothelial cell junctions and insert themselves into the gaps and slowly escape out of the vessel. This process is termed as transmigration. This transmigration is carried out with the help of a protein called **CD31 [platelet endothelial cell adhesion molecule (PECAM-1)]**

A similar movement of the red blood cells is termed as **diapedesis**.

Chemotaxis [Chemo—chemical, taxis—movement]

It is defined as a locomotion oriented along a chemical gradient. It is a process in which the leukocytes are attracted by certain chemicals to reach the site of injury **(Fig. 2.3)**.

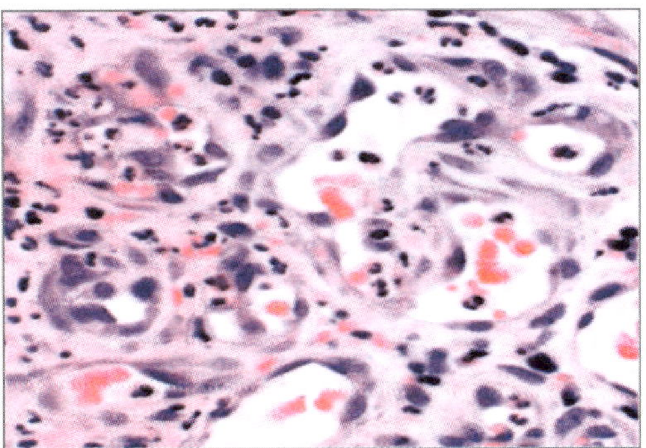

Fig. 2.3: Neutrophils in chemotaxis.

Chemoattractant: The chemicals that attract the leukocytes are called as **chemoattractants**.

They include the following:
- Bacterial products rich in N-Formylmethionine
- Complement fraction 5a
- Leukotriene B4
- Interleukin-8

Mechanism: The leukocytes have cell surface receptors for the chemoattractants and once the receptor is occupied, it leads to sequence of events activating the contractile proteins of the leukocyte which makes the cell to move and reach the site of injury. The contractile proteins are actin, myosin, filamin, gelsolin, calmodulin and profilin. This process not only makes the cell to move but also causes phosphorylation of the cell membranes of the lysosomes. So, the lysosomes become ready to release its contents. This is called priming of the leucocytes.

Phagocytosis: It is an important and critical cellular event in acute inflammation in which the offending pathogen is recognized and killed by the leukocytes.

It comprises of three stages:
1. *Stage of recognition and attachment*: The leukocytes will be able to recognize the offending pathogen only when they are coated with protein substance called **opsonin**. This process is called as opsonization.
   The common opsonin's include **(Table 2.2)**:
   - Fc fragment of immunoglobulin G
   - Complement fraction C3
   - Collections

TABLE 2.2: List of opsonin's and their receptors.

Opsonin	*Receptor on the leukocyte*
Fc fragment of immunoglobulin G	Fc receptor
Complement fraction C3	CR1 and CR3 receptors
Collectins	C1q receptor

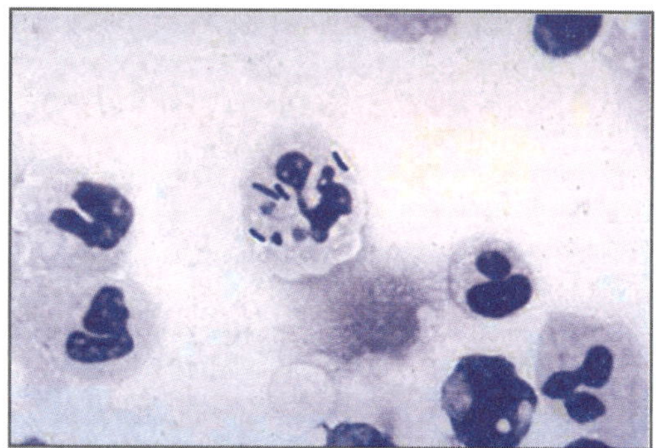

Fig. 2.4: Macrophage with active phagocytosis.

2. *Stage of engulfment*: The leukocytes have cell surface receptors for the opsonins. Once the receptor is occupied by the opsonin, the contractile proteins of the cell gets activated and it put forth cytoplasmic extensions called the pseudopods which slowly engulfs the organism and completely surrounds it. This is called **phagosome (Fig. 2.4)**. By this process, the organism gets internalized within the cytoplasm of the leukocyte. Within the cytoplasm the phagosome is slowly moved close to the lysosome of the leukocyte and they both fuse to form the **phagolysosome**. After the fusion, the contents of the lysosome are released into the phagosome which activates the killing process.
3. *Stage of killing and degradation*: Killing is usually done by two processes. They are
   i *Oxygen dependent mechanism*: The oxygen dependent mechanism is carried out by the generation of free oxygen radicals which undergo a chain reaction to kill the pathogen. The generation of the free oxygen radicals occurs due to the activation of NADPH oxidase which generates a superoxide free radical. This undergoes spontaneous dismutation and gets converted to hydrogen peroxide. The hydrogen peroxide in the presence of an enzyme called Myeloperoxidase gets activated to

another radical called hypochlorite which is a potent microbicidal agent.

Nitric oxide is another free radical generated which can kill the microbes. The nitric oxide combines with superoxide to form peroxynitrite which is a powerful bactericidal agent.

ii. *Oxygen independent mechanisms*: The leukocytes will also be able to kill the offending pathogens without the generation of free oxygen radicals. These are called oxygen independent mechanisms. They include:
   - Bactericidal permeability increasing factor
   - Lysozyme—present in tears and prostatic secretions
   - Lactoferrin
   - Major basic protein of eosinophil—for killing parasites
   - Defensins
   - Cathelicidins

Neutrophil extracellular traps: The neutrophils also secrete extracellular fibrillary networks called traps. These traps contain histone, DNA and antimicrobial peptides which prevent spread of the microbes.

Defects in the Functioning of Leukocytes

The common defects in the functioning of the leukocytes are summarized in **Table 2.3**.

TABLE 2.3: Common defects in the functioning of leukocytes.

Nature of the defect	*Conditions*
Reduced number of leukocytes	♦ Bone marrow aplasia ♦ Radiation ♦ Chemotherapy
Defective Adhesion	♦ Deficiency of adhesion molecules ♦ Diabetes ♦ Chronic alcoholism ♦ Corticosteroids ♦ Long-term hemodialysis
Defective Migration	♦ Microtubular dysfunction ♦ Chediak–Higashi syndrome
Defective chemotaxis and locomotion	♦ Deficiency of chemoattractants ♦ Microtubular dysfunction ♦ Drugs, such as colchicine
Defective opsonization	♦ Deficiency of opsonin
Defective killing	♦ Chronic granulomatous disease of childhood (deficiency of NADPH oxidase), myeloperoxidase deficiency ♦ Lactoferrin deficiency ♦ Lysozyme and G6PD deficiency
Mixed defects	♦ Malnutrition ♦ Diabetes mellitus ♦ Anemia ♦ Neonates ♦ Elderly age ♦ Sepsis ♦ Chediak–Higashi syndrome

Chemical Mediators of Inflammation

These are group of substances that are released endogenously and act at various levels of vascular and cellular events of inflammation.

The **general features** of the mediators include:

- Synthesized by cells and plasma
- Short duration of action
- Acts through the specific receptors on the cells
- Can act on the same cell which has produced it (autocrine)
- Tightly regulated action
- May have harmful effects.

Box 2.1: List of plasma derived mediators.

- Complement system
- Coagulation cascade
- Fibrinolytic system
- Kinins

Classification

The chemical mediators are generally classified as cell derived mediators and plasma derived mediators **(Box 2.1)**.

The cell derived mediators can be further categorized into preformed mediators and newly synthesized mediators. The following are some examples for chemical mediators in **(Table 2.4)**.

Table 2.5 summarizes some of the important components of the chemical mediators.

Table 2.6 summarizes the function of various chemical mediators in inflammation.

TABLE 2.4: List of cell derived chemical mediators.

Preformed cell derived mediators	*Newly synthesized cell derived mediators*
Histamine	Prostaglandins
Serotonin	Leukotrienes
Lysosomal enzymes	Cytokines
	Platelet activating factor
	Free oxygen radicals
	Nitric oxide

Morphological Patterns of Acute Inflammation

There are various morphological patterns of acute inflammatory response. They include the following as shown in **Table 2.7**.

Outcomes of Acute Inflammation

The acute inflammatory process can culminate into one of the following outcomes:

TABLE 2.5: Components of chemical mediators.

Chemical mediators	*Components*
Vasoactive amines	Histamine and serotonin
Lysosomal enzymes	Myeloperoxidase, acid hydrolases, neutral proteases, elastase, proteinase, lactoferrin, defensin, collagenase, and others
Arachidonic acid (cyclooxygenase pathway)	Prostacyclin, thromboxane, prostaglandin D2, E2 and F2 alpha
Arachidonic acid (lipoxygenase pathway)	Leukotriene A4, B4, C4, D4 and E4, Lipoxins
Free oxygen radicals	Superoxide, hydrogen peroxide, singlet oxygen, hydroxyl ion, hypochlorite ion
Free nitrogen radicals	Nitric oxide, peroxynitrites
Cytokines	Interleukin-1, 6, 8, 17, tumor necrosis factor (TNF), interferon gamma
Complement system	C3a, C4a, C5a, C3b, C5b-9
Kinin system	Kallikrein, bradykinin
Coagulation system	Fibrin peptides
Fibrinolytic system	Fibrin split products

TABLE 2.6: Chemical mediators and their specific function.

Chemical mediator	*Source of the mediator*	*Main action of the mediator*
Histamine and serotonin	Mast cell, platelets, basophils	Increased vascular permeability, vasodilatation
Lysosomal enzymes	Neutrophils, monocytes	♦ Microbial killing ♦ Tissue destruction
Thromboxane A2	Arachidonic acid (cyclooxygenase pathway)	♦ Vasoconstriction ♦ Platelet aggregation
Prostacyclin I2	Arachidonic acid (cyclooxygenase pathway)	♦ Vasodilation ♦ Inhibits platelet aggregation
Prostaglandin D2, E2 and F2 alpha	Arachidonic acid (cyclooxygenase pathway)	♦ Vasodilatation ♦ Increased vascular permeability ♦ Edema
Leukotrienes	Arachidonic acid (Lipoxygenase)	♦ Chemotaxis ♦ Leukocyte adhesion ♦ Release of lysosomal granules ♦ Vasoconstriction ♦ Increased vascular permeability
Platelet activating factor	Inflammatory cells	♦ Activation of platelets, increased vascular permeability, vasodilatation ♦ Leukocyte adhesion, ♦ Chemotaxis ♦ Oxidative burst
Nitric oxide	Endothelium, macrophages, neurons	♦ Vasodilatation ♦ Microbicidal
Free oxygen radicals	Inflammatory cells	♦ Microbial killing ♦ Tissue damage
Cytokines	♦ Activated lymphocytes ♦ Macrophages ♦ Endothelial cells ♦ Connective tissue cells	♦ Acute phase reactions—fever, sleep, leukocytosis ♦ Adhesion, chemoattractant ♦ Synthesis of other chemical mediators
Complement system	Plasma derived	♦ C3a, C4a, C5a (anaphylatoxins) ♦ C5a (chemoattractant, leukocyte adhesion) ♦ C3b (opsonin) ♦ C5b-9 (Membrane attack complex—microbicidal)
Kinin system	Plasma	♦ Increases vascular permeability ♦ Pain
Coagulation system	Plasma	♦ Increases vascular permeability ♦ Chemotaxis ♦ Leukocyte adhesion
Fibrinolytic system	Plasma	Increases vascular permeability

TABLE 7: Morphological pattern, features and examples of acute inflammation.

Morphological pattern	*Salient feature*	*Examples*
Serous **(Fig. 2.5A)**	Outpouring of thin watery fluid	♦ Blisters in burns **(Fig. 2.5A)** ♦ Pleural effusion ♦ Ascites
Fibrinous	Deposition of fibrinous material	♦ Pericarditis ♦ Pleuritis ♦ Pneumococcal and staphylococcal infections
Serofibrinous	Serous exudation with fibrinous debris	Rheumatic pericarditis (bread and butter type)
Catarrhal	Outpouring of mucinous material	Common cold
Suppurative **(Fig. 2.5C)**	Accumulation of purulent material (pus)	Abscess, carbuncle
Hemorrhagic **(Fig. 2.5B)**	Vascular damage	Influenza, *Klebsiella* infection
Membranous	Deposition of a true membranous structure	Membranous bronchitis, colitis, e.g., diphtherial infection
Pseudomembranous	Deposition of a fibrinous membrane like material	Pseudomembranous colitis caused by *Clostridium difficile*
Gangrenous	Necrosis with putrefaction	Sepsis, *Clostridium perfringens*
Ulcer	Local defect in mucosa	Acute peptic ulcers, stress ulcers

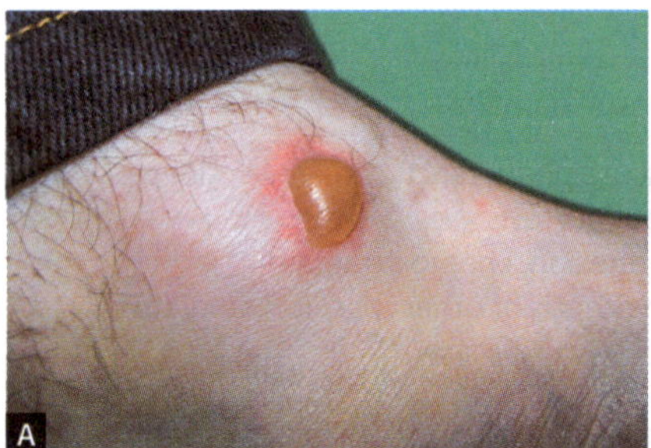
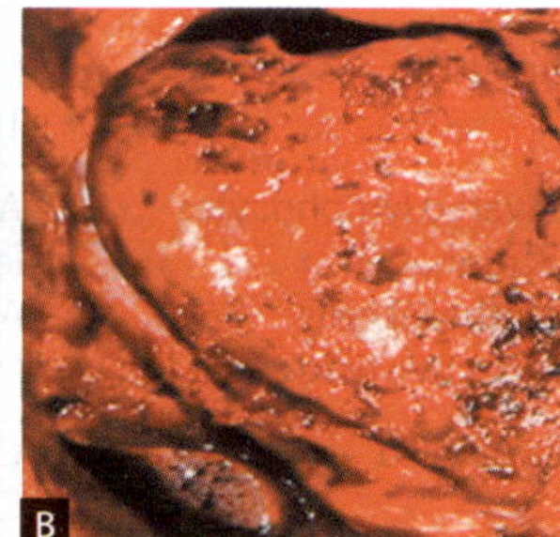
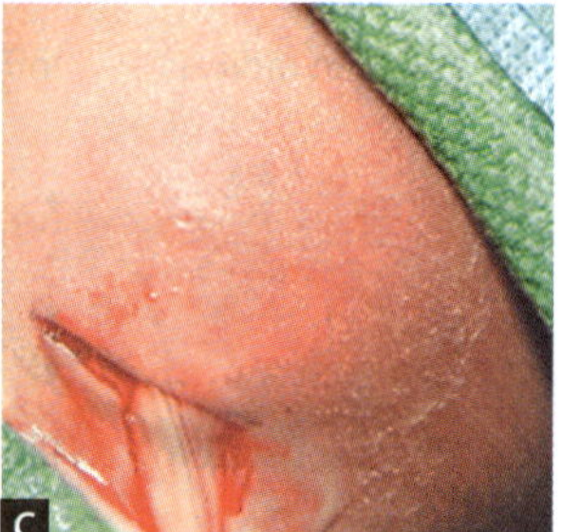

Figs. 5A to C: (A) Blister on the skin—serous inflammation; (B) Hemorrhagic inflammation; (C) Purulent inflammation.

a. *Complete resolution:* Complete return to normalcy with no residual tissue damage, e.g., resolution in lobar pneumonia.
b. *Healing by scarring:* Occurs when there is extensive tissue destruction there will be no regeneration and healing occurs by fibrous scarring, e.g., organizing abscess
c. *Chronic inflammation*: Unresolved acute inflammation or an incomplete phagocytic killing may cause progression of an acute inflammation to chronicity, e.g., chronic cholecystitis, chronic tonsillitis.

Case Scenario

A 35-year-old female patient is having the history of asthma come to OPD with complaints of red, itchy eyes, sneezing, and a runny nose. She reports that these symptoms have been present for the past three days. She has bilateral conjunctival redness and watery discharge with clear nasal discharge and occasional cough. No fever or respiratory distress is noted. She works in a flower shop.

Questions:

1. Based on the presenting symptoms and assessment, what type of inflammation is patient likely experiencing?
   A. Acute inflammation
   B. Chronic inflammation
   C. Allergic inflammation
   D. Infectious inflammation
2. What nursing intervention is appropriate to help alleviate patient symptoms of allergic inflammation?
   A. Prescribe antibiotics
   B. Administer antiviral medication
   C. Recommend rest and hydration
   D. Advise antihistamines and avoidance of allergens.

Answers:

1. (C) Allergic inflammation
2. (D) Advise antihistamines and avoidance of allergens.

Systemic Effects of Acute Inflammation

These are a group of symptoms that occur in cases with acute inflammation. They are also referred to as acute phase responses. These reactions are generally caused by cytokines. The common cytokines include interleukin-1, 6 and tumor necrosis factor alpha (TNF-Alpha). The acute phase responses include:

1. *Fever*: Due to the release of endogenous and exogenous pyrogens.
2. Leukocytosis
3. *Increased erythrocyte sedimentation rate (ESR)*: Due to increase in fibrinogen levels
4. Increased levels of C reactive protein (CRP)
5. Anorexia
6. Malaise

CHRONIC INFLAMMATION

Inflammation of prolonged duration with more tissue destruction and occurrence of parallel healing process is termed as chronic inflammation. A chronic inflammation may—

- Follow an acute inflammation—due to persistence of the injurious stimuli or interference with healing process
- Follow repeated episodes of acute inflammation, e.g., chronic cholecystitis following repeated acute cholecystitis
- Persistence of the microorganism—interference in the process of killing, e.g., tubercle bacilli, *Treponema pallidum*
- Prolonged exposure to non-degradable toxic substances, e.g., silica, talk
- Immune mediated de novo process, e.g., autoimmune diseases.

General Features of Chronic Inflammation

- Infiltration by mononuclear phagocytic cells, lymphoid cells and activated forms of the macrophages (epithelioid cells) and multinucleate giant cells.
- More tissue destruction by the action of the proteolytic enzymes released by the macrophages.
- Repair of the inflamed area by proliferation of blood capillaries and fibroblasts and eventual healing by fibrosis.

Macrophage in Chronic Inflammation

Macrophage in the predominant cell of chronic inflammatory response. It belongs to the mononuclear phagocyte system (MPS).

It is derived from the bone marrow as monoblastic, differentiates into promonocyte and mature monocyte. The monocyte is seen circulating in the peripheral blood. Similar monocytic cells are seen in various tissue and they are referred to as histiocytes. Various

TABLE 2.8: Histiocyte of various organs.

Organ	*Name of the histiocyte*
Liver	Kupffer cells
Spleen	Littoral cells
Lymph node	Interdigitating reticulum cell
Skin	Langerhans cell
Brain	Microglia
Bone	Osteoclast
Lung	Alveolar macrophage
Kidney	Mesangial cell

organs have specific histiocytic cells, which have been enlisted in **Table 2.8**.

When the monocyte is activated, it gets converted into a macrophage. The macrophages appear larger with abundant cytoplasm with many organelles mostly lysosomal enzymes. The metabolic status is very active. The macrophages are capable of secreting a wide range of chemical mediators, such as proteases, free oxygen radicals, arachidonic acid metabolites, growth factors, cytokines, nitric oxide and platelet activating factor. The action of these mediators has been described in detail earlier. The macrophages accumulate in the site of chronic inflammation due to continuous recruitment from circulation, local proliferation and immobilization of macrophages from the site of inflammation.

Other cells, such as the lymphocyte, plasma cells, and mast cells also play role in chronic inflammation.

Chronic Granulomatous Inflammation (Fig. 2.6)

It is a distinct pattern of chronic inflammation characterized by the presence of activated macrophages called epithelioid cells with/without giant cells, necrosis and fibrosis.

Granuloma: It is referred to as a collection of epithelioid cells surrounded by a collar of lymphocytes, occasional plasma cells and fibroblastic cell. It is a tiny lesion about 1 mm in diameter.

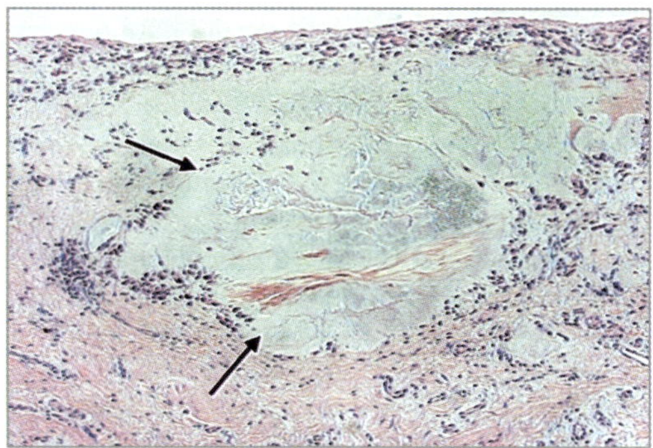

Fig. 2.6: Foreign body (arrows) granulomatous inflammation.

Epithelioid cell: It is an activated macrophage with indistinct cytoplasmic outlines and abundant pale pink granular cytoplasm with oval vesicular nuclei **(Fig. 2.7.)**. The nuclei take the shape of a foot print in cytological preparations. Since, this cell has got a resemblance to that of an epithelial cell it is named so. Under electron microscope, an epithelioid cells have got abundant endoplasmic reticulum, Golgi zone and mitochondria. It is a metabolically active cell but weakly phagocytic than a macrophage.

Pathogenesis: This inflammatory reaction occurs due to presence of a poorly digestible substance by the macrophage of immune mediated reaction by the T lymphocytes. The activation is usually mediated by cytokines like Gamma interferon and interleukin-4.

Giant cells: They are larger cells with multiple nuclei usually formed by the fusion of the epithelioid cells. The number of nuclei may

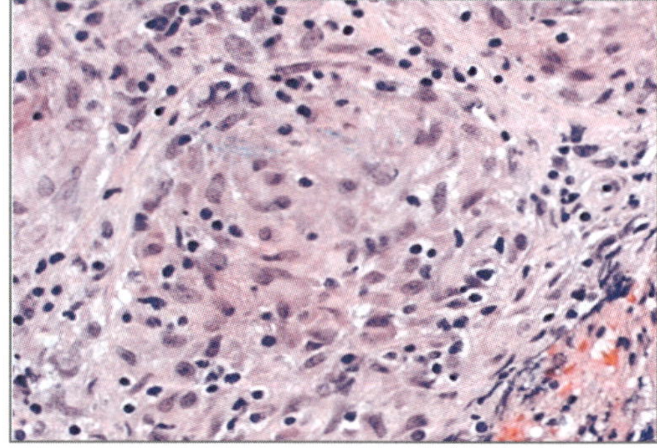

Fig. 2.7: Granuloma composed of epithelioid cells.

vary from 20–40 and the pattern of arrangement of the nuclei also differs. The common types of giant cells are the following:

- *Langhan's giant cell* **(Fig. 2.8)**: The nuclei are arranged along the cytoplasmic outlines on one side of the cells. This pattern is referred to as horse shoe or inverted necklace type. This giant cell is mostly seen in granulomas of tuberculosis.
- *Foreign body type giant cell*: The nuclei are clustered to the central part of the cells.
- *Touton giant cells*: The nuclei are arranged all round the cell membrane like a wreath. These are seen in lipogranulomatosis inflammatory conditions.

Giant cells may also be seen in other conditions, such as neoplasia where they are referred to as the **tumor giant cells** and it is due to abnormality of the cell division of the neoplastic cells and specific type of giant cells like **Reed-Sternberg, Hodgkin's** giant cells seen in Hodgkin's lymphoma. These has to be differentiated from the giant cell seen in chronic granulomatous inflammation.

Examples: The granulomatous inflammation can be grouped into two main categories based on the pathogenesis. They include the immune granulomas and non-immune granulomas.

The various conditions have been summarized in **Table 2.9**.

Special features of individual granulomatous disease conditions have been enlisted in **Table 2.10**.

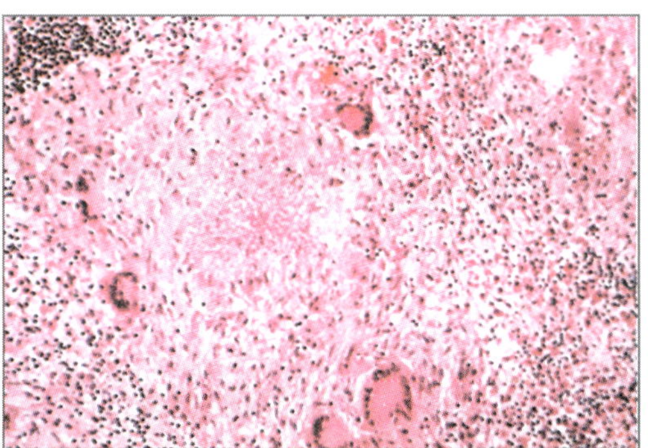

Fig. 2.8: Multiple Langhan's type giant cells.

TABLE 2.9: Examples of immune and non-immune granulomas.

Immune granulomas	***Non-immune granulomas***
Tuberculosis	Foreign body
Hansen's disease	Plastic
Syphilis	Carbon
Schistosomiasis	Silica
Fungal	Iron
Sarcoidosis	Talc
Zirconium	Asbestos
Beryllium	
Cat scratch disease	

TABLE 2.10: Granulomatous diseases and their characteristic features.

Type of granulomatous disease	***Special features***
Tuberculosis	Caseation necrosis and Langhan's giant cell
Hansen disease	Foamy histiocytes (lepra cells) with giant cells
Syphilis	Plasma cell rich lesions with obliterative endarteritis
Sarcoidosis	Non-caseating granulomas without peripheral rimming, giant cells with inclusions
Cat scratch disease	Stellate necrosis, plenty of neutrophils, no giant cells
Fungal	Presence of fungal elements

Points to Ponder

- Inflammation is a reaction of vascularized connective tissue to sublethal injury.
- The two common forms are acute and chronic inflammation.
- The inflammation occurs by a synchronized process of vascular and cellular events.
- Many chemical mediators play a role in mediating the course of inflammation which are categorized as cell derived and plasma derived mediators.
- There are various morphological presentations of acute inflammation.
- Granuloma is a unique type of chronic inflammation.

ASSESSMENT QUESTIONS

Essay Type Questions

1. **Define inflammation. Discuss in detail the various cellular events in acute inflammation.**
2. **Classify chemical mediators of inflammation. Discuss in detail the role of prostaglandins and complement system in inflammation.**
3. **Define granuloma. Describe the mechanism of formation of a granuloma. Enlist common examples for granulomatous inflammation.**

Short Answer Questions

1. **Enumerate the cardinal signs of acute inflammation.**
2. **What are the various steps in phagocytosis?**
3. **What are the functions of nitric oxide?**
4. **What are the major outcomes of acute inflammation?**
5. **Enumerate the characteristic features of chronic inflammation.**
6. **Define granuloma.**
7. **Give examples for adhesion molecules.**
8. **Name the various oxygen independent mechanism of killing.**
9. **Give examples for chemoattractants.**
10. **Enlist the systemic effects of acute inflammation.**
11. **Give examples for common morphological patterns of acute inflammation.**
12. **Enumerate the common defects in the function of leukocytes.**
13. **What is chronic granulomatous disease of childhood?**
14. **What is a giant cell? Give examples.**

MULTIPLE CHOICE QUESTIONS

1. **The predominant cells within 24–48 hours in inflammation are:**
   A. Neutrophils
   B. Lymphocytes
   C. Eosinophils
   D. Monocytes
2. **Which is not an opsonin?**
   A. C3b
   B. IgG-3
   C. IgG-1
   D. IgE
3. **One of the following cytokines is a powerful chemoattractant:**
   A. Interleukin-8
   B. Interleukin-2
   C. Interleukin-6
   D. Interleukin-4
4. **Microglia are macrophages of:**
   A. Brain
   B. Liver
   C. Lymph node
   D. Kidney
5. **Most common type of acute inflammation is:**
   A. Pyogenic inflammation
   B. Catarrhal inflammation
   C. Membranous inflammation
   D. Ulcer
6. **In tuberculosis, the giant cells found are:**
   A. Foreign body type
   B. Langhans cells
   C. Warthin-Finkeldey cell
   D. Reed-Sternberg cells

7. The main bactericidal substance of eosinophils is:

A. Lactoferrin
B. Major basic protein
C. Bactericidal permeability increasing factor
D. Lysozyme

8. The hallmark of inflammation is:

A. Transient vasoconstriction
B. Leukocyte margination
C. Phagocytosis
D. Increased vascular permeability

9. Increased vascular permeability is caused by:

A. LTC4
B. LTD4
C. LTE4
D. LTB4

10. Nitric oxide [NO] is produced in the body by all, *except*:

A. Neurons
B. Macrophages
C. Endothelial cells
D. Lymphocytes

11. Which of the following is a cardinal sign of inflammation?

A. Fever
B. Nausea
C. Dizziness
D. Insomnia

12. What term describes the local application of heat, redness, swelling, and pain during inflammation?

A. Exudation
B. Rubor
C. Infiltration
D. Calo

13. What term describes the accumulation of fluid with a high protein content in the extravascular tissue during acute inflammation?

A. Transudate
B. Exudate
C. Serous fluid
D. Pus

14. Which chemical mediator is responsible for causing pain during acute inflammation?

A. Prostaglandins
B. Histamine
C. Interleukins
D. Tumor necrosis factor (TNF)

15. Which of the following is a local manifestation of acute inflammation?

A. Fever
B. Malaise
C. Edema
D. Leukocytosis

Answer Key for MCQs

1	2	3	4	5	6	7	8	9	10
A	D	A	A	B	B	B	D	D	D
11	**12**	**13**	**14**	**15**					
A	B	B	A	C					

CHAPTER

Wound Healing and Repair

Learning Objectives

At the end of reading this chapter, the student should be able to:

- Define and differentiate regeneration and replacement.
- Describe the mechanisms of wound healing and the types of wound healing.
- Briefly enlist the factors influencing healing of wounds.

INTRODUCTION

Injury to tissue may result in cell death and tissue damage. Healing is one of the body response to injury in an attempt to restore the normal structure and function. The healing can occur by two distinct processes. They are:

1. *Regeneration:* The injured tissue is repaired by the proliferation of similar type cells.
2. *Replacement:* The injured tissue is replaced by a specialized connective tissue called granulation tissue which contains proliferating blood capillaries and myofibroblast cells **(Fig. 3.1)**.

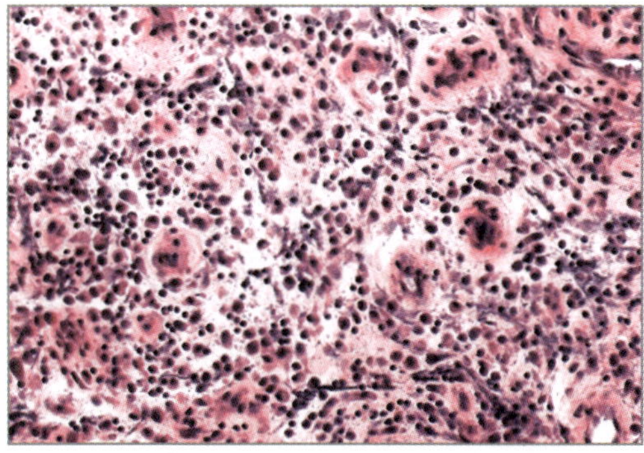

Fig. 3.1: Granulation tissue with capillaries, myofibroblast and inflammatory cells.

REGENERATION

Based on the capacity of regeneration the cells in the body are generally grouped as follows **(Table 3.1)**.

TABLE 3.1: Types of cells based on the capacity of regeneration.

Name of the cell	*Property*	*Sites*
Labile cell	Continuous proliferation all through the life	➢ Bone marrow cells ➢ Epidermal cells ➢ Mucous membrane ➢ GIT ➢ Transitional cell of bladder, etc.
Stable cell	Undergo replication only when stimulated appropriately	➢ Liver ➢ Renal tubules ➢ Fibroblasts ➢ Chondroblasts ➢ Osteoblasts
Permanent cell	Do not replicate after birth	➢ Neurons ➢ Skeletal muscle cells ➢ Cardiac muscle cells

Repair by Connective Tissue

This occurs due to the proliferation of a specialized connective tissue called the granulation tissue. There are three phases in the formation of granulation tissue which are:

1. Phase of traumatic inflammation—indicates the inflammatory responses.
2. Phase of demolition—indicates the extent of tissue damage.
3. Phase of development of granulation tissue—this is further subdivided into a stage of neovascularization and stage of devascularization.

Case Scenario

A male patient of 60 years admitted to hospital with a laceration on his right leg, which he sustained from a fall at home. The wound is 5 cm in length and extends to the subcutaneous tissue. Patient is having the history of type-2 diabetes. During initial assessment, the nurse assess that the wound edges are clean, and there is no evidence of infection, tingling and numbness around the wound site and peripheral pulses and capillary refill are within normal limits.

Questions:

1. What term is used to describe the initial phase of wound healing where bleeding is controlled, and a temporary clot forms?
   A. Proliferation
   B. Inflammation
   C. Hemostasis
   D. Maturation
2. Considering patient condition of tingling and numbness sensation, which nursing intervention is essential to prevent complic-ations during wound healing?
   A. Apply a warm compress to the wound
   B. Elevate the affected leg
   C. Monitor blood glucose levels closely
   D. Administer analgesics for pain relief

Answers:

1. (C) Hemostasis
2. (C) Monitor blood glucose levels closely

Stage of neovascularization: This is characterized by the in growth of new capillaries and proliferation of specialized fibroblastic cells.

New vessels sprout from the parent vessels and migrate towards the area of damage. Initially, these vessels are very weak and leaky and later they get organized and canalized. Due to the leaky capillaries, the injured site appears edematous. Sprouting of the new vessels occurs due to release of various antigenic factors, such as vascular endothelial growth factor (VEGF); Platelet derived growth factor (PDGF) and transforming growth factor—Beta.

Neovascularization is accompanied by the proliferation of plump myofibroblast cells which have more abundant granular cytoplasm and contractility. These cells are responsible for the contraction of the wound area to be repaired.

Stage of devascularization: Once the healing process is over, the new blood vessels gets organized and deposition of collagen replaces the fibroblastic cells.

Healing of Skin Wound

This provides a classic example for both regeneration and replacement responses of healing. Healing of a skin wound can be of two types based on the nature of the wound **(Table 3.2)**.

Healing by Primary Intention

The sequence of events has been illustrated in in **Figure 3.2**. The events include:

TABLE 3.2: Differences between healing by primary and secondary intention.

Healing by primary intention	*Healing by secondary intention*
Clean surgical wounds	Larger wounds
Clean and sharp opposing edges	Gaped opposing edges
Minimal tissue loss	More tissue loss
No contamination	Infected wound

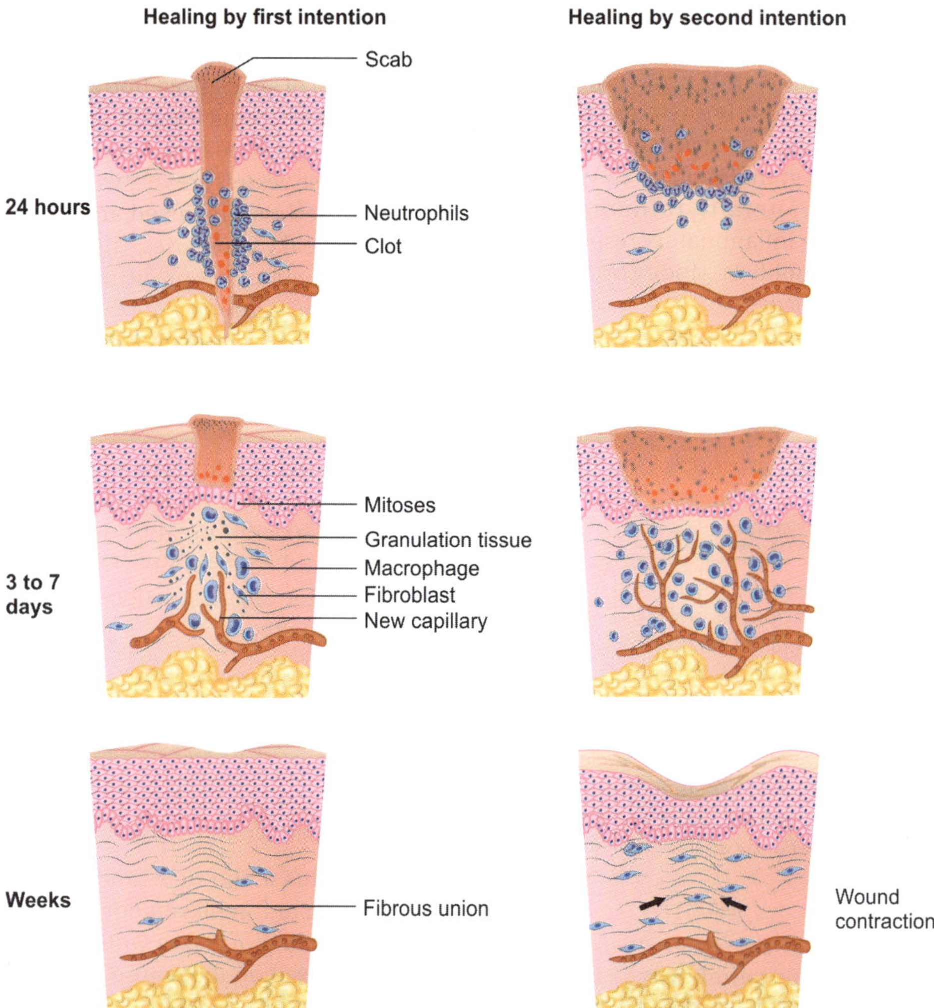

Fig. 3.2: Healing of wound by primary and secondary intention.

- The incision is filled with blood clot. The fibrin bridges the opposing edges. The upper surface of the clot gets dried up and it is called as the scab.
- Within 24 hours neutrophils migrate to the margins of the wound. The basal layer of the skin appears thick at the cut ends. The cells migrate from both the cut ends and unite beneath the scab. The wound continuity is established.
- 1 to 3 days, the epithelial proliferation and differentiation takes place. The neutrophils are replaced by macrophages and there is formation of vascularized granulation tissue **(Fig. 3.3)**.
- 3 to 5 days, there will be abundant proliferation of granulation tissue with deposition of the collagen. The surface epithelium is fully restored **(Fig. 3.4)**.
- By 2 weeks, there will be maximum deposition of collagen with devascularization.
- By 1 month, the scarring the complete and the wound heals by a thin scar.

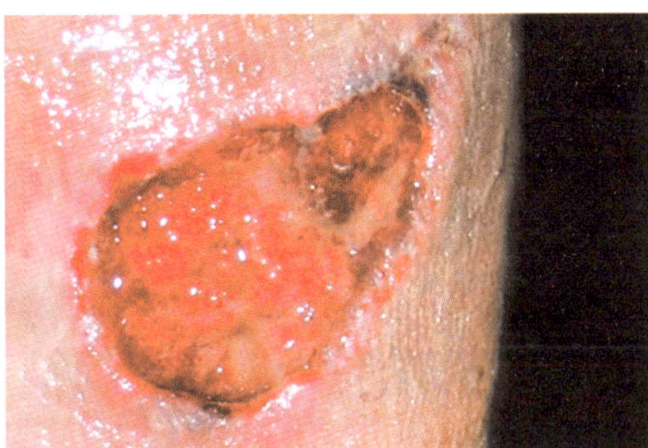

Fig. 3.3: Ulcer with pinkish granulation tissue.

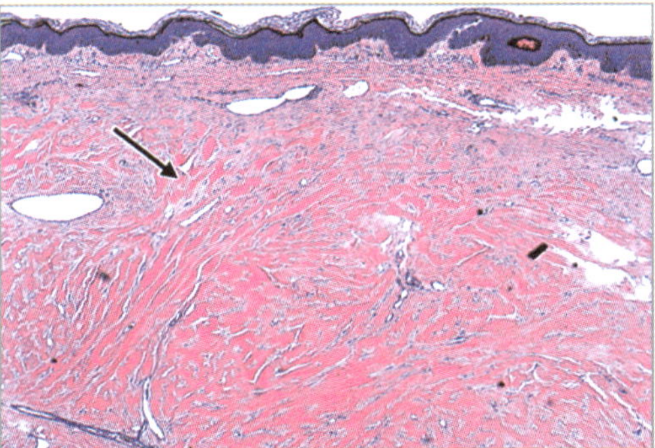

Fig. 3.4: Scar tissue bundles of collagen indicated by arrow.

Healing by Secondary Intention

The sequence of events has been illustrated in **Figure 3.2**.

The basic events in this healing process are similar to that the above process but with the following differences.

There is a larger tissue defect which has to be repaired; amount of granulation tissue generated is more. The major event in this type of healing is the phenomenon of wound contraction. Due to contractile activity of the myofibroblast cells in the granulation tissue, the surface area of the wound gets reduced. This is a protective phenomenon to reduce the scarring.

This healing process is generally slow and results in a thick scar.

Healing of a fracture of bone: This is similar to that of skin wound, where after the formation of granulation tissue, there will be formation of an immature woven bone between the fracture ends which is called the callus. The callus is gradually replaced by mature bone with subsequent calcification and remodeling, the fracture gets healed.

Factors Influencing Wound Healing

The factors influencing wound healing is categorized into local and systemic factors which are summarized in the **Table 3.3**.

TABLE 3.3: Factors influencing wound healing.

Systemic factors	*Local factors*
Age—healing delayed in elderly	Location of wound
Malnutrition	Nature of tissue
Deficiency of methionine and cysteine	Type and size of wound
Vitamin C deficiency	Status of mobility of the site of wound
Deficiency of zinc	Vascularity of the site
Defects in functioning of leukocytes	Presence of infection
Diabetes mellitus	Presence of foreign body
Use of corticosteroids	

Points to Ponder

- Healing of a wound occurs by the process of regeneration and replacement.
- Various tissues of the body have different capacity for regeneration.
- They are categorized as labile cell, stable cells and permanent cells.
- Healing of a clean surgical wound is by primary intention.
- Other skin wounds heal by secondary intention.
- The most common problems in healing are formation of hypertrophic scar and keloid.
- Fracture of bone heals by formation of Callus
- Various local and general factors contribute for the mechanism of healing.

ASSESSMENT QUESTIONS

1. **What are the two major types of healing process?**
2. **What are the various angiogenic growth factors?**
3. **What is callus? Describe its significance.**
4. **What are the common complications of cutaneous wound healing?**
5. **What are the three different phases in cutaneous wound healing?**

MULTIPLE CHOICE QUESTIONS

1. **The characteristic histologic picture of granulation tissue is:**
   A. Transcytosis
   B. Fibroblastic proliferation
   C. Mononuclear infiltration
   D. Angiogenesis
2. **The most important difference between primary and secondary healing is:**
   A. More intense inflammation in secondary
   B. Less granulation tissue is primary
   C. Wound contraction of secondary
   D. Larger defect in secondary
3. **Most of the collagen in the body is of which type:**
   A. Type I
   B. Type II
   C. Type V
   D. Type IX
4. **The single most important cause of delay in wound healing is:**
   A. Steroids
   B. Malnutrition
   C. Infection
   D. Vitamin deficiency
5. **A keloid is:**
   A. Exuberant granulation tissue
   B. Excessive collagen accumulation
   C. Scar due to a burn of seven degree
   D. Recurrent fibroblastic tumor
6. **What is the primary purpose of the inflammatory phase in the process of wound healing?**
   A. Proliferation of new cells
   B. Removal of debris and pathogens
   C. Formation of new blood vessels
   D. Collagen deposition
7. **Which type of tissue is primarily involved in the repair phase of wound healing?**
   A. Nervous tissue
   B. Muscle tissue
   C. Connective tissue
   D. Epithelial tissue
8. **What is the term for the process of replacing damaged tissue with scar tissue?**
   A. Regeneration
   B. Fibrosis
   C. Inflammation
   D. Proliferation
9. **Which of the following is a key cellular component involved in tissue repair?**
   A. Neutrophils
   B. Erythrocytes
   C. Platelets
   D. Lymphocytes
10. **What is the role of fibroblasts in wound healing?**
    A. Phagocytosis of debris
    B. Synthesis of collagen and extracellular matrix
    C. Release of inflammatory mediators
    D. Differentiation into new cells

11. Which factor is essential for the successful healing of a wound?

A. Chronic inflammation
B. Excessive bleeding
C. Adequate blood supply
D. Inhibition of fibroblast activity

12. What is angiogenesis in the context of wound healing?

A. Formation of new blood vessels
B. Removal of damaged tissue
C. Proliferation of immune cells
D. Synthesis of collagen fibers

13. Which vitamin is important for collagen synthesis and plays a crucial role in wound healing?

A. Vitamin A
B. Vitamin B12
C. Vitamin C
D. Vitamin D

14. In which phase of wound healing does tissue remodeling occur?

A. Inflammatory phase
B. Proliferative phase
C. Maturation phase
D. Regeneration phase

15. What is the term for the process by which a tissue returns to its normal structure and function after injury?

A. Fibrosis
B. Regeneration
C. Resolution
D. Maturation

Answer Key for MCQs

1	**2**	**3**	**4**	**5**	**6**	**7**	**8**	**9**	**10**
D	C	A	C	B	B	C	B	A	B
11	12	13	14	15					
C	A	C	C	C					

CHAPTER

Fluid and Hemodynamic Disturbances

Learning Objectives

At the end of reading this chapter, the student shall be able to:

- Define edema, discuss the pathophysiological basis and enumerate the clinical features of renal and cardiac edema.
- Define hyperemia, congestion and hemorrhage.
- Define and describe normal hematosis, etiopathogenesis, pathology and consequences of thrombosis.
- Define and describe embolism and its common types.
- Define and describe infarction and its types.
- Define shock, discuss the pathophysiological basis and enumerate the clinical features and stages of various types of shock.

INTRODUCTION

The normal composition of the internal environment consists of water and electrolytes.

1. *Water:* Principal and essential constituent of the body. The total body water comprises of 50–70% of the body weight. This is distributed into two main compartments, namely the intracellular (33%) mostly within the muscular tissue and extracellular compartments (27%).

   The extracellular fluid compartment is composed of interstitial fluid (12%), intravascular fluid of blood plasma (5%), fluid within the mesenchymal tissue (9%) and transcellular fluid (1%) of the body weight.
2. *Electrolytes*: The distribution of the electrolytes is summarized in **Table 4.1**.

The electrolytes are the main solutes of the body to maintain the acid base equilibrium. They help to maintain the normal osmolality and volume of the body fluids. They are responsible for many specific physiological functions, such as the concentration of calcium ions for neuromuscular contraction.

TABLE 4.1: Composition of intracellular and extracellular fluid.

Nature of the fluid	*Anions*	*Cations*
Intracellular fluid	Phosphates	Potassium
	Proteins	Magnesium
Extracellular fluid	Chloride	Sodium
	Bicarbonate	

The disorders of hemodynamic system can be grouped into three main categories:

1. Disturbances of body fluid and electrolytes—edema
2. Disturbances in the volume of circulating blood—hyperemia, congestion, hemorrhage, shock
3. Disturbances of hemodynamic system of obstructive nature—thrombosis, embolism, infarction.

EDEMA

Definition

It is defined as an abnormal and excessive accumulation of fluid in the interstitial space.

The term is derived from a Greek word *oedema* which means swelling. There are various terms used to describe edema of various sites.

Edema can be further categorized into local and general

The generalized edema is called as Anasarca.

Edema of the serous cavities is examples for localized edema and they are referred according to the space involved:

- Pleura— hydrothorax (Pleural effusion)
- Pericardium—hydropericardium (pericardial effusion)
- Peritoneum—hydroperitoneum (ascites)

Clinically edema can be grouped as pitting and non-pitting edema.

If the edema fluid could be displaced by applying pressure then it is called pitting edema **(Fig. 4.1)**, e.g., cardiac and renal edema and if the fluid could not be displaced it is non-pitting edema, e.g., myxedema, elephantiasis.

Pathogenesis: Edema is caused by mechanism that interferes with the normal balance of the intravascular and extravascular fluid transfer. The two main driving forces for the transfer of fluid in and out of the vessels are the intravascular hydrostatic pressure and the colloid osmotic pressure (plasma oncotic pressure). Normally, at the arteriolar end of vessel fluid escapes into the extravascular space due to increased hydrostatic pressure. This fluid enters the vessel back at the venular end due to the plasma oncotic pressure. A minor proportion of the fluid enters the lymphatics of the interstitium. So normally, there is a perfect balance of the fluid transfer in and out of the vessel. This is referred to as the Starling's Forces.

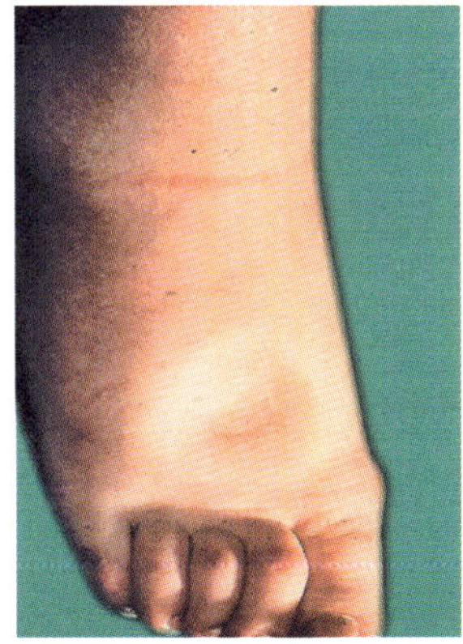

Fig. 4.1: Pitting edema of feet.

Causes for Edema

Table 4.2 describes the causes of edema.

TABLE 4.2: Causes of edema.

Pathophysiologic cause	*Conditions*
Increased capillary hydrostatic pressure	♦ Congestive cardiac failure ♦ Constrictive pericarditis ♦ Mechanical obstruction—thrombosis, mass ♦ Arteriolar dilatation—heat, neurohormonal ♦ Cirrhosis of liver
Reduced colloid oncotic pressure	♦ Nephrotic syndrome (increased loss) ♦ Cirrhosis of liver (reduced synthesis) ♦ Malnutrition (reduced synthesis) ♦ Protein losing Enteropathy
Lymphatic obstruction	♦ Inflammatory—filarial infestation ♦ Neoplastic—tumor emboli ♦ Post-surgical—after axillary dissection ♦ Post-irradiation ♦ Hereditary—Milroy's disease ♦ External pressure
Sodium and water retention	♦ Renal insufficiency ♦ Abnormal secretion of aldosterone ♦ Increased salt intake
Inflammatory	Acute and chronic inflammation

Pathogenesis of Cardiac Edema

The sequences of events of pathogenesis of cardiac edema as described in **Flowchart 4.1**.

Pathogenesis of Renal Edema

The sequences of events of pathogenesis of renal edema as described in **Flowchart 4.2**.

Clinical Profile of Edema

Cardiac Edema

Usually develops in congestive cardiac failure. It is a dependent pitting edema mostly seen in the lower extremities in ambulatory patients and in the sacral area (back) in bed ridden patients. Accumulation of fluid also occurs in serous cavities.

Renal Edema

Seen in patients with nephrotic syndrome, acute glomerulonephritis and acute tubular injury. More severe and marked in the periorbital tissue since it is the tissue of least resistance. Edema also occurs in the ankle area and over the genitalia.

Pulmonary Edema

Most important form of localized edema. It occurs due to elevation of pulmonary hydrostatic pressure and increased vascular permeability of the alveolar capillaries **(Fig. 4.2)**. The common predisposing conditions include left-sided cardiac failure, mitral stenosis, after cardiac surgeries, fulminant infection damaging the alveolar capillaries, Acute respiratory distress syndrome (ARDS) and in high altitudes.

The edema is confined to the basal regions of the lung. Radiograph shows prominent linear lines called the Kerley B lines which indicate the dilated lymphatics. The lungs are heavy, moist and subcrepitant and pinkish frothy fluid escapes on pressing the slice of lung. Microscopically, the alveoli are filled with proteinaceous edema fluid with congestion.

Flowchart 4.1: Sequences of events of pathogenesis of cardiac edema.

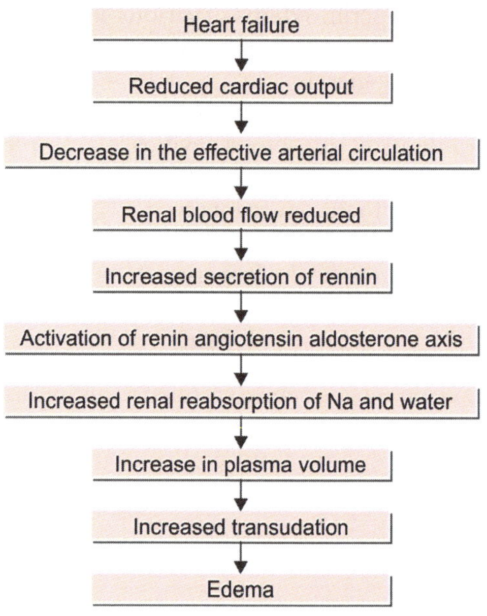

Flowchart 4.2: Sequences of events of pathogenesis of renal edema.

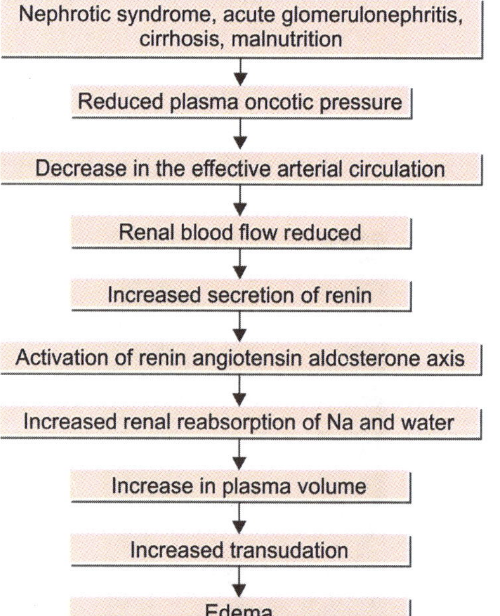

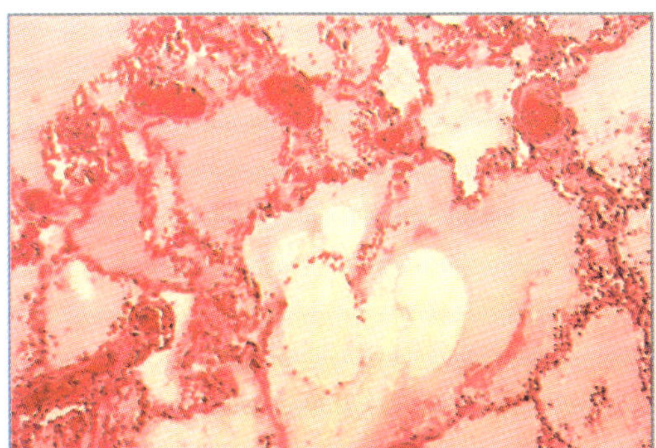

Fig. 4.2: Pulmonary edema, collection of edema fluid in the alveolar spaces.

Cerebral Edema

It is life-threatening condition as the brain is encased in a bony skull cage. There are three types of cerebral edema—vasogenic, cytotoxic and interstitial edema. Vasogenic edema is the most common form and it seen in conditions, such as contusion and infarction of brain, brain abscess and tumors of brain.

HYPEREMIA AND CONGESTION

These are terms used to indicate increased volume of blood in the vessels and organs.

Hyperemia is an active process due to the dilatation of the arterioles, arteries and blood capillaries as a result of inflammation, high fever, strenuous muscular exercise and other conditions.

Congestion is a passive process mainly due to impaired venous drainage and so it is referred to as chronic passive venous congestion. This may be localized or systemic.

Localized congestion is due to venous obstruction by localized pressure and strangulation of hernial contents.

Systemic congestion may be due to right-sided and left-sided heart failure, obstruction of inferior vena cava and portal veins, portal hypertension and other conditions. The major organs involved are the lungs, liver, spleen and kidney. The features are summarized in **Table 4.3**.

HEMORRHAGE

It is described as an abnormal escape of blood from the vessels. It may be external or internal. The internal bleeding can occur within the organs or in the serous cavities. The effects of hemorrhage depends on the amount of blood lost, speed of blood loss and site of blood loss.

TABLE 4.3: Characteristic features of chronic venous congestion in various organs.

Chronic venous congestion	*Predisposing factors*	*Gross morphology*	*Microscopy*
Lung	Left heart failure Rheumatic heart disease	Heavy, firm dark brown indurated lung (Wet lung)	Widened alveolar septae with congestion and hemorrhage, hemosiderin laden alveolar macrophages (heart failure cells)
Liver	Right-sided heart failure, hepatic vein obstruction	Hepatomegaly, tense capsule, nutmeg liver (alternating layers of congested and fatty areas)	Centrilobular congestion, dilated central veins and sinusoids, peripheral zone shows fatty change
Spleen	Right-sided heart failure, portal hypertension, cirrhosis	Splenomegaly, tense capsule, c/s intense congestion seen	Congestion of red pulp, sinusoidal dilatation, hemorrhages with fibrotic reaction—Gamna-Gandy bodies

External hemorrhages may be in the form of a hematoma, ecchymoses (larger bleeding lesions in skin and mucous membrane) of petechiae (pin head to pin point hemorrhagic lesions in the skin and mucosa).

Causes for Hemorrhage

- *Traumatic:* Most common cause
- *Spontaneous:* Bleeding disorders, rupture of aneurysms
- *Inflammatory:* Bleeding from peptic ulcers, typhoid ulcer, and vasculitis
- *Vascular disease:* Atherosclerosis
- *Elevated pressure:* Hypertension
- *Neoplastic*; due to vascular invasion by the tumor cells.

SHOCK

Definition: It is condition characterized by widespread hypoperfusion of the tissues due to reduction in the effective circulating blood volume. This is also termed as circulatory collapse, a serious assault to body's homeostasis.

The critical event is insufficiency in the delivery of oxygen and other nutrients to the cells and inadequate clearance of the metabolites which leads to organ changes.

Etiology and classification: The causes are summarized in **Table 4.4**.

Pathogenesis: The two main basic features in the pathogenesis of shock are:

1. Reduced in the effective circulating blood volume
2. Reduced supply of oxygen and other nutrients to the cells and tissues and the sequence of cell injury due to hypoxia occur as discussed in Chapter 1.

Septic Shock

The pathogenesis of septic shock differs from that of the other types.

Causes: Gram-negative bacteremia—*E. coli*, *Proteus*, *Klebsiella*.

Gram-positive septicemia—streptococci, pneumococci.

The events are triggered by the release of bacterial endotoxins. The endotoxins are lipopolysaccharides and they have a lipid core with polysaccharide coat. The sequence of events in septic shock are:

- Release of endotoxins
- Binding of the endotoxins to the LPS binding protein of the serum
- Activation of CD14 receptor on the surface of leukocytes and endothelial cells
- Release of various chemical mediators and cytokines like (Interleukin 1, 2, 6 and 8), TNF, NO, PAF, arachidonic acid metabolites, complement components, kinins and myocardial depressant factor
- These mediators act on various organ systems and cause multiorgan dysfunction.

TABLE 4.4: Causes and predisposing factors of various types of shock.

Causes and types of shock	*Predisposing factors*
Cardiogenic	♦ Myocardial infarction ♦ Arrhythmias ♦ Extrinsic pressure—cardiac tamponade ♦ Outflow obstruction
Hypovolemic	♦ Hemorrhage ♦ Burns (loss of plasma) ♦ Trauma ♦ Severe dehydration
Septic	♦ Severe gram-negative bacteremia ♦ Sepsis
Neurogenic	♦ Anesthetic accidents ♦ Spinal cord injury
Anaphylactic	♦ Immune mediated hypersensitivity reaction

Organ Changes in Septic Shock

- *Heart*: Chamber dilatation and suppression of myocardial function
- *Lungs*: Diffuse alveolar damage presenting as acute respiratory distress syndrome **(Fig. 4.3)**

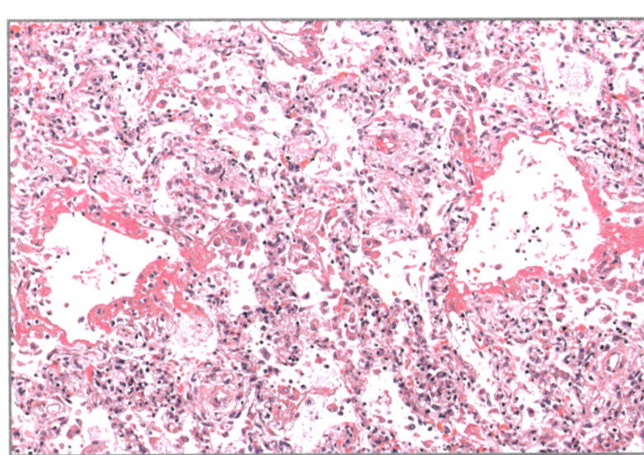

Fig. 4.3: Photomicrograph of lung in shock showing diffuse alveolar damage.

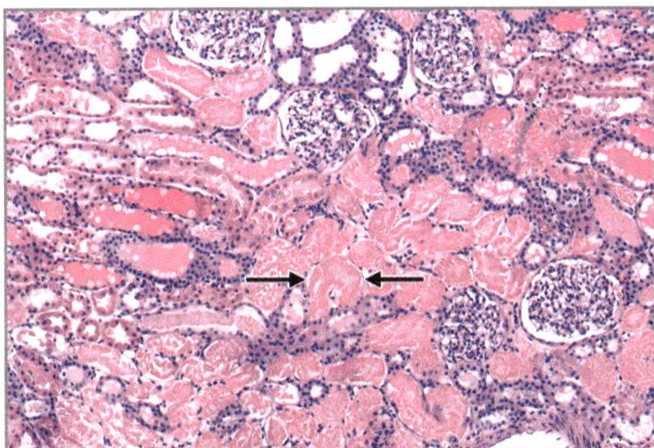

Fig. 4.4: Photomicrograph of renal tubules with acute tubular necrosis.

- *Kidney*: Acute tubular necrosis presenting as acute renal failure **(Fig. 4.4)**
- *Brain*: Features of hypoxic encephalopathy
- *Liver*: Features of acute live cell failure.

Stages of Shock

The evolution of shock can be divided into three different stages. They are:

1. Initial non-progressive phase
2. Progressive decompensated phase
3. Irreversible phase

1. *Initial non-progressive phase*: This is the initial stage of shock where the body tries to compensate for the tissue hypoperfusion by activating the neurohormonal compensatory mechanisms. They include:
   - Activation of baroreceptors
   - Secretion of catecholamine's
   - Activation of renin angiotensin aldosterone axis
   - Release of antidiuretic hormone
   - Stimulation of the sympathetic system

   The blood supply is diverted from the periphery to the brain and kidney to maintain adequate functioning of these organs. It manifests clinically as cool and clammy extremities, thin thready pulse, pallor of skin and tachycardia. Patients with septic shock will have vasodilatation in contrast to vasoconstriction seen in other types of shock.
2. *Progressive decompensated phase*: The shock may progress from the initial phase to this phase due to persistence of the cause of shock and therapeutic in correction. This leads to persistent oxygen deficit. There is a shift from the aerobic metabolism to anaerobic metabolism which results in excessive production of lactic acid and induces intracellular acidosis. There is fall in the pH of the blood which causes vasodilatation. This interferes with the functioning of the vital organs. The clinical manifestations of this phase are fall in the urinary output (oliguria); patient is drowsy and confused, fall in the blood pressure, and bradycardia.
3. *Irreversible phase*: The predisposing factors are mostly severe shock and failure of the compensatory mechanisms. It results in diffuse hypoxic cell injury which produces multiorgan dysfunction. The organ changes are summarized in **Table 4.5**.

TABLE 4.5: Pathological changes in different organs

Organs involved	*Pathology*
Brain (hypoxic encephalopathy)	Edema of the brain, acute neuronal cell death
Heart	♦ Subendocardial hemorrhages ♦ Hypercontraction of myocyte producing zonal lesions
Lungs (ARDS)	Diffuse alveolar damage and pulmonary edema
Kidneys (ARF)	Acute hypoxic tubular injury—acute tubular necrosis
Adrenals	Stress response—depletion of lipids from the adrenal cells
GIT	Hemorrhagic gastroenteropathy
Liver	Centrilobular hemorrhagic necrosis Fatty change

Case Scenario

A male patient of 60 years old with h/o of chronic obstructive pulmonary disease (COPD) admitted to the hospital with a high fever, hypotension (blood pressure 90/60 mm Hg), rapid heart rate (130 bpm), and altered mental status. He is diagnosed with severe sepsis. He is a former smoker and during initial assessment oxygen saturation is 92% and has a productive cough with yellowish—green sputum.

Questions:

1. What is the primary cause of septic shock in Mr Turner, considering his medical history and symptoms?
   A. Respiratory failure
   B. Gastrointestinal bleeding
   C. Urinary tract infection
   D. Bacterial infection in the lungs

Contd...

Contd...

2. Which nursing intervention is a priority in the management of septic shock?
   A. Administering bronchodilators for improved respiratory function
   B. Administering antipyretics to reduce fever
   C. Administering IV fluids and vasopressors to maintain blood pressure
   D. Encouraging ambulation to prevent complications

Answers:

1. (D) Bacterial infection in the lungs
2. (C) Administering IV fluids and vasopressors to maintain blood pressure

Clinical Features

Clinical features of shock are described in **Table 4.6**.

TABLE 4.6: Clinical features of shock.

Stage of shock	*Clinical features*
Stage I	Pallor, cool, clammy skin, thready pulse, tachycardia, tachypnea
Stage II	Renal insufficiency—oliguria, fall in the blood pressure, drowsiness
Stage III	Multiorgan dysfunction with renal shut down, depression of myocardial function, respiratory distress, diffuse cerebral dysfunction—coma

THROMBOSIS

Definition: It is defined as the formation of solid mass or plug from the constituents of blood within an uninterrupted living circulation. This definition was coined by Welch (1887).

Thrombi in the form of a hemostatic plug is useful to arrest the excessive loss of blood. But when it occurs within an uninterrupted living circulation, it leads to pathological consequences. The two most common sequelae of thrombi are:

1. Ischemic injury—due to block in the blood supply
2. Embolism—a portion of thrombi may get dislodged and carried along the blood stream to a distant site.

Normal hemostasis: Before venturing into the pathophysiology of thrombosis, it is a must that we understand the fundamentals of normal hemostasis. There are three important contributors for normal hemostasis. They are:

1. Blood vessel wall
2. Platelets
3. Coagulation system

Sequence of events in normal hemostasis:

1. Injury to vessel wall
2. Brief vasoconstriction
3. Endothelial injury
4. Exposure of thrombogenic subendothelium
5. Adherence of platelets to subendothelium
6. Activation of platelets
7. Release reaction of platelets and aggregation
8. Primary platelet plug
9. Release of tissue factors
10. Activation of the coagulation cascade
11. Formation of fibrin clot (secondary hemostatic plug)

Role of Vessel Wall

The endothelium is a very versatile cell with both procoagulant and anticoagulant properties **(Table 4.7)**. Both are kept in a well-balanced state.

Any disturbance to the normal functioning of the endothelium may tilt the balance and result in formation of thrombi.

TABLE 4.7: Prothrombotic and antithrombotic properties of endothelial cell.

Prothrombotic functions	*Antithrombotic functions*
Synthesis of von Willebrand factor (vWF) which binds platelets of subendothelium	Antiplatelet function by secretion of prostacyclin, nitric oxide and ADPase
Secretion of tissue factor which activates extrinsic pathway	Secretion of anticoagulant proteins, such as antithrombin III, thrombomodulin and protein C
Inhibits plasminogen activator which prevents fibrinolysis	Synthesis of tissue plasminogen activator which promotes fibrinolysis

Role of Platelets

The platelets are tiny anucleate cells of the blood which play a vital role in hemostasis. The platelets contain two types of granules—alpha and delta granules which mediate their function. The functions of platelet in hemostasis includes:

- *Adhesion:* The platelets adhere to the subendothelial through the vWF. The surface glycoprotein Ib (Gp Ib) binds with the von Willebrand's factor (vWF).
- *Activation and secretion:* After adhesion, the platelets undergo activation by the release of ADP, calcium and other substances and actively secrete the contents of the granules which cause recruitment of more platelets to the site and its activation.
- *Platelet aggregation:* Due to release of ADP, the platelets adhere well to form a primary hemostatic plug in the site of endothelial damage. It also leads to the expression of the phospholipid complex in its surface which activates the intrinsic pathway of coagulation.

Role of the Coagulation System

The main function of this system is to convert soluble fibrinogen to solid fibrin. It comprises of three pathways—intrinsic, extrinsic and common. The intrinsic pathway is activated by the surface contact and it leads to the sequential activation of factor XII, XI, IX, and VIII and X.

The extrinsic pathway is activated by the release of tissue factors which act on factor VII and subsequently on factor X. The common pathway starts with factor X and sequentially activates factor V, II and finally converts fibrinogen to fibrin. The fibrin is laid between the platelets of the primary plug, such as the cement layering between the bricks and forms the secondary (permanent) hemostatic plug **(Fig. 4.5)**.

The fibrin plug seals the vascular damage until there is regeneration of the endothelial cell. Once the regeneration is complete, the intrinsic fibrinolytic system gets activated and released plasmin which acts of the fibrin and breaks fibrin into fibrin degradation products and the vessel wall returns to normalcy.

Thrombogenesis

The three most important predisposing factors for thrombogenesis are:

1. Endothelial injury
2. Alterations in the flow of blood
3. Hypercoagulability of blood

These are referred to as Virchow's triad. We shall now discuss the causes for the abovesaid predisposing factors which leads to formation of thrombi.

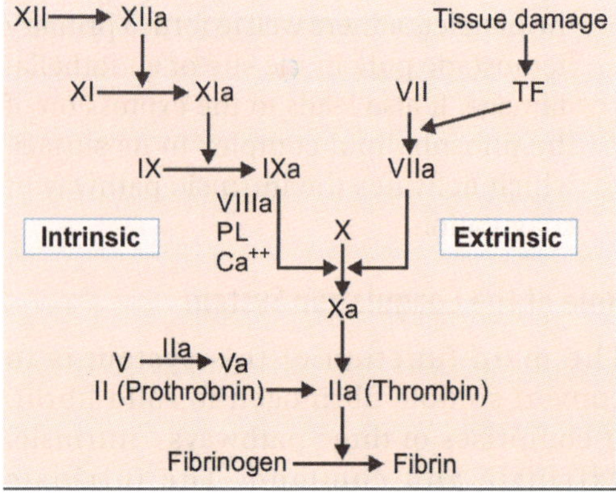

Fig. 4.5: Sequence of events in coagulation cascade.

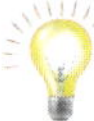

Case Scenario

A 26-year-old women with third degree burns developed septic shock. With 24 hours, she was bleeding from all needle puncture sites, with extensive ecchymoses and petechiae and GI bleeding. Lab studies showed Hb 6 g/dL, platelet count 64,000/cu mm, PT 20 seconds, PTT 50 seconds and D-dimer positive.

Question:

What is your probable diagnosis?

Answer:

Disseminated intravascular coagulation

Endothelial Injury

It is a dominant factor in thrombogenesis. The most common causes for endothelial injury are:

- Atherosclerosis
- Myocardial Infarction
- Valvulitis
- Vasculitis
- Traumatic—indwelling catheters, extremes of temperature
- Hemodynamic stress—hypertension
- Toxins—homocysteine
- Hypercholesterolemia
- Smoking
- Radiation

Alterations in the Flow of Blood

The two main alterations in the flow of blood are turbulence and stasis:

1. Turbulence—abnormal haphazard flow of blood within the vessel
2. Stasis—abnormal pooling of the blood within the vessel.

Any alteration in the flow of blood leads to the disruption of the axial flow of blood. It brings the platelets close to the endothelium, promotes endothelial cell activation, prevent dilution of the activated clotting factors and retard the inflow of clotting factor inhibitors.

Turbulence usually causes arterial and cardiac thrombi and stasis leads to venous thrombi. The common predisposing factors for alterations in flow of blood is hypertension, ulcerated atheromatous plaque, aneurysms and dilated cardiomyopathy.

Hypercoagulability of Blood

There is increased predisposition to hypercoagulability in these groups of disorders. They can be classified as primary and secondary causes. Some important disorders are summarized in **Table 4.8**.

TABLE 4.8: Primary and secondary hypercoagulability disorders.

Primary hypercoagulability disorders	*Secondary hypercoagulability disorders*
Mutations of factor V	Prolonged immobilization
Deficiency of antithrombin III	Myocardial Infarction, atrial fibrillation
Deficiency of protein C and S	Massive tissue damage
Hereditary homocystinuria	Malignancies
	Prosthetic valves
	Disseminated Intravascular coagulation
	Antiphospholipid syndrome
	Cardiomyopathy
	Nephrotic syndrome
	Oral contraceptive pills
	Sickle cell disease
	Smoking

Pathology of Thrombus

Sites of thrombi: Thrombi can occur anywhere in the cardiovascular system mostly in the cardiac chambers, valve cusps, arteries, veins and capillaries. They are located at the sites of endothelial damage.

Morphology: Thrombi can be grouped into red thrombi, white thrombi and mixed thrombi (**Table 4.9**) based on the morphology.

Cardiac thrombus: Thrombi can be seen in the cardiac chambers and on the valve leaflets. The thrombi of the cardiac chambers are referred to as mural thrombi and of the valve leaflets are referred to as thrombotic vegetations.

Cut section of a mural thrombi shows alternating layering of dark red and pale white areas which are called as the **lines of Zahn** (**Fig. 4.6**).

Thrombi are usually seen over an infracted area and thrombi of the left atrium may cause sudden obstruction to the outflow tract and it is called as *Ball Valve Thrombi*.

The thrombi seen in the cardiac chambers have to differentiate from the clots formed in the chambers after death which are called as postmortem clots.

The salient differences between them are summarized in **Table 4.10**.

Arterial thrombi: The predisposing factors included—atherosclerosis, aneurysms,

TABLE 4.9: Features of the various types of thrombus.

Nature of thrombi	*Site of thrombi*	*Morphology of thrombi*	*Composition*
Pale thrombus	Rapidly flowing arterial blood, left atrium	Firm and pale	Platelets and fibrin
Red thrombus	Stagnant venous blood, right atrium	Soft, dark red, smooth and gelatinous	Fibrin with blood cells.
Mixed thrombus	Cardiac chambers	Alternating layers of dark red and pale areas	Platelets, fibrin and blood cells

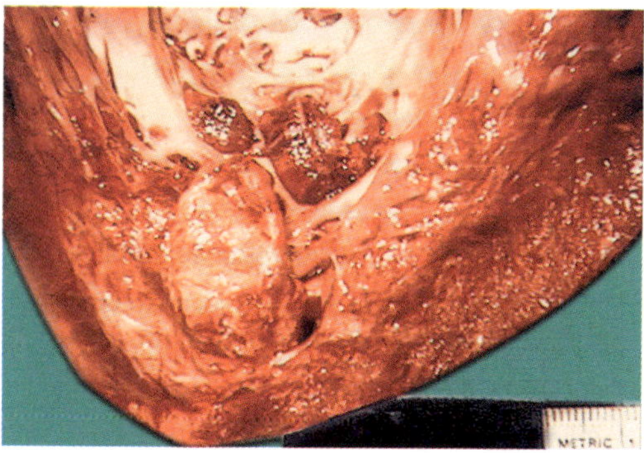

Fig. 4.6: Mural thrombi within cardiac chamber.

TABLE 4.10: Comparison between antemortem and postmortem clots.

Antemortem thrombi	*Postmortem clots*
Granular, pale and firm	Soft, gelatinous, reddish brown
Attached well to the endocardium	Not attached to the endocardium
Presence of lines of Zahn	Lines of Zahn are absent
No chicken fat appearance	The red cells settle down the clot with a superficial yellowish fatty material—chicken fat appearance
Underlying infracted area	Normal endocardium

hypertension, vasculitis, peripheral vascular diseases and others.

Morphology; Usually a pale thrombus **Table 4.9**.

Sites: Aorta, coronaries, cerebral, mesenteric, renal and other vessels

Effects: Mostly ischemia leading to infarction

Venous thrombi: The most common predisposing factors include prolonged immobilization, chronic debilitating illness (marantic thrombus), malnutrition, myeloproliferative disorders, puerperium, pregnancy, malignancies, such as adenocarcinoma pancreas (migratory thrombophlebitis—Troisier's sign) and thrombophlebitis.

Morphology: Usually a red thrombus **Table 4.9**.

Sites: Most commonly in the deep veins of the leg **(Fig. 4.7)**. Other sites include varicose veins, popliteal, femoral, iliac and pelvic veins. splenic vein, mesenteric vein, pulmonary veins, superior vena cava, inferior vena cava **(Fig. 4.8)** and renal veins.

Effects: Source of embolism, skin ulceration and poor wound healing.

Fate of thrombi:

- *Resolution:* Complete dissolution of the thrombi by the activity of fibrinolytic system.
- *Organization:* The thrombi are invaded by the neutrophils and macrophages with the onset of an inflammatory reaction and the thrombi are converted into a fibrovascular inflammatory tissue attached to the wall of the vessel and may get resorbed later.

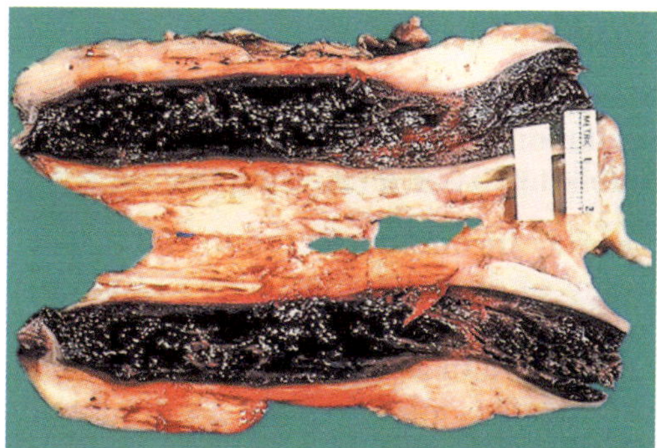

Fig. 4.7: Venous thrombosis in deep veins of the leg.

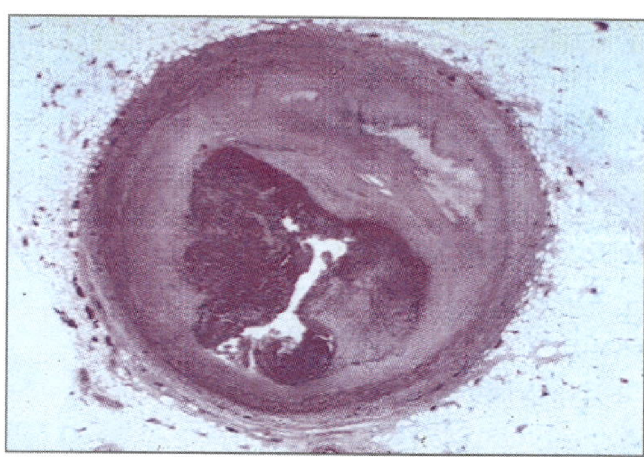

Fig. 4.8: Photomicrograph of thrombi with calcification.

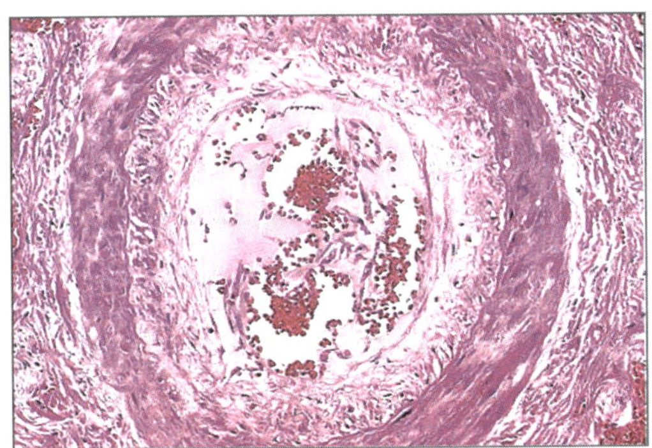

Fig. 4.9: Photomicrograph of thrombi with recanalization.

- *Recanalization* **(Fig. 4.9)**: This occurs in an organized thrombus. Newer lumina may evolve in the organized tissue to restore the continuity of the blood supply.
- *Propagation:* Slow growth of the thrombi through the vessels, seen mostly in venous thrombi.
- *Embolization:* Fragmentation of thrombi leads to detachment of a portion which is carried to a distant site for lodgment—thromboembolism.

EMBOLISM

Definition: It is defined as a detached intravascular solid, liquid or gaseous mass, i.e., carried in the circulation to a site distant from the site of origin.

Types of embolism: The most common types of embolism are:

- Thromboembolism (most common type) lodges in the pulmonary circulation
- Arterial Embolism (Systemic embolism)
- Fat embolism
- Air embolism
- Amniotic fluid embolism

Other causes:

1. Disseminated tumor cells
2. Radiocontrast media

We shall now discuss the salient features of the various types of embolism.

Pulmonary Thromboembolism

Seen in 20–25/1,00,000 hospitalized patients.

Pathogenesis: About 96% of the emboli originate from the deep veins of the leg. The fragmented thrombi are carried by the venous channels into the right side of heart, from which it enters the pulmonary arteries.

The course of the embolism depends on the size of the embolus. If it is very small, it passes through the smaller branches and gets lodged in the alveolar vessels. If it is very big it can occlude the bifurcation of the pulmonary trunk like a saddle and cause sudden death. This embolism is called *saddle embolism* **(Fig. 4.10)**.

In persons with intra-arterial septal defect of interventricular septal defect the emboli pass from the right side of the heart to the left side and thereby enters the systemic circulation. This is called a *paradoxical embolism* (a venous embolus entering systemic arterial circulation).

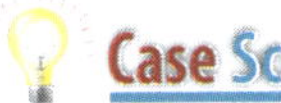

Case Scenario

A 60-year-old male was bedridden following surgery. He complained of pain in the calf muscles on squeezing. He suddenly developed breathlessness and died.

Question:

What is the probable cause of death?

Answer:

Deep vein thrombosis with acute pulmonary embolism

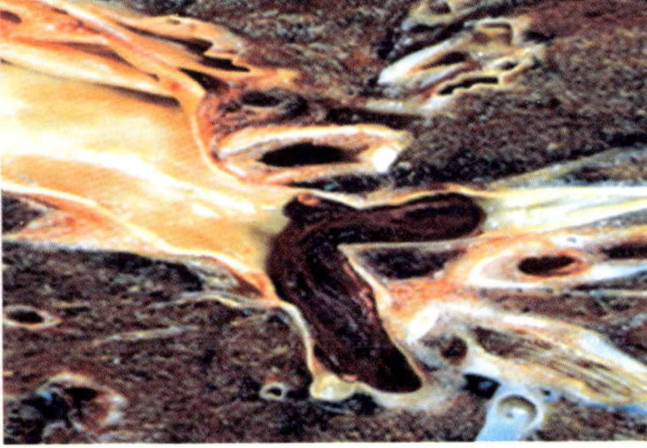

Fig. 4.10: Saddle embolism in pulmonary trunk.

Pathology

Only 10% of the emboli causes pulmonary infarction, because lungs have double vascular supply from the pulmonary and bronchial system. Saddle embolus causes sudden death due to acute dilatation of the right heart (acute cor pulmonale).

Morphology: It involves the lower lobes of lung. Produces a wedge-shaped infarct which is grayish brown and hemorrhagic. The overlying pleura is thick and fibrinous. The infracted are later undergo fibrosis and forms a scar tissue. Rarely infection may occur on an infracted area producing an abscess.

Clinical Features

Patients present with chest pain, difficulty in breathing, shock, cough, tachycardia, tachypnea, hemoptysis and pleural pain.

Prevention

Pulmonary thrombosis is a preventable condition. It can be avoided by early ambulation of the bed ridden patients, giving isometric leg exercises and prophylactic therapeutic measures.

Arterial Embolism (Systemic Thromboembolism)

About 80% arises from an underlying mural thrombi. The emboli enter the systemic circulation and gets lodged in the brain, kidney, mesentery and lower extremities. The effects depend on the vessel occluded and tissue vulnerability to ischemia.

Fat Embolism (Fig. 4.11)

Obstruction of the capillaries by globules of fat.

Most common predisposing factors include:
- Multiple fracture of long bones
- Soft tissue trauma
- Extensive burns
- Pancreatitis
- Diabetes mellitus

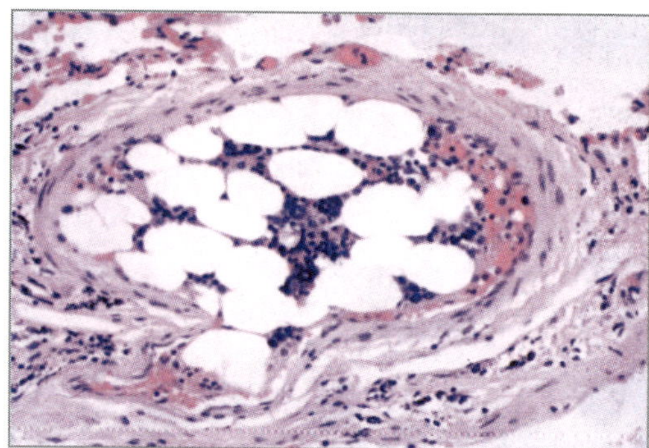

Fig. 4.11: Photomicrograph of fat embolism.

The traumatic causes are more common than the non-traumatic causes.

Pathogenesis: Mechanical obstruction induced by the microaggregates of fat or release of free fatty acids from the fat causes toxic damage to the endothelium and thereby induces a thrombus and subsequent embolization.

Clinical profile: This is a common occurrence in multiple skeletal injuries but only 1% of the affected patients suffer from *fat embolism syndrome*. This occurs 24 to 72 hours after the initial injury and may be fatal in 10% of cases. Fat embolism syndrome is characterized in **Table 4.11**.

Amniotic Fluid Embolism

It is an extremely grave complication during labor which causes significant maternal mortality. The incidence is 1 in 50,000 deliveries. But now, it has become a very rare complication due to the advances in the obstetric care.

TABLE 4.11: Characteristics of fat embolism syndrome.

Features	*Manifestations*
Pulmonary insufficiency	Dyspnea, tachypnea
Neurological symptoms	Irritability, restlessness, coma
Anemia	Tachycardia
Thrombocytopenia	Petechial rashes

Pathogenesis: The amniotic fluid enters the circulation through tear in the placental membranes or rupture of the uterine or cervical venous sinuses. Once the amniotic fluid enters the circulation, it causes widespread thrombosis due to the release of thromboplastic substances in the fluid.

Clinical profile: It is characterized by profound respiratory difficulty, deep cyanosis, pulmonary edema, massive bleeding and shock.

Air Embolism

It is condition in which bubbles of the air are trapped within the circulation producing obstruction. This is also referred to as Barotrauma.

Causes: The common causes which predispose to air embolism are decompression sickness, penetrating injuries to lung and chest wall, due to rupture of uterine venous sinuses during delivery and in cases of pneumothorax.

At least about 100cc of air is required to produce symptoms.

Decompression sickness: These are group of disorders seen in persons who work in deep sea in a pressurized cabin (Scuba/Deep sea divers).

When the person ascends up to the surface to rapidly the gases comes out of the blood vessels and these gases mostly nitrogen and helium persist in the circulation and causes obstruction. This occurs in two clinical forms—acute and chronic.

Acute decompression sickness: This occurs due to sudden obstruction of the small blood vessels of the joints and skeletal muscle and produces severe pain and severe respiratory distress. These symptoms are referred to as Bends and Chokes. (The patient bends with pain and has respiratory difficulty).

Chronic decompression sickness: This is also referred to as Caisson's disease. There is an obstruction of the blood vessels of long bones, such as femur, tibia and humerus leading to severe ischemia.

INFARCTION

Definition: It is defined as an area of ischemic necrosis within the tissue or organ produced by occlusion of either the arterial supply or venous drainage.

Causes: The common causes include thrombotic occlusion of vessels, twisting of blood vessels, compression of vessels and trapping of blood vessel.

Types: Infarction is classified into two types white and red infarct (based on the color), septic and bland (based on microbial contamination).

The characteristic features of the types of infarct are summarized in **Table 4.12**.

The following are the features on which the effect of infarction depends. They are:

1. Nature of blood supply—endarterial, dual supply
2. Rate of development of occlusion—acute/gradual
3. Vulnerability of the tissue to hypoxia
4. Oxygen content of the blood
5. Rate of development of collaterals

TABLE 4.12: Types of infarct and its characteristic features.

Type of infarct	*Characteristic features*	*Common organs*
White	♦ Due to arterial occlusion ♦ Solid organs ♦ Organs with end arterial blood supply	♦ Heart ♦ Spleen ♦ Kidney
Red	♦ Venous occlusion ♦ In loose tissues ♦ Organs with double circulation ♦ In previously congested tissue	♦ Loop of bowel ♦ Lung ♦ Ovary
Bland infarct	Infarct without microbial contamination	
Septic infarct	Infarct with superadded microbial contamination	Abscess

Morphology of infarct: The infract is usually wedge shaped **(Fig. 4.12)**. The apex of the wedge points to the point of occlusion and the base lies on the external surface of the organ. Initially, the infarct is poorly defined, later it becomes slightly darker, firm and sharply demarcated. The margins of the infarcted area are hyperemia due to inflammatory response.

Histologically, the infarction of all organs is characterized by coagulative necrosis except brain which manifests with liquefactive necrosis **(Fig. 4.13)**.

Infarcts of clinical significance: The following infarcts are of great clinical significance. They are myocardial infarction, cerebral infarction and ischemic necrosis of the extremities.

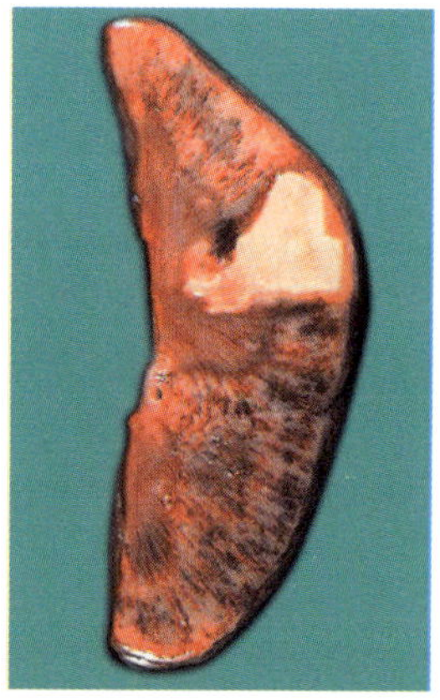

Fig. 4.12: Wedge-shaped white infarct of spleen.

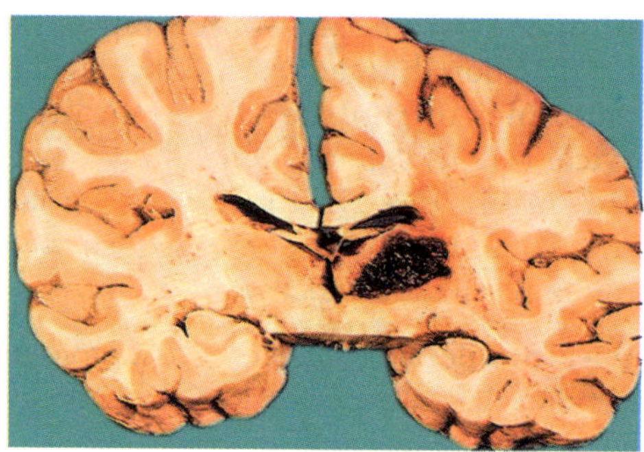

Fig. 4.13: Hemorrhagic infarct of brain.

Points to Ponder

- The most common forms of hemodynamic disturbances include: Edema, congestion, hyperemia, thrombosis and shock.
- Various forms of edema have different pathophysiological mechanisms.
- Shock is a state of tissue hypoperfusion due to various causes. It is a multisystem disease.
- Thrombosis occurs due to defect in the normal hemostatic balance. There are two main forms of thrombi—arterial and venous. Thrombosis is important for the clinical implications.
- Embolism is the most common complication of thrombosis. There are various forms of embolism.
- Infarction is a form of ischemic necrosis due to arterial and venous obstruction.

ASSESSMENT QUESTIONS

Essay Type Questions

1. **Define edema. Discuss in detail the pathogenesis, pathology and clinical features of cardiac edema and renal edema.**
2. **Define thrombosis. Discuss in detail the mechanism of thrombogenesis, morphology and clinical implications of thrombosis.**
3. **A 45-year-old male was admitted to the casualty services of hospital following a road traffic accident. He has multiple lacerated wounds with active bleeding. On examination,**

he was confused. His pulse rate was 110/mt, feeble and thread. His blood pressure was 90/60 mm of Hg. He had tachycardia .

a. What is your clinical diagnosis?
b. Describe in detail the pathogenesis and pathology of this condition.
c. Mention the stages of progression of this condition.
d. Briefly mention the organ changes you see in this condition.

Short Answer Questions

1. **Enumerate the causes for chronic venous congestion of lung.**
2. **Define shock. Enumerate the common types of shock.**
3. **What is nutmeg liver? Enumerate the common causes .**
4. **Define embolism.**
5. **Enumerate the differences between antemortem thrombi and postmortem clot.**
6. **What are the common sequelae to a thrombi?**
7. **What are the common causes for fat embolism?**
8. **Enumerate the various stages of shock.**
9. **What are the GAMNA GANDY BODIES? In which organ do you see them?**
10. **Define paradoxical embolism.**

MULTIPLE CHOICE QUESTIONS

1. **Maximum body water is present:**
   A. Extracellularly
   B. Intracellularly
   C. Intravascular
   D. Equal in A and B
2. **Dependent edema is seen in:**
   A. Cirrhosis
   B. Malnutrition
   C. Nephrotic syndrome
   D. Congestive cardiac failure
3. **Heart failure cells usually occur in chronic venous congestion of:**
   A. Liver
   B. Lymph node
   C. Lung
   D. Spleen
4. **Main mediator of platelet adhesion is:**
   A. von Willebrand's factor
   B. Thromboxane A
   C. ADP
   D. Fibronectin
5. **Lines of Zahn in a thrombus are found when thrombus forms in:**
   A. Peripheral veins
   B. Heart
   C. Brain
   D. Muscular arteries
6. **Most common source of embolism is:**
   A. Atheromatous debris
   B. Thrombus
   C. Bone fragment
   D. Air bubbles
7. **White infarcts are seen in all, *except*:**
   A. Spleen
   B. Lung
   C. Kidney
   D. Heart
8. **Ischemia produces coagulative necrosis in infarcts of all organs, *except*:**
   A. Lung
   B. Brain
   C. Small intestine
   D. Kidney

9. **Septic shock can be due to:**
   A. Gram negative bacilli
   B. Gram positive bacteria
   C. Fungi
   D. All of the above
10. **In platelets calcium and ADP are present in:**
   A. Alpha granules
   B. Dense bodies
   C. Ribosomes
   D. None of the above
11. **What is the primary function of the lymphatic system in fluid balance?**
   A. Oxygen transport
   B. Nutrient absorption
   C. Fluid drainage and immune response
   D. Blood clotting
12. **Which of the following is a characteristic of hypovolemic shock?**
   A. Increased blood volume
   B. Decreased cardiac output
   C. Elevated blood pressure
   D. Constricted blood vessels
13. **Which of the following is a manifestation of edema?**
   A. Increased urine output
   B. Pitting of the skin
   C. Hypotension
   D. Decreased respiratory rate
14. **What is the term for the force exerted by blood against the walls of the arteries during cardiac contraction?**
   A. Diastolic pressure
   B. Systolic pressure
   C. Pulse pressure
   D. Mean arterial pressure
15. **Which of the following conditions is characterized by an accumulation of excess fluid in the pericardial sac surrounding the heart?**
   A. Pericarditis
   B. Myocardial infarction
   C. Endocarditis
   D. Aortic stenosis

Answer Key for MCQs

1	2	3	4	5	6	7	8	9	10
B	D	C	A	B	B	B	C	D	B
11	**12**	**13**	**14**	**15**					
C	B	B	B	A					

5

CHAPTER

Neoplasia

Learning Objectives

At the end of reading this chapter, the student shall be able to:

- Define and classify neoplasia. Describe the fundamental characters of benign and malignant neoplasms and differentiated between them.
- Describe the molecular basis of neoplasia.
- Enumerate the carcinogens and describe the process of carcinogenesis.
- Enlist the common clinical presentation of neoplasia.
- Describe the common laboratory methods for diagnosis of neoplasia.

INTRODUCTION

Literal meaning of the term neoplasia is **"new growth" (neo—new, plasia—growth)**. Oncology **(oncos—tumor, logos—study)** is the scientific study of neoplasms. The mostly widely used terminology for indicating neoplasia is *cancer* **(meaning crab—as the disease infiltrates the organs like the crab)**.

Definition: It is an abnormal mass of tissue, the growth of which exceeds and is uncoordinated with that of normal tissue and persists in the same excessive manner even after the cessation of the stimuli which has evoked the change. In simple terms, it is an autonomous and purposeless proliferation of cells.

Nomenclature: The common terminologies used in neoplasia are benign tumors and malignant tumors. The features of these are discussed in the forthcoming columns.

Every tumor has got proliferating cells with a supporting stroma. Most of the benign tumors are labeled according to the nature of the proliferating cells with a suffix of *oma*. For example, a tumor of fibroblast is called as **fibroma**.

The malignant tumors of the epithelia are called as *carcinoma* and that of the mesenchymal tissue is *sarcoma*. For example, malignant tumor of squamous cells—squamous cell carcinoma and osteocytes—osteosarcoma. Apart from the above, there are other terminologies used in neoplasia they are:

Teratoma: These are neoplasms which arise from totipotent cells and represent tissue from more than one germ layer. They are commonly seen in ovaries and testis **(Fig. 5.1)**.

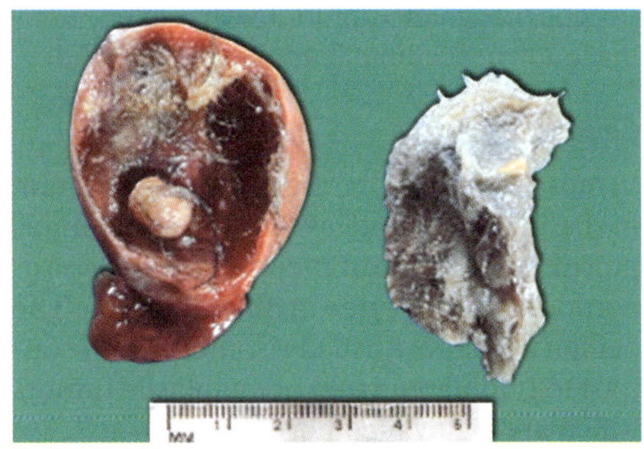

Fig. 5.1: Cystic teratoma with tuft of hair and teeth.

Hamartoma: It refers to a condition characterized by disorganized proliferation of cells native to the particular site. For example, hemangioma (proliferation of blood vessels). This is considered to be a tumor like condition.

Choristoma: Ectopic rest of a normal tissue is called choristoma. For example, presence of adrenal tissue within the renal capsule.

CHARACTERISTICS OF BENIGN AND MALIGNANT TUMORS

The following are the characters on which the tumors are categorized into benign and malignant. They include:

1. Differentiation and cellular features
2. Rate of growth
3. Local invasion
4. Metastasis

Differentiation

This is defined as the extent to which the neoplastic cells look like that of the normal parenchymal cells. There are generally four forms of differentiation, well differentiated, moderately differentiated, poorly differentiated and undifferentiated. The undifferentiated form is called as ***anaplasia***.

Most of the benign tumors are well differentiated and malignant tumors may be well differentiated, moderately differentiated, poorly differentiated or undifferentiated. Presence of anaplasia is a marker of malignancy.

The malignant tumors are characterized by the following cellular features. They include:

Cellular Features

In most of the tumors, there is a vast variation in size of the cell and it is termed as pleomorphism. The extent of pleomorphism is proportional to the degree of differentiation. The benign tumors are usually isomorphic in contrast to undifferentiated or anaplastic tumors which are highly pleomorphic.

There will be irregular enlargement of the cell and the nuclei. The size of the nuclei increases abnormally to that of the cytoplasm. The normal nuclear cytoplasmic ratio is **1:4–1:6**. In a neoplastic cell, it gets converted to **1:1**. The variation in the nuclear size is referred to as anisonucleosis or anisokaryosis.

Other nuclear changes include condensation of nuclear chromatin, it makes the nuclei to stain darker than normal and this is referred to as **hyperchromasia**. The nuclear membrane appears thick and with prominent nucleoli.

There will be abnormal cohesion among the tumor cells which leads to the formation of multinucleated tumor giant cells, which are large cells with above said nuclear features **(Fig. 5.2)**.

Mitotic Activity

Other important feature of a neoplasia is presence of visible mitotic activity. As there is increased rate of cell division, the mitotic figures look prominent in neoplasia. In malignant tumors, the mitotic division will be irregular and atypical, so it produces atypical mitotic **(Fig. 5.3)**. There will be increase in the number of normal mitotic figures or presence of abnormal mitotic figures which appear due to aberrant cell division.

Cellular Arrangement (Polarity)

There may be lack of orientation of the arrangement of the cells in neoplasia and it is termed as *dyspolarity*. The malignant neoplastic cells usually grow in a disorganized pattern.

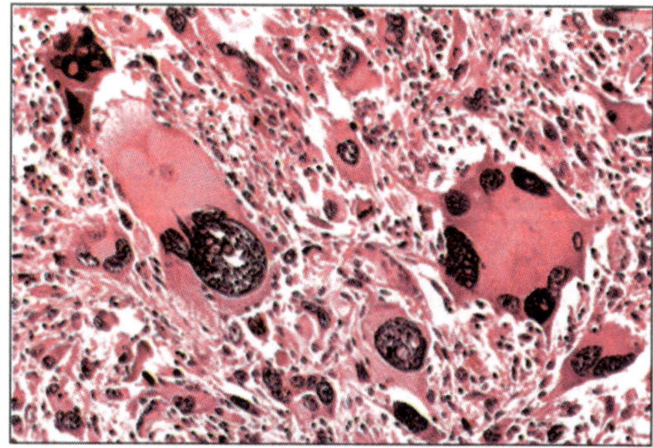

Fig. 5.2: Large abnormal cells and tumor giant cells.

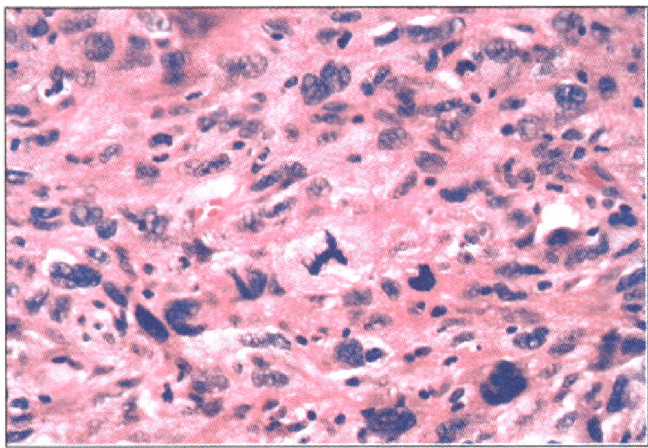

Fig. 5.3: Photomicrograph showing an atypical tripolar mitotic figure in the center.

Functional characters: The neoplastic cells may retain their normal function, show increased or decreased functional activity or secrete fetal proteins or abnormal hormones.

Rate of Growth

The growth rate of tumor depends on the blood supply and hormonal status. Generally, benign tumors have a slow rate of growth and malignant tumors grow very rapidly because the malignant cells have an increased mitotic rate and slower death rate (the cells are immortal). The other important factor is the degree of differentiation. The more undifferentiated the tumor is, higher will be the rate of growth. The rate of growth of tumors is controlled by various growth factors.

Local invasion

Benign tumors generally are encapsulated with a fibrous capsule. The tumor cells are cohesive with no capacity to invade. Malignant tumors do not have a true capsule and they invade the least resistant surrounding tissue. They have infiltrative margins and they produced ulceration and fungation **(Figs. 5.4 and 5.5)**.

The differentiating features of benign and malignant tumors are summarized in the **Table 5.1**.

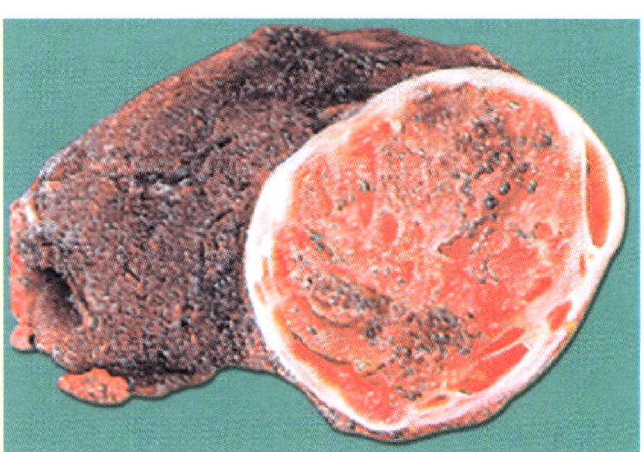

Fig. 5.4: Benign tumor of thyroid with encapsulation.

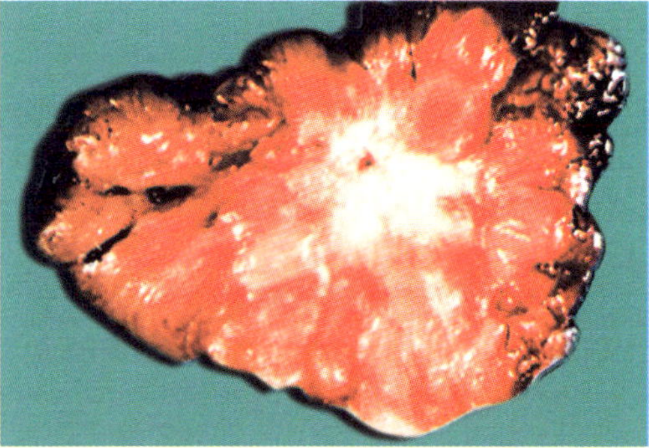

Fig. 5.5: Malignant tumor with infiltrating borders.

TABLE 5.1: Differentiating features of benign and malignant tumors.

Features	*Benign tumors*	*Malignant tumors*
Differentiation	Well differentiated	Well differentiated, moderately differentiated, poorly differentiated and undifferentiated
Pleomorphism	Usually, isomorphic	Often pleomorphic
N/C ratio	Normal	Increased
Mitotic activity	Not prominent	Increased with normal/abnormal mitotic figures
Polarity	Retained	Lost

Contd...

Contd...

Features	*Benign tumors*	*Malignant tumors*
Rate of growth	Slow growth	Rapid growth rate
Surrounding tissue	Usually compressed	Usually infiltrated
Local invasion	Encapsulated with true capsule	Not encapsulated with local infiltration
Metastasis	Absent	Present
Secondary changes	Less common	More common

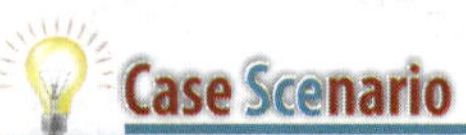

A male patient of 62 years visited the clinic with complain of persistent cough, unintentional weight loss and occasional blood-tinged sputum. The patient is having history of hypertension and type 2 diabetes. He is non-smoker and occasionally consume alcohol and has history of working in a factory with asbestos exposure. During initial assessment, the respiratory examination reveals decreased breath sounds on the right side and chest X-ray shows a mass in the right lung.

Question:

Given the presenting complaint and assessment findings, what should the nurse prioritize during the initial care of patient, and what is a key nursing intervention?

A. Prioritize pain management: Administer analgesics as prescribed.
B. Monitor blood glucose levels: Adjust insulin dosage accordingly.
C. Address respiratory distress: Administer oxygen therapy and assist with a sputum sample collection.
D. Focus on blood pressure control: Administer antihypertensive medications.

Answer:

C. Address respiratory distress: Administer oxygen therapy and assist with a sputum sample collection.

Metastasis

Metastatic deposits are tumor implants discontinuous from the primary tumor, which are carried by the blood vessels or lymphatics to distant sites. Malignant tumors usually undergo metastatic spread and benign tumors generally do not metastasize.

Routes of Metastasis

- *Lymphatic invasion:* This pattern is seen mostly in carcinomas. The tumor cells may form emboli within the lymphatics (lymphatic emboli) or may grow within the lymphatics (lymphatic permeation). The tumor cell is carried to the nearest regional lymph node. This is the reason for the enlargement of the regional lymph node in cases of neoplasia and examination of the regional lymph node is very important in every case of neoplasia carcinoma breast—axillary lymph nodes, carcinoma lung—hilar nodes, etc.
- *Hematogenous invasion:* This pattern is mostly seen in sarcomas. The tumor cells usually invade larger and smaller veins. Spread of tumor is less likely in thick-walled elastic arteries.
- *Other patterns of invasion:* Invasion of tumor cells can occur through the perineural lymphatic spaces, through the serous cavities leads to malignant effusion in the serous cavities, transcoelomic spread, subarachnoid spaces and along epithelial lined spaces.

The most common site for metastasis is regional lymph nodes, lungs, liver, bone, brain and adrenals **(Figs. 5.6 and 5.7)**. Rarer sites for metastasis are skeletal muscle, cardiac muscle and spleen. Metastasizing power of tumors vary widely. Soft tissue sarcomas, carcinoma of lung and breast have increased risk of metastasis.

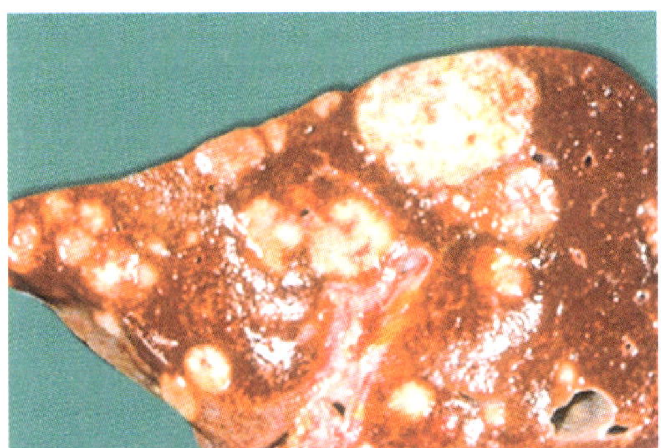

Fig. 5.6: Slice of liver with multiple metastatic deposits.

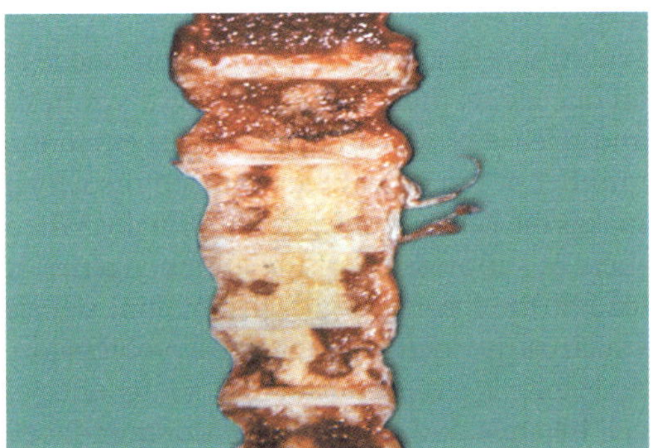

Fig. 5.7: Vertebrae with metastatic deposits.

Flowchart 5.1: Various events in metastasis.

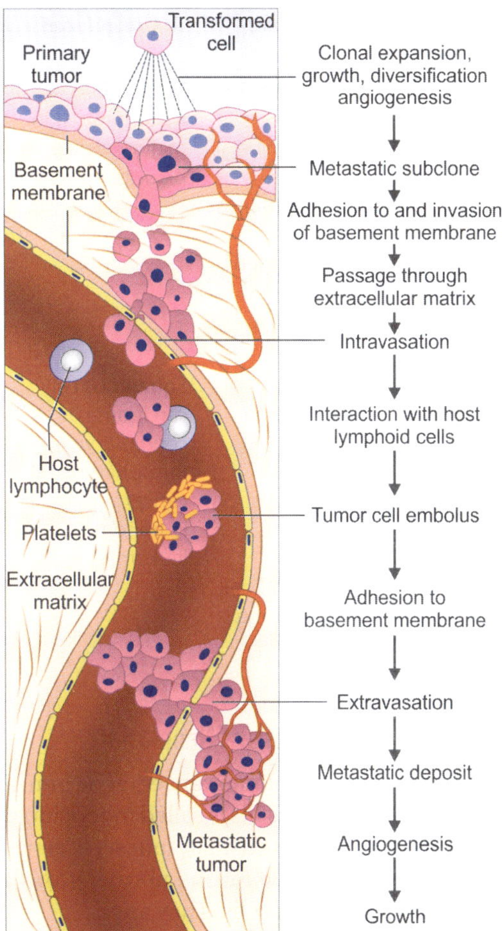

Mechanism of Metastasis

Invasion and metastasis are biological hallmarks of malignancy. The following are the sequence of events that lead to metastasis **(Flowchart 5.1)**.

CARCINOGENESIS

(Synonym: Oncogenesis)

This refers to the process of development of neoplasia. The agents which induce the formation of tumors are called as *carcinogens* **(Table 5.2)**. Initially, the mechanism of carcinogenesis was not clear and various theories and hypothesis were described to explain carcinogenesis. The increasing knowledge in the molecular biology and genetics made the concept of oncogenesis clearer.

TABLE 5.2: Types of carcinogens with examples and tumors induced by them.

Type of carcinogens	*Examples*	*Tumor induced*
Physical agents	Radiation, Ionizing radiation, ultraviolet rays, particulate radiation	Skin cancers, leukemia, visceral cancers

Contd...

Contd...

Type of carcinogens	*Examples*	*Tumor induced*
Chemical agents	Anticancer drugs, aromatic amines, nitrosamines, natural carcinogens, asbestos, polyvinyl chloride	Leukemia, lymphoma, skin malignancies, bladder tumors
Biological agents	Human papilloma virus, Epstein-Barr virus, hepatitis B virus, human T cell lymphoma leukemia virus	Squamous cell carcinoma of cervix, larynx, nasopharyngeal cancer, lymphoma, leukemia

Molecular Pathogenesis of Neoplasia

It was found that all human cancers arise from a single abnormal cell. This is called monoclonal proliferation. There are usually four set of genes which are responsible for the normal growth and differentiation of cells. They are:

1. Proto-oncogenes—genes that promote normal growth and differentiation of the cells.
2. Antioncogenes—genes that normally inhibit growth of a tumor.
3. Apoptosis regulatory genes—these are genes which normal regulate the process of apoptosis.
4. DNA repair genes—these are set of genes which help in the repair of the damaged DNA.

Neoplasia can occur due to any one of the following mechanisms:

1. Activation of a proto-oncogene to an oncogene.
2. Deletion or absence of an antioncogene.
3. Abnormalities in genes that regulate apoptosis may retard cell death.
4. Absence of DNA repair genes—so damage in the DNA is not repaired.

The above changes can be induced either by physical agents, such as radiation rays or chemical agents, such as anticancer drugs, polycyclic aromatic amines of biological agents like few viruses.

The main target of action of these carcinogens is the loci of proto-oncogene, antioncogene, apoptotic gene or the DNA repair gene.

Mechanism

When there is activation of a proto-oncogene to an oncogene, there will be excessive synthesis and release of growth factors or excess in the number of the growth factor receptors which makes the cell to proliferate abnormally. When there is suppression of the antioncogenes, it leads to the absence of growth inhibiting signals which causes increased abnormal proliferation. Apoptosis is a mechanism for maintenance of cell balance and if there is retardation of cell death, it leads to abnormal accumulation of cells which causes neoplasia. DNA repair genes are a set of genes which regulate the repair of DNA. In normal individuals due to influence of many environmental factors, damage can occur to the DNA structure. These genes recognize the DNA damage and repair it immediately with the help of a set of enzymes, such as exonuclease, endonuclease, polymerase and ligase. When there is deficiency of these enzymes produced by these genes, it leads to accumulation of DNA damage which may culminate as neoplasia. This is seen in conditions, such as xeroderma pigmentosum, ataxia telangiectasia, Bloom's syndrome and Fanconi's syndrome. Patients with the above disorders have an increase chance of developing neoplasia.

The carcinogens are generally grouped into physical, chemical and biological agents.

Table 5.3 summarizes the various types of tumors induced by the individual carcinogens.

TABLE 5.3: List of common carcinogens and the tumors caused by them.

Type of carcinogens	*Tumor induced*
Radiation	Visceral malignancies, leukemia
Ultraviolet rays	Malignant melanoma, basal cell carcinoma, squamous cell carcinoma
Anticancer drugs—alkylating agents, acylating agents	Leukemia, lymphoma
Polycyclic aromatic hydrocarbons	Bladder tumors, tumors of lung, sarcomas
Aflatoxins	Hepatocellular carcinoma
Nitrosamines	Gastric carcinoma
Asbestos	Mesothelioma Bronchogenic carcinoma
Polyvinyl chloride	Angiosarcoma
Chromium, nickel	Carcinoma lung
Human papilloma virus	Papilloma of larynx, squamous cell carcinoma larynx, cervix, genital warts
Epstein-Barr virus	Nasopharyngeal carcinoma, Burkitt's Lymphoma, Hodgkin's lymphoma
Hepatitis B virus	Hepatocellular carcinoma
Human T cell lymphoma/leukemia virus (HTLV)	T cell lymphoma, leukemia

Clinical Features of Neoplasia

The clinical features depend on the following factors:

- Location of tumor, e.g., pituitary tumor produces visual disturbances
- Involvement of adjacent structures
- Functional activity due to release of hormones—endocrine tumors
- Bleeding—erosion of vessels
- Secondary infection
- *Cancer cachexia:* Progressive loss of weight, weakness and wasting
- *Paraneoplastic syndromes:* These are group of syndromes induced by the elaboration of hormones indigenous to the tissues. **Table 5.4** summarizes the features of various paraneoplastic syndromes.

Laboratory Diagnosis of Neoplasia

There are various laboratory methods available for the diagnosis of neoplasia. They are:

1. *Histological methods*: It is process of microscopic study of tissue sampled from the suspected site to confirm the nature of malignancy. There are various types of biopsy methods—incision biopsy, trucut biopsy and excision biopsy.
2. *Cytological methods*: This method involves the study of the cytological features of individual tumors to make a diagnosis. There are various methods of cytopathological studies which includes:
   - *Exfoliative cytology:* Study of exfoliated cells from the tumor tissue, e.g., study of cells in malignant effusions, exfoliated cells from cervix to detect cervical cancers, bronchial brush cytology from tumor of lung.
   - *Fine needle aspiration cytology:* Here a fine needle is introduced into the mass and cells are aspirated and studied. This is a very ideal, rapid and cheap diagnostic tool for the detection of neoplasia.
3. *Newer laboratory methods for diagnosis*:
   - Immunohistochemistry
   - Molecular diagnostic methods
   - Study of tumor markers
   - Flow cytometry

TABLE 5.4: Features of paraneoplastic syndromes.

Name of the syndrome	*Hormone elaborated*	*Tumors involved*
Cushing's syndrome	ACTH like substance	Small cell carcinoma lung
Hypercalcemia	Parathormone	Squamous cell carcinoma, renal cell carcinoma
Hypoglycemia	Insulin like substance	Fibrosarcoma, hepatocellular carcinoma
Carcinoid	Serotonin, bradykinin	Bronchial adenoma, gastric cancer
Polycythemia	Erythropoietin	Renal cell carcinoma Cerebellar hemangioblastoma
Neuromuscular syndromes	Immunologic	Bronchogenic carcinoma
Dermatologic	Immunologic	Gastric cancers
Hypertrophic osteoarthropathy (clubbing)	Unknown	Bronchogenic carcinoma
Venous thrombosis	Tumor products	Pancreatic cancer
Anemia	Unknown	Thymic neoplasms
Nephrotic syndrome	Tumor antigens	Visceral cancers

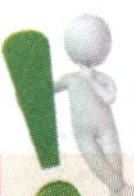

Points to Ponder

- Neoplasia is an autonomous new growth of tissue which is grouped as benign and malignant types.
- Rapid infiltrative growth and metastasis are the hallmarks of malignancy.
- The tumor spreads through various routes, such as veins, arteries and serous cavities.
- The basic molecular mechanism is an activation of a growth regulating proto-oncogene. This activation may be due to primary genetic anomalies, radiation, chemicals or oncogenic viruses.
- The clinical features of neoplasia is varied and diverse. Paraneoplastic syndromes are group of symptoms not directly related to the primary location of the neoplasia.
- The various methods of laboratory diagnosis includes biopsy, cytological methods, immuno-histochemistry and tumor markers.
- The newer methods include genomic studies and study of tumor cell kinetics by flow cytometry.

ASSESSMENT QUESTIONS

Essay Type Questions

1. **Define neoplasia. Describe the features of a malignant cell. Enumerate the common differences between benign and malignant neoplasms.**
2. **Define metastasis. Describe the process of metastasis in detail.**
3. **Define carcinogenesis. Enlist the common chemical and biological carcinogens with suitable examples.**

Short Answer Questions

1. **Define carcinoma and sarcoma.**
2. **What is carcinoma in situ?**

3. **Enumerate the common pathways of spread of a tumor.**
4. **Enumerate few precancerous conditions.**
5. **Name the four classes of genes that regulate cell growth.**
6. **How do you classify carcinogenic agents?**
7. **What are paraneoplastic syndromes? Give two examples.**
8. **Give example for tumor markers.**
9. **Name the newer methods in the diagnosis of cancer.**
10. **What is a hamartoma?**

MULTIPLE CHOICE QUESTIONS

1. **Maligant tumor of mesenchymal origin is:**
   A. Carcinoma C. Teratoma
   B. Sarcoma D. Hamartoma
2. **Pathological hallmark of malignant transformation is:**
   A. Anaplasia C. Local invasion
   B. Metastasis D. Rapid growth rate
3. **Perineural lymphatic spread is more common with tumor of:**
   A. Prostate C. Ovary
   B. Liver D. Colon
4. **Beta-naphthylamine is carcinogenic for:**
   A. Pleura C. Skin
   B. Colon D. Urinary bladder
5. **Carcinogen present in cigarette smoking is:**
   A. Aromatic amine C. Polycyclic aromatic hydrocarbon
   B. Nitrosamines D. Direct acting alkylating agent
6. **Which virus is carcinogenic for liver?**
   A. HPV 16 C. Epstein-Barr virus
   B. Hepatitis B virus D. HTLV
7. **Skin cancer is caused by:**
   A. Asbestos C. Nitrosamine
   B. Arsenic D. Vinyl chloride
8. **The organ to which metastasis very rarely occurs in:**
   A. Ovary C. Adrenal
   B. Spleen D. Colon
9. **Which is not a hereditary neoplasm?**
   A. Retinoblastoma C. Multiple endocrine neoplasia
   B. Familial polyposis coli D. Carcinoid tumor
10. **The most common paraneoplastic syndrome is:**
    A. Polycythemia C. Hypercalcemia
    B. Neuropathy D. Clubbing
11. **What is the primary characteristic of neoplasia?**
    A. Inflammation C. Dysplasia
    B. Hyperplasia D. Uncontrolled cell growth

12. Which term is used to describe a benign tumor of glandular origin?
- A. Sarcoma
- B. Carcinoma
- C. Adenoma
- D. Lymphoma

13. What is the difference between a benign tumor and a malignant tumor?
- A. Benign tumors are cancerous, and malignant tumors are non-cancerous.
- B. Benign tumors are encapsulated, and malignant tumors are invasive.
- C. Benign tumors metastasize, and malignant tumors do not.
- D. Benign tumors grow faster than malignant tumors.

14. What is metastasis in the context of cancer?
- A. The initial formation of a tumor
- B. The spread of cancer cells to distant sites
- C. The process of angiogenesis
- D. The encapsulation of a tumor

15. Which of the following is a risk factor for the development of cancer?
- A. Regular exercise
- B. Healthy diet
- C. Tobacco smoking
- D. Adequate sleep

Answer Key for MCQs

1	2	3	4	5	6	7	8	9	10
B	B	A	D	C	B	B	B	D	C
11	**12**	**13**	**14**	**15**					
D	C	B	B	C					

2

UNIT

Systemic Pathology

Section Outline

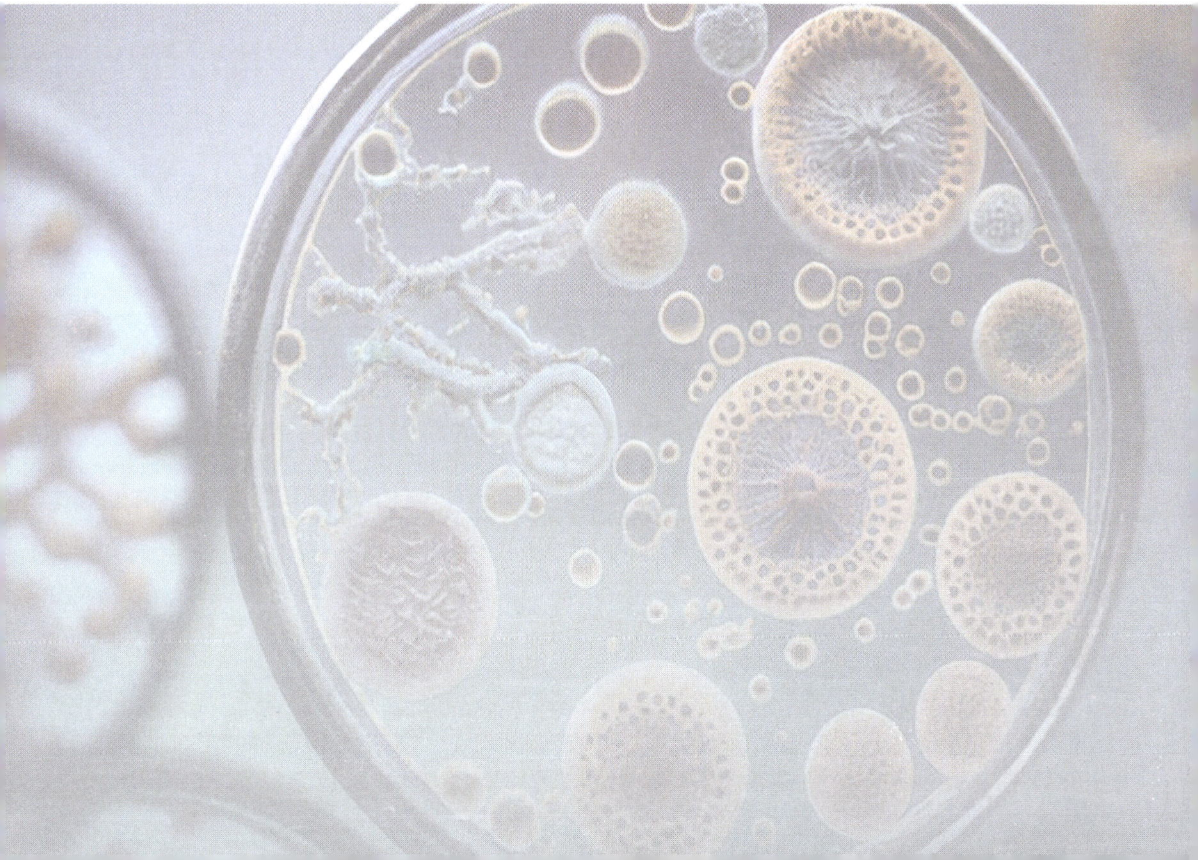

CHAPTER

Cardiovascular System

Learning Objectives

At the end of reading this chapter, the student shall be able to:

- Define arteriosclerosis and atherosclerosis and differentiate both of them.
- Describe the risk factors, pathogenetic mechanisms, pathology and clinical implications of atherosclerosis.
- Define aneurysm and discuss the various causes and manifestations of aortic aneurysms.
- Describe the epidemiology, risk factors, etiology, pathogenesis, pathology, clinical features, diagnosis and complications of ischemic heart disease.
- Describe the etiology, pathogenesis, pathology, and complications of rheumatic heart disease.
- Describe the risk factors, etiology, pathogenesis, pathology, clinical features and complications of infective endocarditis.
- Define cardiomyopathy. Enlist the causes for cardiomyopathy.
- Describe the etiology and pathology of the pericardial diseases.

NORMAL STRUCTURE

The blood vessels are closed circuits for the transport of blood and other nutrients. They are composed of arteries, arterioles, capillaries, venules and large veins. The anterior view of the heart with coronary arteries is shown in **Figure 6.1**.

Based on the caliber and histological features, the arteries are grouped into large elastic arteries, medium-sized muscular arteries and smaller arterioles.

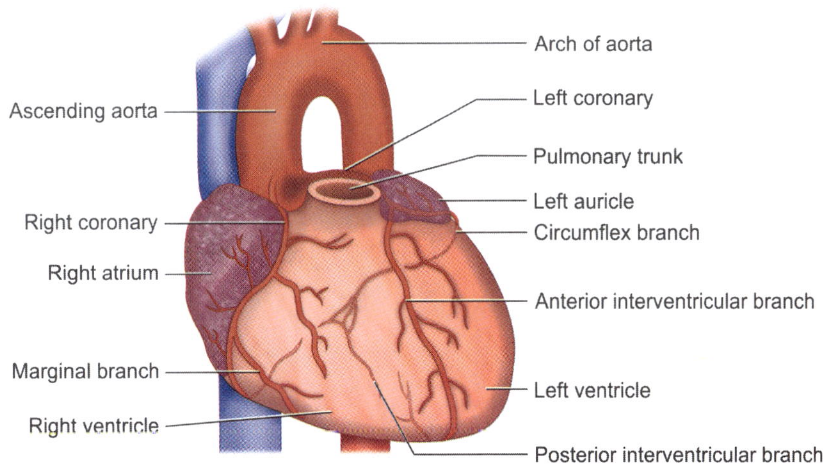

Fig. 6.1: Anterior view of coronary arteries.

Type of artery	*Examples*
Large elastic	Aorta, common carotid, common iliac
Medium muscular	Cerebral, coronary, uterine, mesenteric
Arterioles	Smaller branches of arteries

Histologically, the arteries have three layers in their wall. They are:

1. *Tunica intima:* It is the inner most layer and composed of lining endothelial cells and subendothelial collagen. It also contains the myointimal cells. It is bounded externally by the fenestrated internal elastic lamina.
2. *Tunica media:* It is the middle layer and is composed of smooth muscle cells elastic fibers and amorphous ground substance. This is the thickest of all the three layers and is limited by the external elastic lamina. This layer is responsible for vasomodulation.
3. *Tunica adventitia:* It is the outermost layer of the vessel composed of connective tissue. This layer is rich in vessels and nerves like the vasa vasorum and vasa nervosum.

   Capillaries have a similar architecture without tunica media. The veins also have a similar histomorphological pattern. The endothelium of the vein is thrown into valvular folds and the media layer is very thin and poorly developed.

PATHOLOGY OF BLOOD VESSELS

Arteriosclerosis

Definition

It is defined as a process of thickening and hardening of the vessel wall due to various conditions. The common causes are the following:

- Atherosclerosis
- Senile arteriosclerosis
- Hypertensive arteriosclerosis
- Monckeberg's arteriosclerosis.

Atherosclerosis

Definition

It is a disease of large and medium-sized muscular arteries and elastic arteries characterized by the formation of an atheromatous plaque which is a raised intimal lesion composed of lipid core and fibrous cap (**Fig. 6.2**).

It is one of the leading causes of morbidity and the major consequences of atherosclerosis are the following:

- Myocardial infarction
- Cerebrovascular accidents
- Peripheral vascular occlusive disorders—gangrene
- Abnormal dilatation and rupture of the vessel—aneurysm

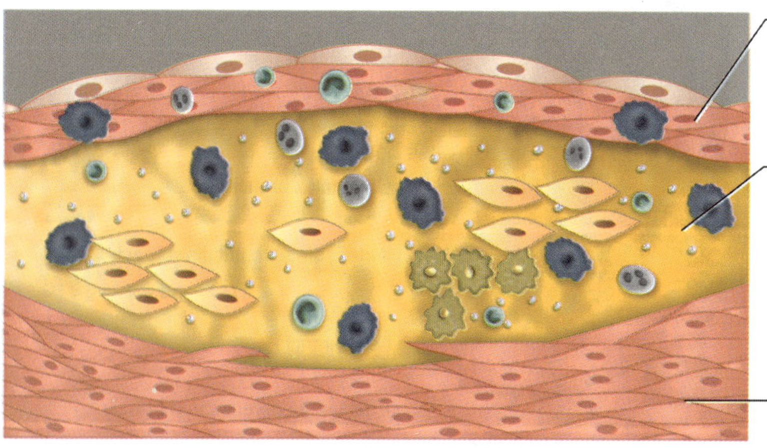

Fig. 6.2: Atheromatous plaque.

Epidemiology

There are various risk factors which contribute to atherosclerosis and they are grouped into modifiable (soft), potentially modifiable and non-modifiable (hard) risk factors.

Non-modifiable risk factors	*Potentially modifiable risk factors*	*Modifiable factors*
Age	Diabetes mellitus	Reduced physical activity
Gender	Hypertension	Stress
Familial hyperlipidemias	Obesity	Drugs—contra-ceptive pills
Family history		Smoking
Homocystinemia		Type A personality
		Hyperuricemia

Role of the Important Risk Factors in the Evolution of Atherosclerosis

- *Age:* The incidence of atherosclerosis increases with increase in age of the individual.
- *Gender:* Up to the menopause women have a lesser chance for atherosclerosis due to the protective action of estrogen, but after menopause the incidence is same.
- *Familial hyperlipidemia and obesity:* It is one of the most important risk factors for atherogenesis. The atheromatous plaques are generally rich in lipids and a strict control of the level of the lipoproteins reduces the risk of atherosclerosis.
- *Diabetes mellitus:* It is an important predisposing factor for atherosclerosis due to following reasons. Patients with diabetes mellitus have elevated levels of triglycerides, low levels of high-density lipoproteins (HDL), reduced levels of prostacyclin and risk of endothelial cell dysfunction. All these factors play a vital role in the formation of an atheroma.
- *Hypertension*: It produces significant damage to the endothelium which is the initiating event in many forms of atherogenesis.
- *Smoking:* It increases the risk by lowering the levels of high-density lipoproteins and increasing the levels of fibrinogen.
- *Physical inactivity:* Lack of physical activity reduces the level of high-density lipoproteins which in turn contributes to atheroma formation.
- *Type A personality:* Atherosclerosis is more common in individuals who are highly

Primary Events

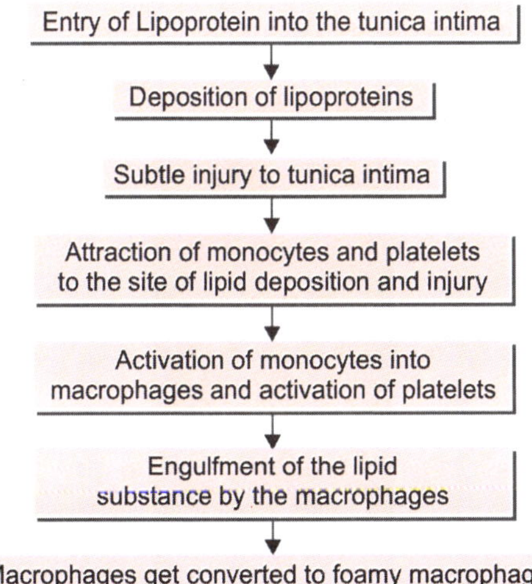

Secondary Events

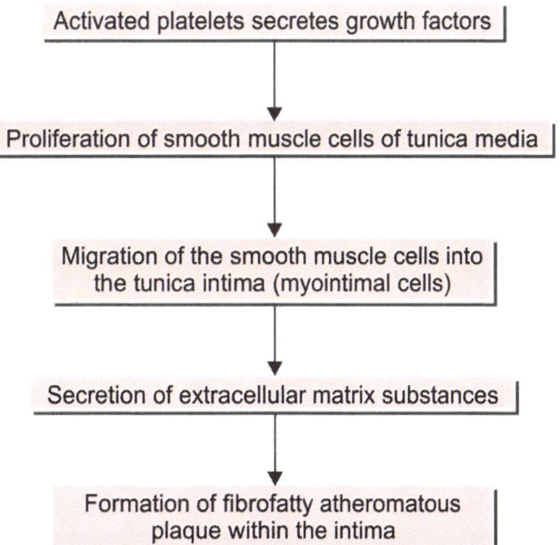

aggressive, ambitious, bustling, impatient and short tempered.

Pathogenesis of Atherosclerosis

There are various theories and hypothesis that contribute to the formation of atheroma. The most widely accepted theory is **modified reaction to injury hypothesis**. We shall now discuss briefly the salient features of this mechanism.

Modified reaction to injury hypothesis: The mechanism is depicted in the below flowcharts:

To conclude, the four major events in atherogenesis are:

1. Endothelial cell injury
2. Hyperlipidemic state
3. Proliferation of smooth muscle cells
4. Formation of foamy macrophages

Morphology

There are various morphological forms of atherosclerosis (**Fig. 6.3**). The lesions are:

- *Fatty streak:* It is the earliest lesion characterized by the presence of multiple thin yellowish spots within the intima **(Fig. 6.3)**.
- *Gelatinous elevation:* It is the next transient lesion characterized by soft raised gelatinous lesions within the intima and is composed mostly of macrophages filled with lipid.
- *Fibrofatty plaque* (**Fig. 6.4**)*:* It is the fundamental lesion of atherosclerosis. This is a raised intimal whitish yellow lesion 3–15 mm in size which protrudes into the lumina. Each plaque has a fibrous cap and fatty core. Histologically, the fibrous cap is composed of proliferating fibroblastic cells, smooth muscle cells and extracellular matrix proteins. The inner lipid core consists of cholesterol debri, foamy macrophages, and extracellular lipid.

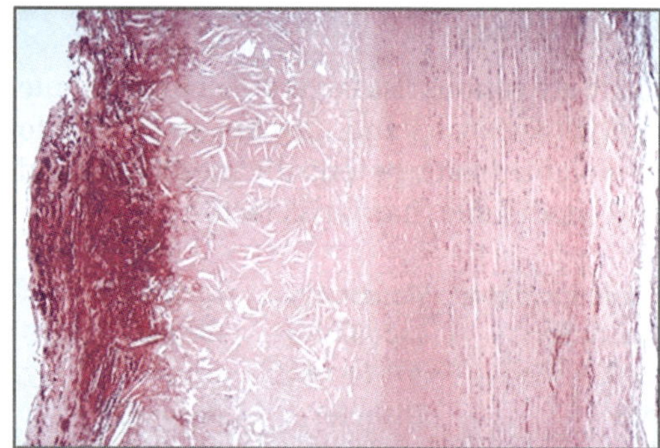

Fig. 6.4: Histomicrograph of fibrofatty atherosclerotic plaque.

Common sites for the location of atheromatous plaque:

- Abdominal aorta
- Thoracic aorta
- Ostia of the coronaries
- Popliteal
- Internal carotid
- Circle of Willis

- *Complicated plaque* (**Fig. 6.5**): This indicates advanced lesion of atherosclerosis.

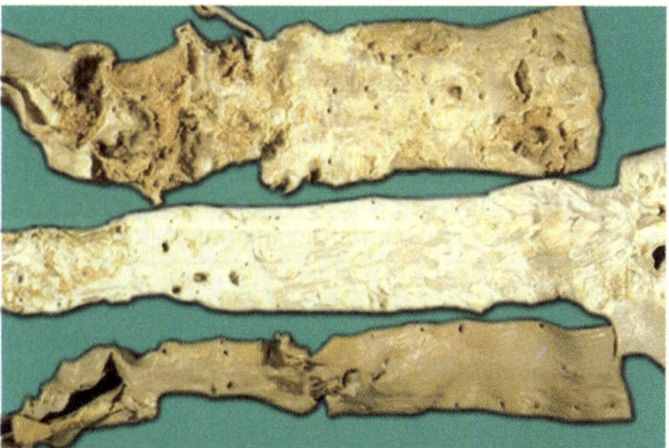

Fig. 6.3: Gross photographs of aorta showing various grades of atherosclerotic lesions.

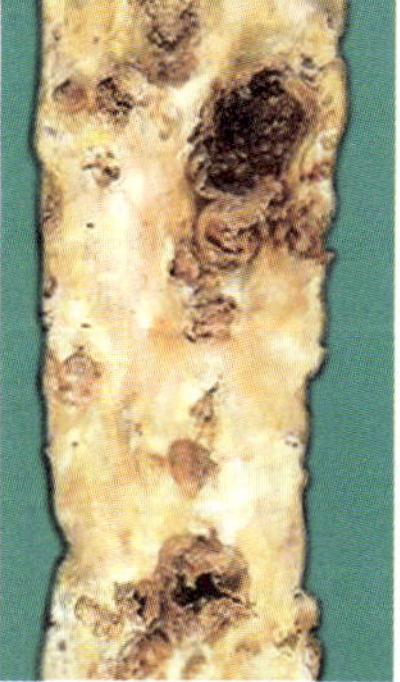

Fig. 6.5: Ulcerated atheromatous plaque.

The changes that occur includes:
- Fibrosis of the plaque
- Ulceration of the plaque
- Formation of thrombosis
- Hemorrhage within the plaque
- Calcification of the plaque
- Thinning of the underlying vessel wall leading to formation of aneurysm.

Clinical Implications of Atherosclerosis

The various clinical implications of Atherosclerosis are summarized below:

Site of atherosclerosis	*Clinical implications*
Coronaries	♦ Myocardial Infarction, angina pectoris ♦ Cardiac arrhythmias, sudden death
Cerebral vessels	♦ Transient ischemic attack, hemiplegia ♦ Neurological dysfunction
Peripheral vessels	Intermittent claudication, gangrene
Mesenteric vessels	Bowel infarction, malabsorption
Renal vessels	Renal ischemia
Abdominal aorta	Aneurysmal dilatation

ANEURYSMS

Definition

Aneurysms are defined as localized abnormal permanent dilatation of blood vessels due to weakness of the tunica media. **Figure 6.6** depicted the types of aneurysm.

Classification criteria	*Examples*
Nature of the wall	♦ True (lined by vessel wall) ♦ False (lined by fibrous tissue)
Morphology	♦ Berry (small 1–10 mm) ♦ Saccular (sac like) ♦ Fusiform (spindle shaped) ♦ Cylindrical ♦ Cirsoid (irregular)
Etiology	♦ Atherosclerosis ♦ Syphilis ♦ Aortic dissection ♦ Traumatic ♦ Inflammatory (vasculitis) ♦ Congenital ♦ Infective (mycotic)

Classification

The aneurysms are classified based on the composition of the lining, morphology and etiology.

We shall now discuss the salient features of the most common forms of aneurysms.

❖ *Atherosclerotic aneurysms:* These are the most common forms of aneurysms. Usually seen in men above the age of 50 years.
Site: Abdominal aorta (below the origin of renal arteries and above the bifurcation of aorta) is the most common site (**Fig. 6.7**). Other vessels include superior and inferior mesenteric vessels.
The shape may be fusiform or cylindrical. The basic underlying mechanism for these

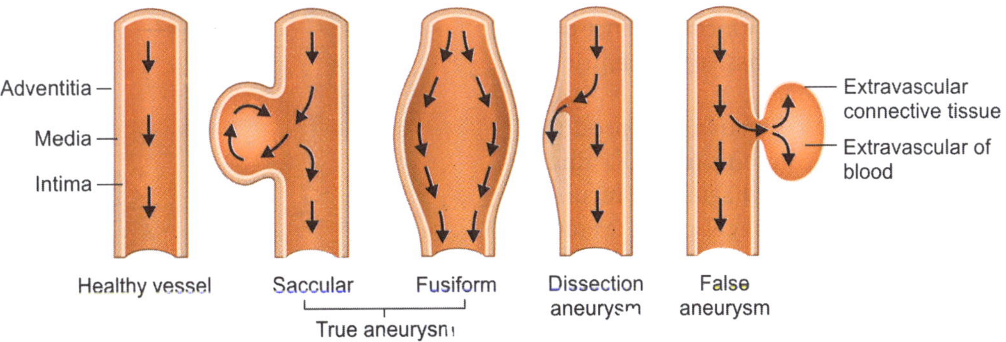

Fig. 6.6: Types of aneurysm.

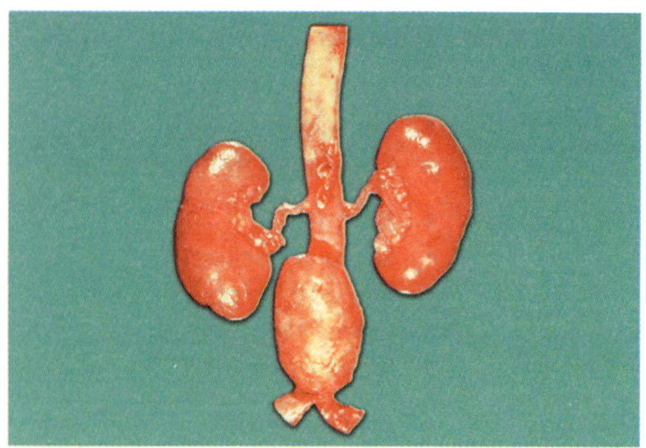

Fig. 6.7: Gross photograph of atherosclerotic aneurysm of abdominal aorta.

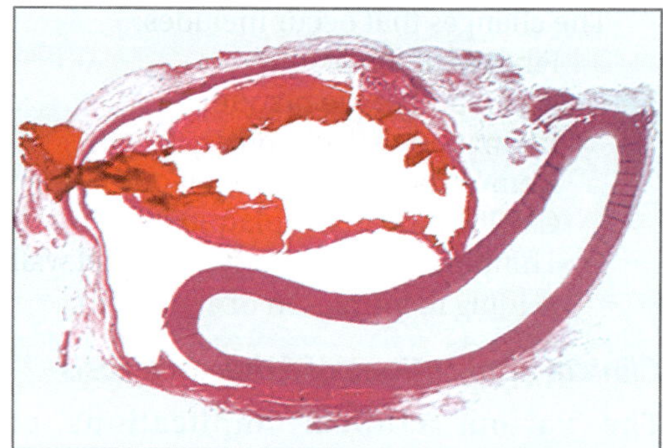

Fig. 6.8: Cross-section of aorta showing dissection.

aneurysms is the thinning and weakening of the tunica media by long standing atheromatous lesions.

Complications: Most common complication is rupture of the aneurysm leading to massive hemorrhage, pressure effect on adjacent vital organs, thrombosis and embolization.

- *Syphilitic aneurysm:* These aneurysms are seen in the tertiary stage of syphilis and are confined to thoracic aorta. The aneurysmal sac is usually saccular or fusiform in shape. The most common underlying cause for the aneurysmal dilatation is inflammation mediated thinning of the tunica media. The basic inflammatory reaction in syphilis is obliterative endarteritis and when this involves the vasa vasorum of the vessel it leads to ischemia of the tunica media and thereby thinning. These aneurysms are often accompanied by other cardiovascular lesions of syphilis like incompetence of the aortic valve and massive left ventricular hypertrophy.

  Complications: It usually produces compressive symptoms of mediastinum, adjacent lung, esophagus and recurrent laryngeal nerve. It may also lead to erosion of the underlying bone.
- *Dissecting aneurysm:* This is a special type of aneurysm affecting the ascending and descending aorta, in which a column of blood enters into the tunica media and dissects the media, which leads to dilatation of the vessel wall **(Fig. 6.8)**.

  The initial event is a tear in the tunica intima (**Fig. 6.9**). This is mostly due to a hemodynamic stress induced by hypertension. The smooth muscle cells of tunica media of the affected vessels are replaced by an amorphous basophilic material with focal cystic dilatation. This change in referred to as cystic medial necrosis. This change is due to an underlying biochemical defect in the cross-linking of collagen molecule which occurs in Marfan's syndrome. There is a mutation of a gene (fibrillin gene) in the long arm chromosome 15 (15q21) which leads to aberrant collagen cross linking.

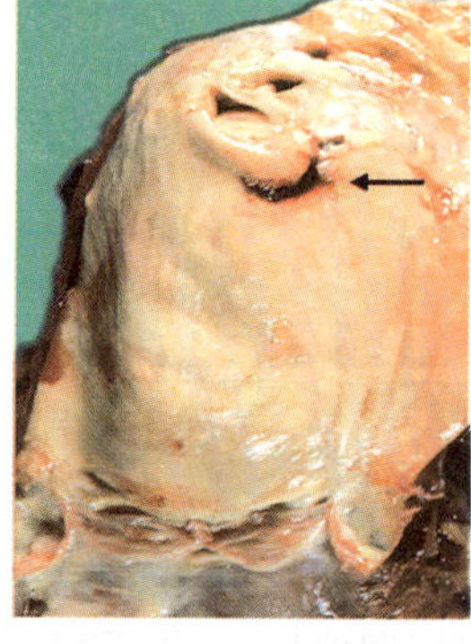

Fig. 6.9: Gross photomicrograph of aortic dissection with an intimal tear (arrow).

In few of the cases, the blood that enters into the media reenters into the lumina due to a second tear in the intima which leads to a change called "Double barrel aorta".

Clinical profile: This condition presents with sudden onset of excruciating chest pain with increase blood pressure.

INTRODUCTION

The heart is a special type of muscular pump which ejects blood into the arterial tree to maintain optimum circulation. It is divided into four chambers—the right and left atrium and ventricles. These chambers are separate by muscular partition called interatrial septa and interventricular septa **(Fig. 6.10)**.

The flow of blood occurs in the following manner within the heart:

- Venous blood from circulation
- Right atrium
- Right ventricle
- Pulmonary artery
- Lungs—alveoli
- Pulmonary veins

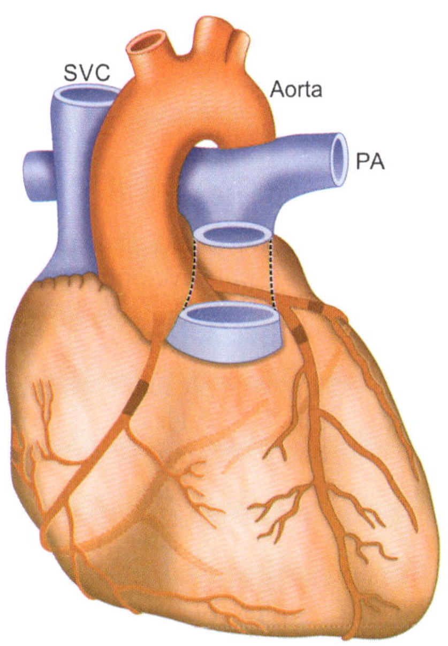

Fig. 6.10: Heart.
(SVC: superior vena cava; PA: pulmonary artery)

- Left atrium
- Left ventricle
- Aorta
- Systemic arterial circulation

The transport of blood is regulated by a set of four cardiac valves. The atrioventricular valves are the tricuspid (right) and mitral (left). The semilunar valves are the pulmonary (right) and aortic (left).

Histologically, the heart consists of an external thin layer—pericardium, a muscular myocardium (**Fig. 6.11**) composed of the specialized cardiac muscle which has the property of conduction and inner thin endocardium, which is a specialized endothelial tissue. The endocardium that lines the valve is referred to valvular endocardium and that of the chambers, mural endocardium.

BLOOD SUPPLY

The heart is a richly vascular organ supplied by right and left coronary artery which are direct branches of aorta. The left coronary artery further divides into left anterior descending and left circumflex which supplies a major portion of heart. The right coronary artery supplies right atrium and posterior third of interventricular septum (**Fig. 6.12**). Coronary veins run parallel to the arteries and drain into coronary sinus.

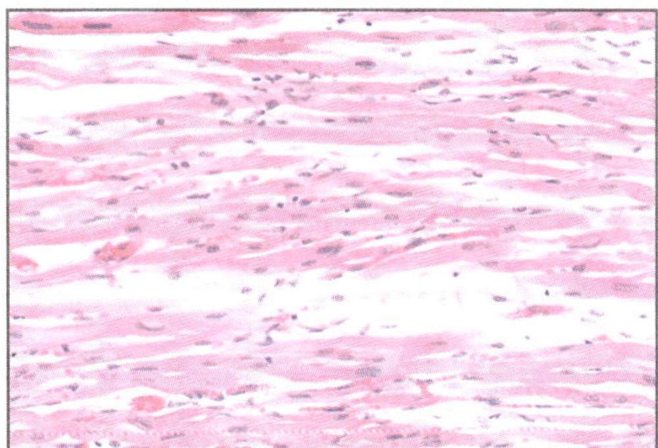

Fig. 6.11: Photomicrograph of normal myocardium.

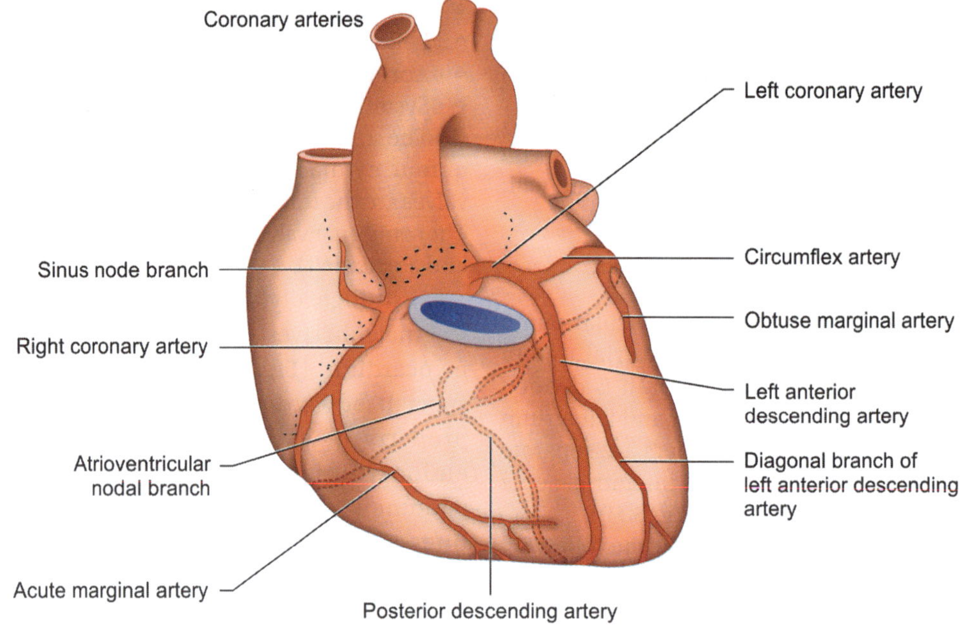

Fig. 6.12: Pattern of distribution of the coronary arteries.

DISEASES OF HEART

The diseases of the heart are categorized on the basis of the anatomic region involved and the nature of functional impairment. They are:

- *Congenital heart disease*: Due to congenital anomalies in the structure of the heart, e.g., atrial septal defect, ventricular septal defect, tetralogy of Fallot, patent ductus arteriosus, transposition of great vessels and others.
- *Ischemic heart disease*: Due to impaired blood supply to the myocardium, e.g., myocardial infarction, angina pectoris, etc.
- *Heart failure*: Due to impairment of the pumping function of the heart, e.g., left-sided and right-sided congestive cardiac failure.
- *Rheumatic heart disease*: Most common acquired immune mediated disorder of the cardiac valves, e.g., rheumatic mitral stenosis.
- *Infective endocarditis*: Valvular diseases of infective origin.
- *Cardiomyopathy*: Disorder of the cardiac musculature of unknown etiology leading to functional impairment, e.g., hypertrophic CMP, dilated CMP and restrictive CMP.
- *Hypertensive heart disease*: The changes in the heart due to hypertension.
- *Disease of pericardium*: Pericarditis, pericardial effusion.
- *Cor Pulmonale*: Disease state of the heart secondary to a chronic lung disease.
- Tumors of the heart.

Ischemic Heart Disease

It is one of the leading causes of death in both sexes in developed and developing countries.

Definition

These are group of closely related conditions resulting from myocardial ischemia. There is an imbalance between the supply and demand of oxygenated blood to the heart.

Most common causes include:

- Coronary atherosclerosis (> 90%)
- *Others*: Coronary vasospasm, coronary thromboembolism, arteritis, severe anemia, cyanotic heart diseases, advanced lung diseases.

The most common conditions included in this category of heart disease include:

1. Myocardial infarction
2. Angina pectoris
3. Chronic ischemic heart disease
4. Sudden cardiac death

Pathogenesis of Ischemic Heart Disease

The major underlying pathogenetic mechanisms that lead to ischemic heart disease are:

- Fixed coronary obstruction
- Acute changes in plaque morphology and superadded thrombi formation
- Platelet aggregation and vasospasm

Fixed Coronary Obstruction

When > 75% of the cross-sectional area of the vessel is involved by the atherosclerosis, it is called as fixed obstruction. It is mostly seen in left anterior descending, left circumflex and right coronary artery. This mostly leads to subendocardial ischemia.

Acute Changes in Plaque Morphology and Superadded Thrombi Formation

In this, a change occurs in the morphology of the plaque, such as fissuring, erosion or ulceration. This triggers thrombogenesis and a coronary thrombus is formed over the preexisting atheromatous plaque. It converts a partial obstruction into a complete one and causes transmural ischemia.

Platelet Aggregation and Vasospasm

These play a minor role in causing obstruction to the coronary circulation in association with a preexisting coronary atherosclerosis.

We shall now discuss the salient features of the various clinical entities included as ischemic heart diseases.

Angina Pectoris

Definition

It is defined as paroxysmal and recurrent attacks of substernal or precordial chest pain/discomfort due to transient myocardial ischemia that falls short of inducing an infarction and is usually relieved by rest.

The pain is usually described as constrictive, squeezing or chocking pain.

Types of Angina

There are three different types of angina—stable, variant and unstable.

1. *Stable angina*: It is the most common form of angina. Patient experiences the pain due to exertion, such as physical exercise and emotional excitement. There is an underlying chronic stenosing coronary atherosclerosis which produces subendocardial type of myocardial ischemia due to increased demand. The pain is relieved by rest or medication. Electrocardiogram shows depression of the ST segment.
2. *Variant angina* (Syn: Prinzmetal's angina): In this type of angina, the pain occurs even at rest and is not related to physical exertion. This is due to vasospasm of the coronary vessels. Electrocardiogram shows elevation of the ST segment, which indicates a transmural ischemia.
3. *Unstable angina*: This pattern is characterized by progressive increase in the pain even at rest. The duration of pain is also prolonged. It is due to acute changes in the morphology of the plaque and is a harbinger of subsequent myocardial infarction and so it is referred to as "preinfarction angina".

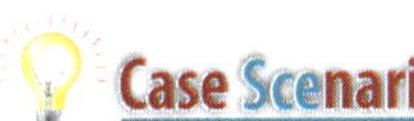

A 48-year-old male working as a marketing executive complaints of chest pain on and off. The pain is squeezing and choking in nature and gets relieved by rest. Today he is seen in the cardiology casualty with severe chest pain of similar kind.

Question:

What is your provisional diagnosis?

Answers:

Stable angina pecrotis

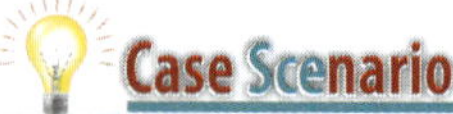

A 54-year-old business man complaints of progressively increasing chest pain since morning. No radiation of pain seen. Not associated with sweating, nausea and vomiting. The pain is not relieved by rest and is progressive in nature.He had similar episodes earlier and was on medication. He was found to have elevated levels of LDL cholesterol and triglycerides and was advised medications and lifestyle changes.

Question:

What is your provisional diagnosis?

Answers:

Unstable angina pectoris

Myocardial Infarction

It is one of the leading causes of death. Around 1.5 million individuals die due to myocardial infarction and its complications. It accounts for one-third of total mortality.

Epidemiology

The risk factors and major etiopathogenetic factors have already been discussed in the chapter on Atherosclerosis and Ischemic Heart Disease.

Types of Myocardial Infarction (MI)

There are two patterns of myocardial infarction—subendocardial and transmural.

Features	*Transmural*	*Subendocardial*
Incidence	Most common	Less common
Area involved	Full thickness of myocardium	Inner third of myocardium
Pathogenesis	Acute change in plaque morphology—with formation of thrombi on a prep-existing atheroma	Chronic stenosing atheromatous lesion. No change in plaque morphology

Myocardial Response to Ischemia

The myocardium undergoes various biochemical, morphological and functional alterations in response to ischemia.

Biochemical changes: The myocardial cell is a very sensitive to hypoxia. The changes seen are cessation of aerobic respiration, onset of anaerobic glycolysis, fall in the level of ATP and accumulation of lactic acid leading to lactic acidosis.

Functional changes: Loss of contractility is seen within 60 seconds of myocardial ischemia and cell death occurs within 20–40 minutes.

Morphological changes: Various alterations can be seen at the gross level **(Fig. 6.13)**, light microscopic level and ultrastructural level. The changes are summarized in below table.

Factors influencing the morphological changes are the following:

- Location, severity, duration and rate of development of occlusion
- Metabolic need of the myocardium
- Nature of the coronary vessel involved
- Extent of formation of collateral vessels
- Underlying cardiovascular status

Clinical Features

Patients with myocardial infarction experiences sudden excruciating chest pain of retrosternal

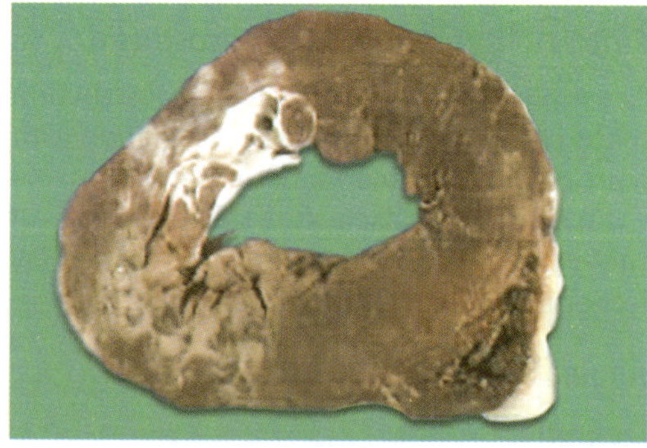

Fig. 6.13: Gross photomicrograph of myocardial infarction.

Duration after ischemia	*Gross changes*	*Light microscopic changes (Figs. 6.14A to E)*	*Ultrastructural changes*
0–30 min	None	None	Swelling of mitochondria, loss of glycogen, relaxed myofibrils
30–4 hrs	Triphenyltetrazolium chloride imparts pale color to the infarcted zone and dark brown to the normal myocardium	Waviness of the myocardial fibers (**Fig. 6.14A**)	Disruption of the sarcolemma, amorphous densities of mitochondria, irreversible cell death
12–24 hrs	Dark mottled area	Onset of coagulative necrosis	
24–92 hrs	Dark mottled area with central yellowish areas	Prominent coagulative necrosis with contraction band necrosis and neutrophilic infiltration	
3–7 days	Hyperemic border delineates infarcted area	Early phagocytosis of the dead myofibers by macrophages	
7–10 days	Central yellow area with reddish-gray borders	Formation of granulation tissue	
10–14 days	Grayish tan depressed area	Deposition of collagen	
2–8 weeks	Grayish white scar	Dense collagenized scarring	
8–10 weeks	Complete scarring		

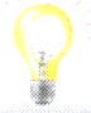

Case Scenario

A female patient of 65 years had a history of type 2 diabetes and hypertension. The patient arrives at the emergency room complaining of a squeezing chest pain that has lasted for the past hour. She rates the pain as 8/10 and describes it as radiating to her jaw. She also feels nauseous and dizzy. During initial assessment, she looks anxious, blood pressure 160/95 mm Hg, heart rate 100 bpm, respiratory rate 22/min, oxygen saturation 95% on room air. The ECG reveals ST-segment elevation in the inferior leads.

Question:

Considering the patient medical history and the ECG findings, which part of the heart is most likely affected in this myocardial infarction?

A. Left atrium
B. Right ventricle
C. Left ventricle
D. Right atrium

Answer:

B. Right ventricle

or precordial nature with radiation of the pain to the left shoulder accompanied by rapid thready weak pulse, sweating and difficulty in breathing. In 10–15% of the individuals, it can be asymptomatic, and they are referred to as silent myocardial infarction and are seen in patients with diabetes mellitus.

Diagnosis

Diagnosis of myocardial infarction is usually based on clinical examination along with ECG.

ECG changes: Elevation of depression of ST segment and appearance of new Q waves are the most common findings seen in an ECG.

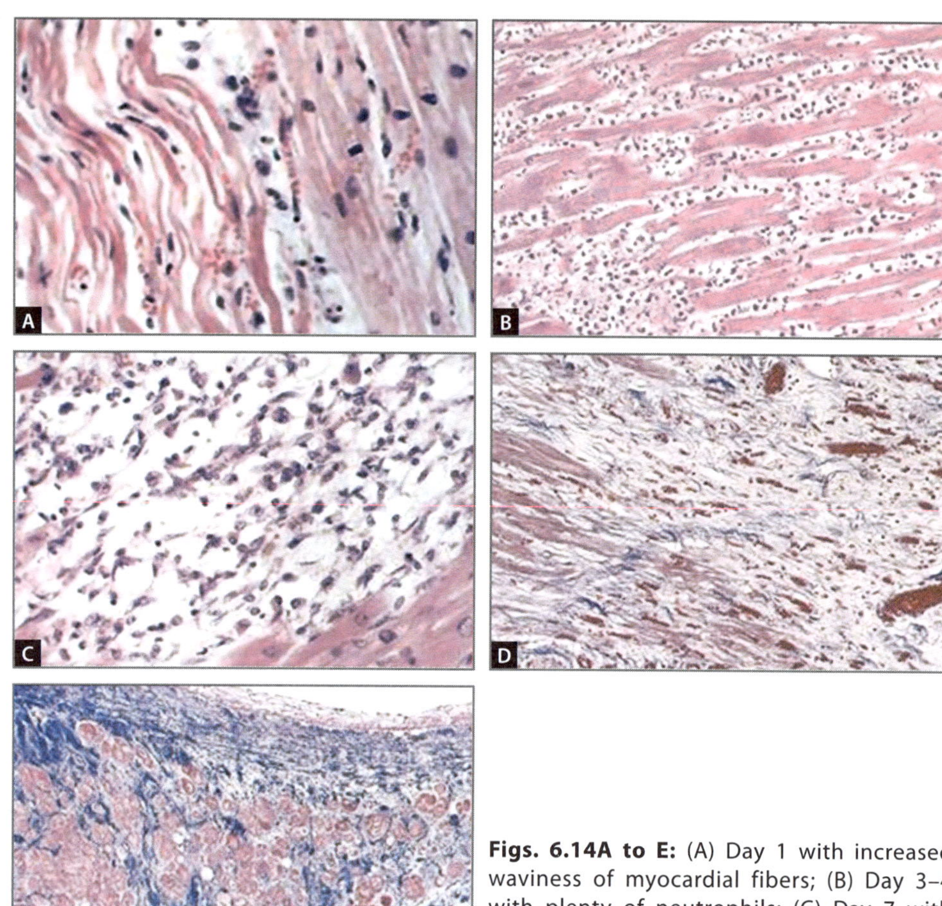

Figs. 6.14A to E: (A) Day 1 with increased waviness of myocardial fibers; (B) Day 3–4 with plenty of neutrophils; (C) Day 7 with many macrophages; (D) Second week with predominant fibrosis; (E) Stained with a special stain for connective tissue.

Laboratory tests: The myocardium is rich in various enzymes and its damage is accompanied by the release of these enzymes into the circulation. Estimation of these levels are very useful in the diagnosis of myocardial infarction. The common enzyme levels that are elevated are:

- *Creatine kinase-MB:* Estimation of the levels of CK MB is useful to diagnose myocardial infarction in the early phase. The level of this enzyme rises within 4–8 hours of infarction and reaches peak level by 18 hours and disappears within 72 hours.
- *Troponin I and T (TnI and TnT):* These are cardiac specific proteins and are released into the circulation following damage to the myocardium. The levels of troponins rise along with that of CK-MB and it remains elevated for up to 7–10 days.
- Other enzymes that are elevated in myocardial infarction are lactate dehydrogenase, aminotransferase and aspartate transferase.

The following factors are associated with poor prognosis. They include advanced age, previous history of myocardial infarction, patients with diabetes mellitus and in female gender.

Complications of Myocardial Infarction

- *Contractile dysfunction*: Lead to hypotension, pulmonary congestion and edema and cardiogenic shock.
- *Cardiac arrhythmias*: Most common lethal complication of myocardial infarction. They include ventricular tachycardia, ventricular fibrillation, sinus and bradycardia.
- *Myocardial rupture syndromes*: Massive infarction may lead to rupture of the ventricular wall producing ventricular aneurysm leading to massive hemopericardium, rupture of the interventricular septum leading the septal defect and rupture of the papillary muscle leading to mitral regurgitation.
- *Pericarditis*: Inflammation of the pericardium may occur 2–3 days after infarction and it leads to a fibrinohemorrhagic pattern of inflammation.

Rheumatic Heart Disease

Rheumatic Fever

It is defined as a multisystem non-suppurative inflammatory disease that affects the joints, tendons, arteries, connective tissue, heart, lungs, brain and serous membranes as a sequelae of infection due to group A beta-hemolytic streptococci.

The most common consequences of rheumatic fever in acute carditis and chronic deforming fibrotic valvular disease which causes permanent dysfunction of the valves.

This is usually seen in developing and under developed economically deprived regions due to poverty and overcrowding.

Rheumatic fever is diagnosed by a constellation of clinical findings which are grouped into major and minor criteria by Jones 1944. This was later modified by the American Heart Association in 1992 and the findings are:

Major criteria	*Minor criteria*
♦ Migratory polyarthritis	♦ Arthralgia
♦ Carditis	♦ Fever
♦ Subcutaneous nodules	♦ Raised ESR
♦ Erythema marginatum	♦ Raised C reactive protein levels
♦ Sydenham's chorea	♦ Raised ASO titer
	♦ Prolonged PR interval in ECG
	♦ Previous history of rheumatic fever
	♦ Positive throat culture for streptococci

The diagnosis is made based on the presence of any two major criteria or one major and two minor criteria.

Pathogenesis of Rheumatic Heart Disease (Fig. 6.15)

This disease usually begins as a pharyngitis due to group A beta hemolytic-streptococci. About 3% of the individuals with this form of pharyngitis may show features of acute rheumatic carditis.

The major pathogenetic factor involved is an immune-mediated tissue injury due to the cross-reacting antibodies. The antistreptococcal antibodies which are generated by the individual cross reacts with the tissue glycoprotein antigens of the cardiac valves, tendons, joints and other tissue and induces an inflammatory reaction. The lesions are usually sterile and the organism cannot be demonstrated in these tissues. Other causes could be a hypersensitivity reaction to the streptococcal antigens or an autoimmune process triggered by the infection.

Pathology (Acute Cardiac Lesions)

This usually causes inflammation of all the three layers of the heart (pancarditis).

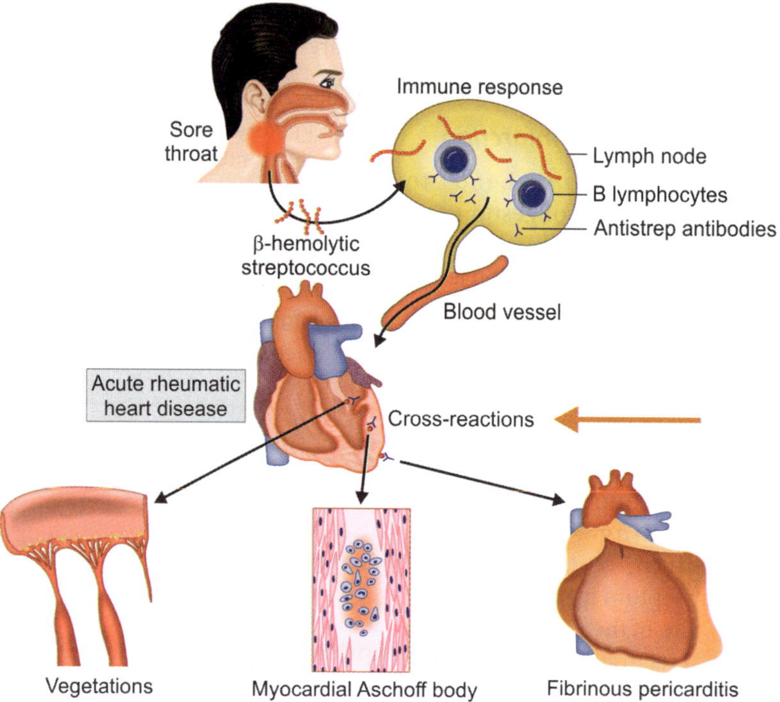

Fig. 6.15: Pathogenesis of rheumatic heart disease.

Rheumatic pericarditis: In acute phase, it produces an exudative effusion of the pericardium with deposition of fibrin, which gives a shaggy appearance to the inner surface of pericardium often referred to as the bread-and-butter type pericarditis (as it resembles the inner surface of a sandwich pulled apart).

Rheumatic myocarditis: Formation of structures called Aschoff bodies are pathognomonic of this lesion.

Aschoff body (Fig. 6.16A): It is an inflammatory lesion composed of central area of fibrinoid necrosis rimmed by plump cardiac histiocytes (Syn: Aschoff cell/Anitschkow cell), with a thread-like chromatin (Syn: Caterpillar cells) and multinucleated Anitschkow giant cells with peripheral fibrosis (**Fig. 6.16B**). There are three phases in the process of evolution of an Aschoff body. They are exudative phase, proliferative phase and fibrotic phase.

Rheumatic endocarditis: This causes inflammation of both the valvular and mural endocardium and is characterized by the presence of Aschoff bodies mostly in the posterior wall of the left atrium **(McCallum's plaque)** and left atrial appendage.

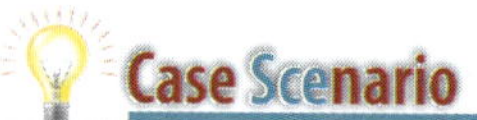

A 10-year-old boy was seen in the department of pediatrics with difficulty in breathing, on and off chest pain, cough with expectoration. He had similar episodes before and was on medications. The person had fever with painful joints two years back and was treated in the same hospital. On examination thin built boy, mild anemia, not jaundiced. Pulse and BP within normal limits.

Question:

What is your provisional diagnosis?

Answers:

Rheumatic heart disease

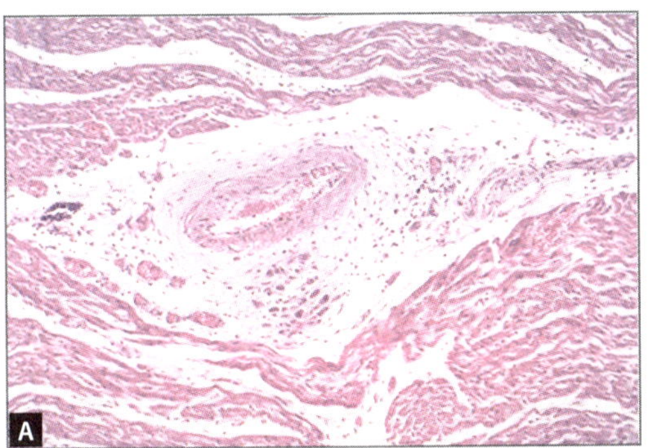

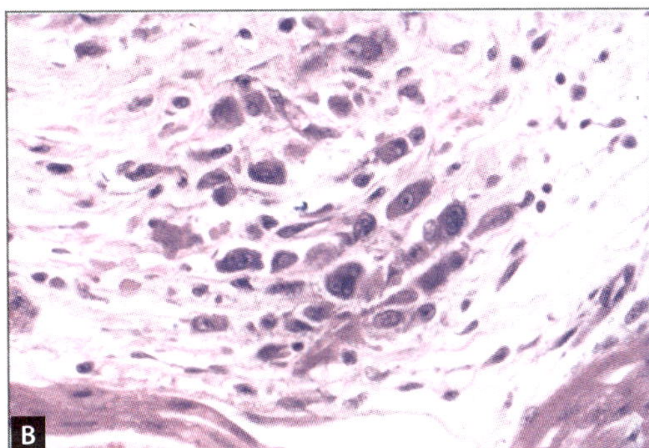

Figs. 6.16A and B: (A) Photomicrograph of as Aschoff body within the myocardium; (B) Picture showing prominent Anitschkow cells.

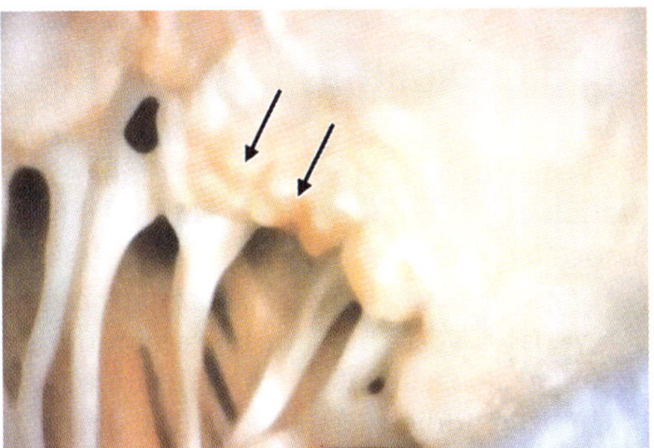

Fig. 6.17: Rheumatic valvular vegetations.

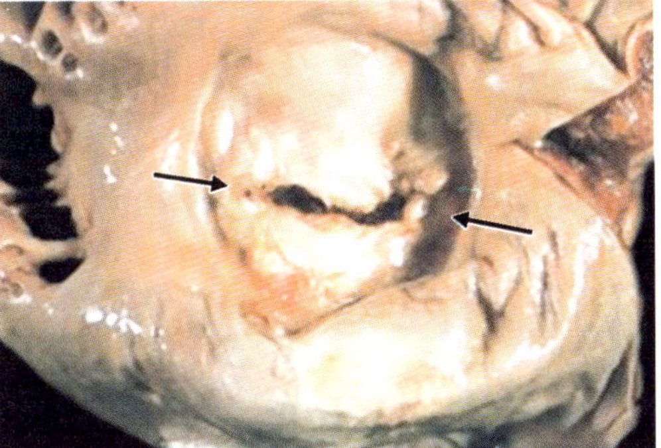

Fig. 6.18: Mitral valve with fish moth/button hole type stenosis.

The Aschoff bodies over the cardiac valves takes the form of fine grayish-pink spiky deposits along the line of closure of the valve leaflets and they are called the vegetations **(Fig. 6.17)**. Similar vegetations can be seen in the chordae tendineae and the papillary muscle.

Chronic Cardiac Lesions

Pericardium: In chronic phase of the disease, the pericardium develops fibrosis with adhesions.

Myocardium: It shows variable areas of myocardial fibrosis and degeneration.

Endocardium: After the acute phase of carditis, there will be ingrowth of the capillaries and fibroblastic proliferation in the sites of inflammation followed by fibrosis. This causes thickening of the valve leaflets and may lead to bridging of the valve leaflets producing narrowing of the opening leading to stenotic lesions **(Fig. 6.18)**. The fibrosis may also involve the chordae tendineae and papillary muscles which leads to shortening of them causing valvular incompetence. The common valves affected are the mitral valve and mitral and aortic valves. Involvement of the pulmonary and tricuspid valves are rare in rheumatic heart disease.

Other Lesions of Rheumatic Fever

The findings are summarized below:

Lesions	*Features associated with the lesions*
Arthritis	Migratory in nature, involves major joints, produces synovial inflammation, no residual deformity

Contd...

Contd...

Lesions	*Features associated with the lesions*
Subcutaneous nodule (**Fig. 6.19**)	Seen against bony prominences of arm and elbow, painless nodules. microscopy shows lesion similar to Aschoff body
Erythema marginatum (**Fig. 6.20**)	Erythematous skin lesions, margins are raised, trunk of the body involved (bath suit pattern), extremities spared
Sydenham's chorea	Involvement of basal ganglia, fine purposeless involuntary movements

Infective Endocarditis

Definition

Inflammation of the endocardium due to infective organisms.

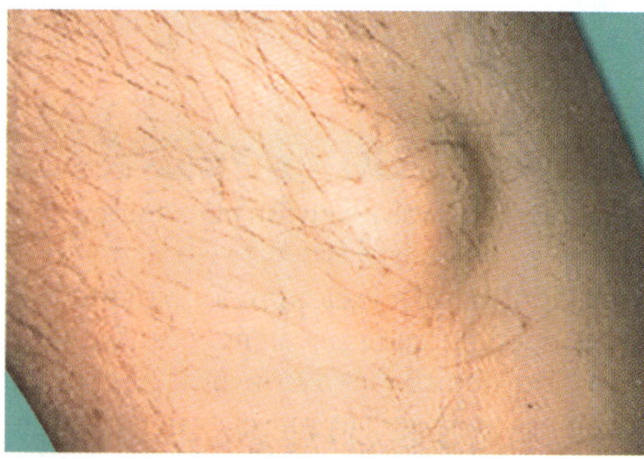

Fig. 6.19: Subcutaneous nodule of rheumatic fever.

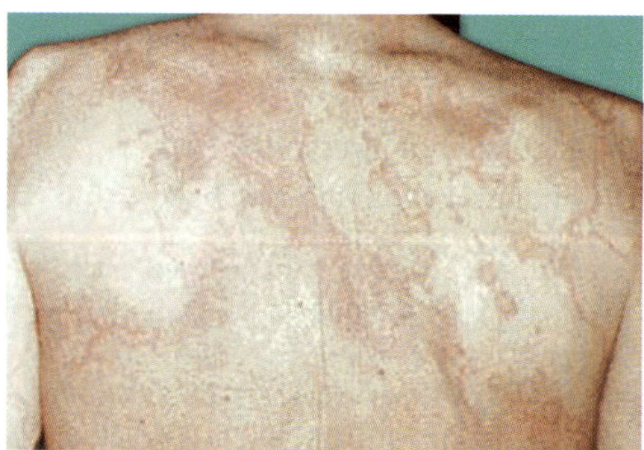

Fig. 6.20: Clinical picture of erythema marginatum.

Classification

It is usually classified into acute and subacute forms. The salient features are summarized in the table below:

Acute infective endocarditis	*Subacute infective endocarditis*
More fulminant disease	Less fulminant disease
Highly virulent organisms	Less virulent organisms
Occurs in a normal heart	Occurs usually in a diseased heart
Usually, fatal course	Clinical course in mild

Causative Organisms

A wide range of organisms ranging from bacteria, fungi and viruses can cause this pathology. Some of the common organisms associated are given here:

- *Staphylococcus aureus and Staphylococcus epidermidis:* They are more commonly associated with infective endocarditis seen in drug addicts (narcotic carditis) and in case of prosthetic valve implants.
- Streptococci viridans and bovis
- *Escherichia coli*
- Group of bacteria called the HACEK which includes *Haemophilus, Actinobacillus, Cardiobacterium hominis, Eikenella corrodens* and *Kingella*
- *Salmonella* and *Listeria* group of bacteria
- Fungi, such as *Candida, Aspergillus* and mucormycosis
- Polymicrobial—combination of more microorganisms
- Culture negative—in which no organism could be demonstrated.

Predisposing Factors

A wide range of factors predispose to the occurrence of the disease, which include:

- *Bacteremia and septicemia*: Most common conditions include severe dental sepsis, severe pneumonia, lung abscess, genitourinary infections and others

- *Underlying heart disease*: Conditions like rheumatic heart disease, congenital cardiac anomalies, such as tetralogy of Fallot, atrial septal defect, ventricular septal defect and others
- *Intravenous drug abuse*: Narcotic carditis
- Individuals with implanted prosthetic valves and other devices.

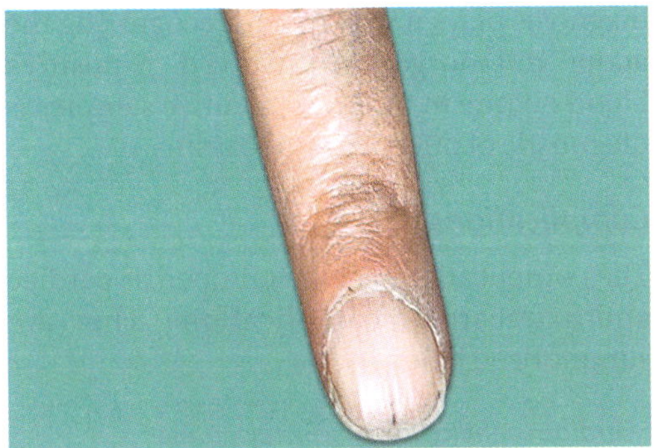

Fig. 6.21: Splinter hemorrhages in the nail.

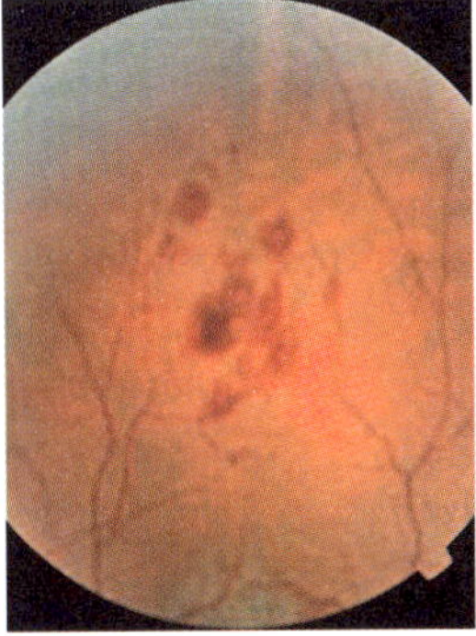

Fig. 6.22: Roth spots (hemorrhagic spots in the retina).

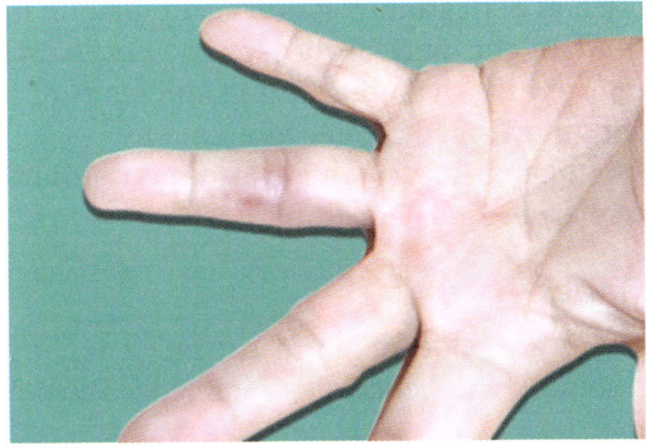

Fig. 6.23: Oslers nodes in the palm.

Pathology

It is characterized by the presence of friable, bulky, irregular vegetations that project from the surface of the valve leaflets. These vegetations are composed of microorganisms, fibrin, platelets, acute and chronic inflammatory cell infiltration. These vegetations causes destruction of the leaflets producing serious valvular dysfunction. Mitral and aortic valves are more commonly involved. The adjoining myocardium shows localized abscess formation. The infection may also involve the valve ring producing ring abscess, mostly seen in individuals with prosthetic valves.

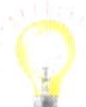

Case Scenario

A 22-year-old person was seen in the medical OPD with high fever for the past one week. The fever was irregular with spikes and he had local medication. On examination the patient is febrile, anemic, spleen is palpable. No hepatomegaly. He was diagnosed to have a cardiac valvular disease and was on irregular follow up with the cardiology department.

Question:

What is your provisional diagnosis?

Answers:

Infective endocarditis

Clinical Features

This disease is characterized by irregular high fever, malaise, palpable spleen, change in the pattern of cardiac murmurs and other lesions, such as splinter hemorrhage (**Fig. 6.21**) within the nail bed (Roth's spots in retina) (**Fig. 6.22**), painful raised lesions in the hand and feet (Osler's node) (**Fig. 6.23**) and painless hemorrhagic lesions in the palm and sole (Janeway's lesion). Fever is the most consistent sign for the diagnosis of infective endocarditis. The diagnosis is usually established on clinical examination based on Duke's criteria which has major and minor signs. Laboratory diagnosis plays a vital role in recognizing the actual microorganism involved. A positive blood culture in three consecutive samples is diagnostic of infective endocarditis.

Complications

The complications can be grouped as cardiac and extracardiac complications. They are summarized below:

Cardiac complications	*Extracardiac complications*
Perforation of valve cusps	Septic embolization—cerebral abscess, renal abscess, lung abscess
Ring abscess and myocardial abscess	Systemic sepsis—osteomyelitis
Suppurative pericarditis	Immune mediated—glomerulonephritis
Valve dehiscence (artificial valves)	Infarcts of brain, spleen and kidney

Pericardial Diseases

Pericardium is a fibrous sac that surrounds the heart. It has two layers—the parietal and visceral pericardium. Rapid accumulation of fluid in the pericardial space (**Fig. 6.24**) interferes with cardiac filling and leads to a condition called cardiac tamponade.

Inflammatory condition of the pericardium is referred to as pericarditis.

Causes

There are wide range of causative factors associated with pericarditis, summarized below:

Causes	*Conditions*
Infections	Viral, bacterial, fungal infections
Malignancy	Bronchogenic carcinoma, esophageal cancer
Metabolic	Uremia, hypothyroidism
Ischemia	Myocardial infarction
Immune mediated	Rheumatic fever, rheumatoid arthritis, systemic lupus erythematous
Iatrogenic	Post-radiation, drug induced
Idiopathic	

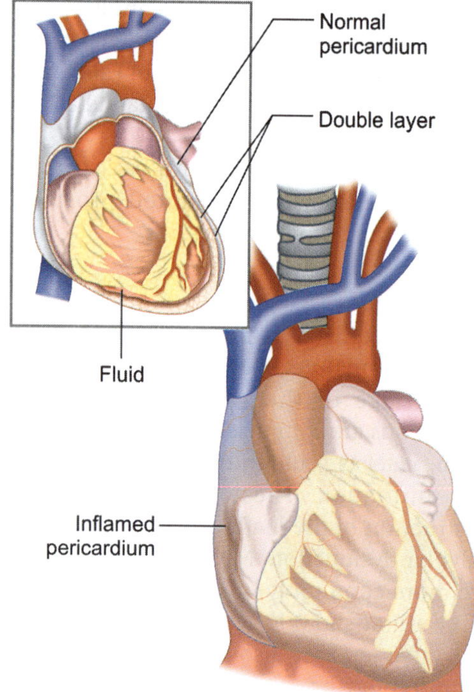

Fig. 6.24: Inflammation reaction with effusion with pericardial space.

Types of Pericarditis

The pericarditis is grouped into various morphological patterns based on the type of inflammatory response and pathology. They are as follows:

Type	*Pathological features*	*Causative factors*
Serous	Collection of thin serous fluid	Post-viral, immune mediated

Contd...

Type	*Pathological features*	*Causative factors*
Serofibrinous/ fibrinous **(Fig. 6.25)**	Accumulation of serous fluid with deposition of fibrinous material	Rheumatic fever, uremia, post-myocardial infarction
Purulent	Accumulation of pus like material	Suppurative inflammation
Hemorrhagic	Accumulation of hemorrhagic fluid material	Tuberculosis, bleeding disorders, tumors
Chronic adhesive pericarditis	Healing of the acute inflammation by fibrosis and organization with dense adhesions into adjacent structures	Tuberculosis
Chronic constrictive pericarditis	Dense fibrocalcific thickening leading to mechanical impedance of cardiac function—concretio cordis	Tuberculosis, complication of suppurative pericarditis

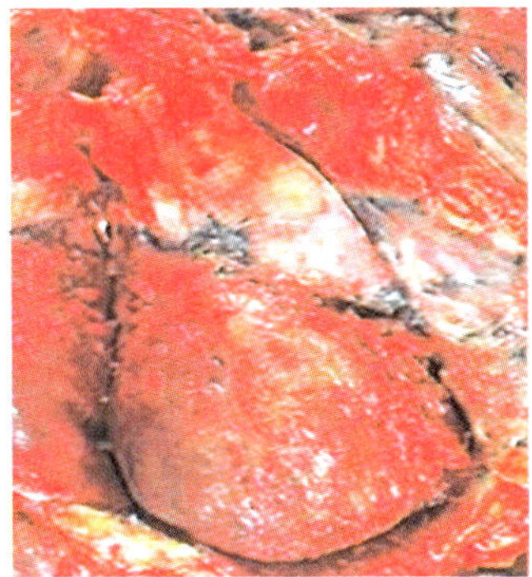

Fig. 6.25: Heart with fibrinous pericarditis.

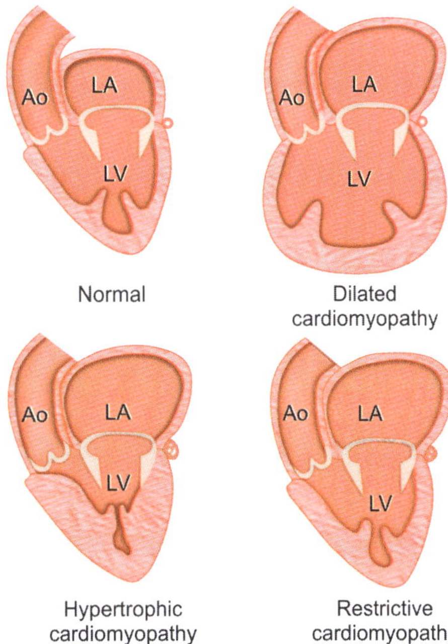

Fig. 6.26: Common types of cardiomyopathy.

Cardiomyopathy

These are heterogenous group of conditions in which there is a chronic myocardial dysfunction of uncertain cause.

They are generally grouped as primary and secondary cardiomyopathy.

There are three forms of primary cardiomyopathy (**Fig. 6.26**):

1. *Hypertrophic*: Diastolic function is defective.
2. *Dilated*: Systolic function is defective (**Fig. 6.27**).
3. *Restrictive*: Both systolic and diastolic functions are defective.

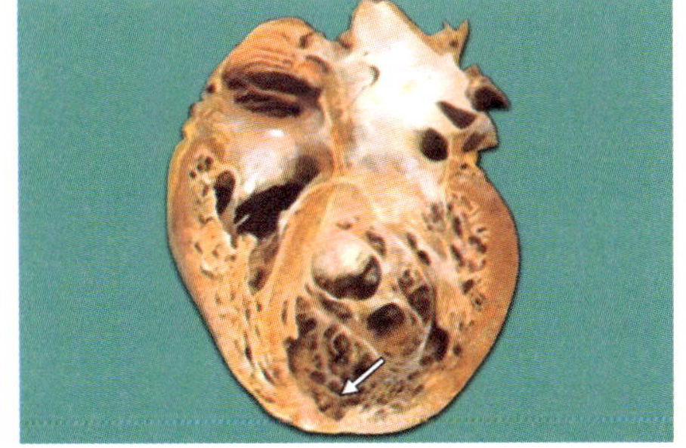

Fig. 6.27: Heart in dilated cardiomyopathy (all the chambers are dilated).

There are numerous secondary factors associated with cardiomyopathy which include causes for secondary cardiomyopathy.

Causes	Examples
Nutritional	Beriberi, alcoholism, vitamin E deficiency
Toxins	Cobalt, arsenic, lithium, serotonin
Drugs	Adriamycin, cyclophosphamide
Metabolic	Amyloidosis, hemochromatosis, storage disorders
Neuromuscular	Friedreich's ataxia, muscular dystrophy
Connective tissue disorders	Systemic lupus erythematosus, rheumatoid arthritis, dermatomyositis
Malignancy	Leukemia
Geochemical	Deficiency of magnesium and increased levels of cerium in soil

The diagnosis of cardiomyopathy is made based on the clinical examination and echocardiographic findings. Endomyocardial biopsy is very useful in rendering a tissue diagnosis in case of cardiomyopathy.

Points to Ponder

- Arteriosclerosis is defined as a process of thickening and hardening of the vessel wall due to various conditions.
- Atherosclerosis is a disease of large and medium-sized muscular arteries and elastic arteries characterized by the formation of an atheromatous plaque which is a raised intimal lesion composed of lipid core and fibrous cap.
- Aneurysms are defined as localized abnormal permanent dilatation of blood vessels due to weakness of the tunica media.
- The diseases of the heart are categorized on the basis of the anatomic region involved and the nature of functional impairment. They are:
  - Congenital heart disease—due to congenital anomalies in the structure of the heart, e.g., atrial septal defect, ventricular septal defect, tetralogy of Fallot, patent ductus arteriosus, transposition of great vessels and others.
  - Ischemic Heart disease—due to impaired blood supply to the myocardium, e.g., myocardial infarction, angina pectoris, sudden cardiac death and chronic ischemic heart disease.
  - Heart failure—due to impairment of the pumping function of the heart, e.g., left-sided and right-sided congestive cardiac failure.
  - Rheumatic heart disease—most common acquired immune mediated disorder of the cardiac valves, e.g., rheumatic mitral stenosis
  - Infective endocarditis—valvular diseases of infective origin.
  - Cardiomyopathy—disorder of the cardiac musculature of unknown etiology leading to functional impairment, e.g., hypertrophic, dilated and restrictive.
  - Hypertensive heart disease—the changes in the heart due to hypertension.
  - Disease of pericardium—pericarditis, pericardial effusion.

ASSESSMENT QUESTIONS

Essay Type Questions

1. **Define atherosclerosis. Enlist the common risk factors for atherosclerosis. Describe in detail the pathogenesis and pathology of atherosclerosis. Add a note on the clinical implications.**
2. **A 22-year-old person was rushed to the casualty with excruciating chest pain radiating to the back with excessive sweating and palpitation. His pulse rate was 102/mt. His blood pressure was 180/100 mm Hg. He was tall for his age with tall and lax fingers. He also had ophthalmic problems. One of his uncle also had a similar problem.**
   a. What is your provisional diagnosis?
   b. Substantiate your answer.
   c. Enlist the differential diagnosis in this case.
   d. Mention the brief pathogenesis of this condition.
   e. What are the common predisposing factors of this condition?
3. **A 59-year-old CEO of a multinational company was rushed to the medical emergency room with severe chest pain. The pain was acute and radiating to the left shoulder. He had a bout of vomiting and has nausea now.**

   Past history: The patient had similar episodes before and was on medications.

   On examination the patient is in shock with weak thready pulse, blood pressure is 90/60 mm Hg.
   a. What is your provisional diagnosis?
   b. Substantiate your answer.
   c. Enlist the differential diagnosis in this case.
   d. List the investigations that will help you to arrive at the correct diagnosis.
   e. Mention in brief the pathogenesis of this condition.
   f. Enumerate the complication of this condition ?
4. **A 10-year-old boy was seen in the department of pediatrics with difficulty in breathing, on and off chest pain, cough with expectoration. He had similar episodes before and was on medications. The person had fever with painful joints two years back and was treated in the same hospital.**

   On examination thin built boy, mild anemia, not jaundiced. Pulse and BP within normal limits.
   a. What is your provisional diagnosis?
   b. Substantiate your answer.
   c. Enlist the differential diagnosis in this case.
   d. Mention in brief the pathogenesis of this condition.
   e. What are lesions you will see in the heart of this person?
   f. List the common investigations you do in this case.
   g. Enumerate the complication of this condition?

5. **A 22-year-old person was seen in the medical OPD with high fever for the past one week. The fever was irregular with spikes and he had local medication.**
   On examination, the patient is febrile, anemic, spleen is palpable. No hepatomegaly. He was diagnosed to have a cardiac valvular disease and was on irregular follow up with the cardiology department.
   a. What is your provisional diagnosis?
   b. Substantiate your answer.
   c. Enlist the differential diagnosis in this case.
   d. Mention the common predisposing factors for this pathology.
   e. What are lesions you will see in the heart of this person?
   f. What is the diagnostic criteria for this condition?
   g. Enumerate the complication of this condition.

Short Answer Questions

1. **Name the nonmodifiable risk factors for atherosclerosis.**
2. **Enumerate the functions of oxidized low density lipoproteins.**
3. **What are the common sites of occurrence of atheromatous plaque?**
4. **Enumerate the common etiological factors for aneurysm.**
5. **Enumerate the four anatomical changes that define tetralogy of Fallot.**
6. **Enlist the various disease entities included in IHD.**
7. **Enumerate the differences between subendocardial and transmural infarct.**
8. **Enlist the common complications of acute myocardial infarction.**
9. **What is acute rheumatic fever?**
10. **What is an Aschoff body?**
11. **Enumerate the differences between acute and subacute infective endocarditis.**
12. **Enumerate the common causes for serofibrinous pericarditis.**
13. **Define cardiomyopathy.**
14. **Name the diagnostic modalities available for the diagnosis of cardiomyopathy.**
15. **Enlist the causes for hemorrhagic pericarditis.**

MULTIPLE CHOICE QUESTIONS

1. **Fixed stenosis of a coronary refers to occlusion of __________ in its cross-section.**
   A. 25%
   B. 35%
   C. 60%
   D. 75%
2. **Sudden death in acute myocardial infarction is mostly due to:**
   A. Pulmonary edema
   B. Ventricular fibrillation
   C. Cardiogenic shock
   D. Ventricular rupture
3. **The most common type of pericarditis in acute rheumatic fever is:**
   A. Serous
   B. Fibrinous
   C. Serofibrinous
   D. Purulent
4. **McCallum's patch is seen in:**
   A. Rheumatoid arthritis
   B. SLE
   C. Rheumatic fever
   D. Polyarteritis nodosa

5. Anitschkow cells in RHD are derived from:
A. Lymphocytes
B. Plasma cells
C. Histiocytes
D. Neutrophils

6. Roth's spots are pathognomonic of:
A. Infective endocarditis
B. Rheumatic heart disease
C. Cardiomyopathy
D. Carcinoid heart disease

7. The type of cardiomyopathy seen in alcoholism is:
A. Dilated
B. Hypertrophic
C. Restrictive
D. None of the above

8. Marfan's syndrome most often causes:
A. Atherosclerotic aneurysm
B. Luetic aneurysm
C. Aortic dissection
D. Traumatic aneurysms

9. Berry aneurysms are usually seen in:
A. Brain
B. Lung
C. Heart
D. Liver

10. The vessel most commonly involved in coronary atherosclerosis is:
A. Right coronary
B. Left circumflex
C. Left anterior descending
D. Marginal artery

11. The medical term for a heart attack is:
A. Myocarditis
B. Arrhythmia
C. Myocardial infarction
D. Atherosclerosis

12. What is the role of the coronary arteries in the cardiovascular system?
A. Pumping blood to the lungs
B. Supplying oxygen and nutrients to the heart muscle
C. Regulating blood pressure
D. Draining deoxygenated blood from the heart

13. Which of the following chambers of the heart pumps oxygenated blood to the body?
A. Right atrium
B. Left atrium
C. Right ventricle
D. Left ventricle

14. What is the main component of blood responsible for carrying oxygen?
A. Plasma
B. Platelets
C. Red blood cells (RBCs)
D. White blood cells (WBCs)

15. The pulmonary circulation involves the flow of blood between:
A. Heart and brain
B. Heart and lungs
C. Heart and liver
D. Heart and kidneys

Answer Key for MCQs

1	2	3	4	5	6	7	8	9	10
D	B	C	C	C	A	A	C	A	C
11	**12**	**13**	**14**	**15**					
C	B	D	C	B					

Respiratory System

Learning Objectives

At the end of reading this chapter, the student shall be able to:

- Describe the etiology, types, pathogenesis, stages, clinical features and complications of pneumonia.
- Describe the etiology, types, pathogenesis, clinical features, complications and laboratory diagnosis in a case of pulmonary tuberculosis.
- Describe the etiology, types, pathogenesis, clinical features and complications of chronic obstructive lung disorders.
- Describe the etiology, types, pathogenesis, clinical features and complications of interstitial lung diseases.
- Describe the etiology, types, pathogenesis, clinical features of bronchogenic carcinoma.
- Discuss the etiology and pathology of common pleural disorders.

GENERAL FEATURES

Lungs are paired organs—right and left, which are responsible for the purpose of ventilation and perfusion. The right lung weighs around 375–500 g and the left 325–450 g.

The arrangement of the air tree network in the lung is as follows:

- Trachea (main windpipe)
- Main bronchi
- Bronchioles
- Terminal bronchiole
- Respiratory bronchiole
- Alveolar duct
- Alveolar sac

Histologically, the air passages are lined by pseudostratified ciliated columnar epithelium with many mucus secreting glands and neuroendocrine cells **(Fig. 7.1)**.

The alveolar spaces are lined by two types of cells—type I pneumocytes and type II pneumocytes.

- *Type I cell*: These are very thin cells lining 95% of the alveolar surface area and are very sensitive to hypoxia.
- *Type II cell*: Sparsely distributed and are called granular pneumocytes. They secrete substances called surfactants which lowers the surface tension of the alveolar space.

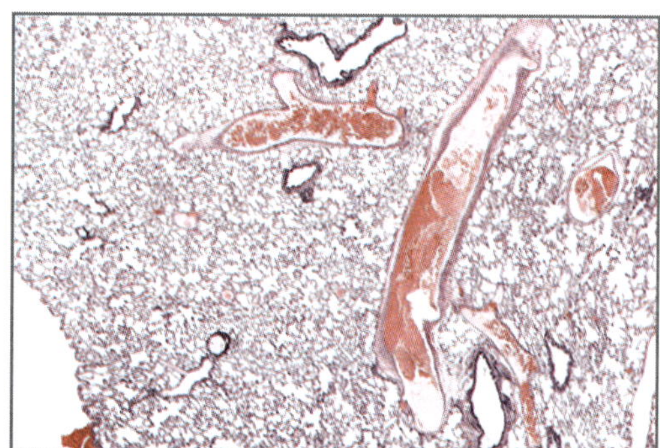

Fig. 7.1: Histology of lung with alveoli, bronchioles and pulmonary capillaries.

Other cells in the alveoli include the alveolar macrophages which are the native phagocytic cells of the lung and play a vital role in pulmonary defense mechanism.

DISORDERS OF LUNG

The disorders of lung can be grouped conveniently into the following headings:

- Congenital anomalies and pediatric lung diseases

- Infections of lung
- Chronic obstructive lung disorders
- Interstitial lung disorders
- Disorders of pulmonary vasculature
- Tumors of lung
- Diseases of pleura

We shall now discuss some of the common lung disorders and their pathological significance.

Pulmonary Infections

Infections of lung are very common in all age groups and they are one of the main causes for morbidity. They are caused by a wide range of microorganism including bacteria, viruses and fungi. Due to the prevalence of the immunocompromised states the risk of infections with fungi have now emerged to be a serious public health issue. We shall now discuss the pathological features of some of the important pulmonary infections.

Bacterial Pneumonia

Definition

It is defined as an inflammatory condition of lung caused by bacterial organisms resulting in consolidation of the lung **(Fig. 7.2)** parenchyma due to presence of an inflammatory exudate within the alveolar spaces.

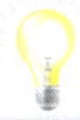

Case Scenario

Mrs X 70-year-old female patient with history of hypertension, type 2 diabetes. She presents to the OPD with complaints of cough, shortness of breath, and fever for the past five days. She also mentions chest pain that worsens with deep breaths. Her RR: 26/min, oxygen saturation: 92%. During chest auscultation reveals crackles in the right lower lobe and chest X-ray confirms the presence of a right lower lobe infiltrate.

Questions:

1. Based on the presenting symptoms and assessment findings, what is the likely diagnosis for Mrs X?
   a. Acute bronchitis
   b. Pleuritis
   c. Pneumonia
   d. Asthma exacerbation

Contd...

2. What nursing intervention is crucial for Mrs X to improve oxygenation and assist with respiratory comfort?
   a. Administering oral antibiotics as prescribed.
   b. Encouraging deep breathing exercises and incentive spirometry.
   c. Providing a heating pad to alleviate chest pain.
   d. Administering antipyretics to reduce fever.

Answers:

c. Pneumonia

b. Encouraging deep breathing exercises and incentive spirometry

Classification

It is classified based on the anatomic location and etiological agents (e.g., pneumococcal pneumonia, *Legionella pneumonia*).

Anatomic classification

There are two anatomic forms of pneumonia: (1) Bronchopneumonia (lobular pneumonia) and (2) Lobar pneumonia.

1. *Bronchopneumonia (Syn: Lobular pneumonia):* Inflammatory condition of the lung due to the colonization of

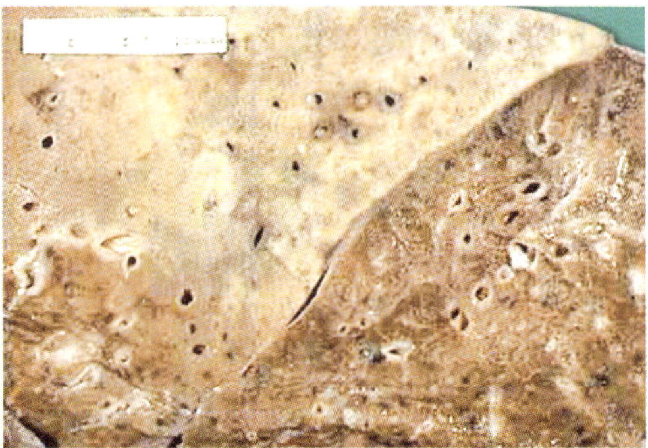

Fig. 7.2: Gross appearance of lung in consolidation.

the microorganisms within the terminal bronchioles and extension of the infection into the adjacent alveoli producing patchy consolidation.

Organisms: The common organisms responsible are Staphylococci, Pneumococci, *Klebsiella, Haemophilus, Pseudomonas* and *Legionella*.

Predisposing factors: The following are the common predisposing factors:

- *Extremes of age*: Infancy and old age
- Persons with prolonged hospitalization (nosocomial infection)
- Chronically ill and debilitated patients
- Patients with chronic end stage renal disease
- Coexistent with other lung diseases, such as chronic bronchitis, bronchiectasis, viral infections and cystic fibrosis.

Pathology: It more commonly involves the lower lobe of lung. On gross examination, it produces focal dark grayish red mottled areas of size < 1 cm firm in consistency. Pus like material is expressed out when the affected area is gently squeezed.

Microscopically, it shows acute inflammation of the bronchioles (acute bronchiolitis) with extension of the inflammation into the adjoining peribronchial alveoli. The lesion heals with minimal damage to the wall of the bronchiole with fibrosis of the alveolar wall **(Fig. 7.3)**.

Clinical profile: Patient presents with irregular fever with productive cough. Clinical examination shows features of consolidation and a chest radiograph reveals mottled opacifications in lower lobe of lung **(Fig. 7.4)**.

Complications: The more common complications include: Lung abscess, empyema, suppurative pericarditis and bacteremia.

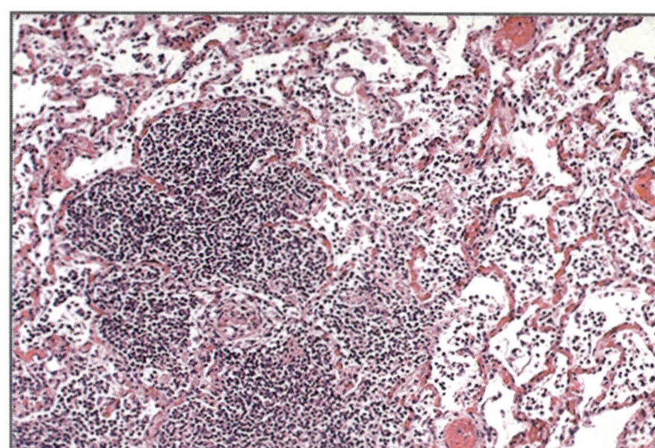

Fig. 7.3: Histomicrograph of bronchopneumonia.

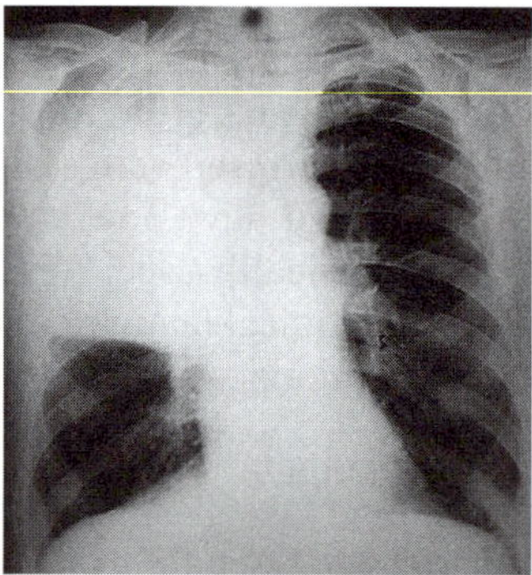

Fig. 7.4: Chest X-ray of pneumonic consolidation.

2. *Lobar pneumonia:*

   Definition: It is an inflammatory condition of lung caused by bacterial organisms resulting in consolidation of the lung parenchyma **(Fig. 7.5)** due to presence of a watery exudates filling the alveoli. The consolidation is diffuse and sharply confined to one affected lobe.

   Etiology: More than 90% of all lobar pneumonia is caused by streptococci pneumonia (Pneumococci). Other causative organisms include staphylococci, *Klebsiella, Pseudomonas, Proteus*, and other gram-negative aerobic bacteria.

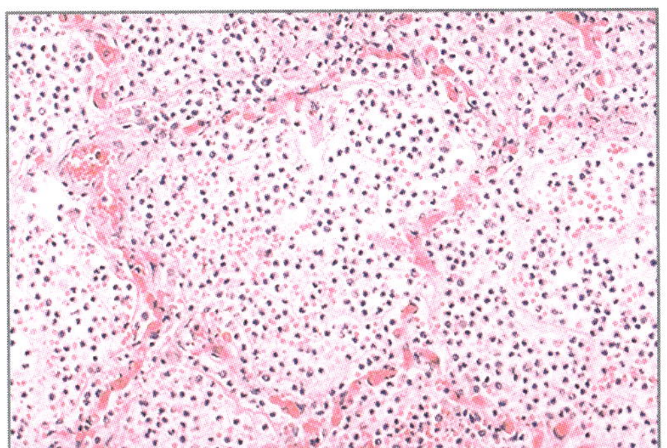

Fig. 7.5: Histomicrograph of lobar pneumonia. Alveoli filled with inflammatory exudates.

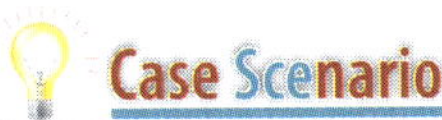

A 45-year-old male patient presented to the OPD with features of fever with chills, cough with production of rusty sputum, chest pain.

On examination, the patient was toxic, febrile.

Pleural friction rib was heard on auscultation.

Question:

What is your provisional diagnosis?

Answer:

Lobar pneumonia

Pathology: The pathological changes are grouped into four stages according to the main pathological event (**Fig. 7.6**). The features are summarized below:

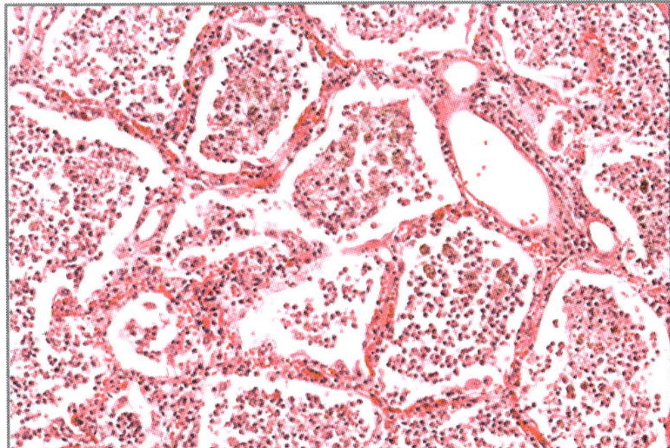

Fig. 7.6: Histomicrograph of lobar pneumonia. Alveoli with organizing inflammatory exudates.

Stage of disease and duration	*Gross morphological changes*	*Microscopic changes*
Congestion 1–2 days	Affected lobe is dark red, heavy and firm	Dilated and congested alveolar capillaries, alveolar spaces filled with edema fluid and RBCs, numerous demonstrable microorganisms
Red hepatization 2–4 days	Affected lobe is dry, granular firm, dark red with pleural thickening	Inflammatory exudation with neutrophils, RBCs and edema fluid. Less prominent alveolar septa
Gray hepatization 4–8 days	Affected lobe is firm, heavy, dull gray and thickened pleura	Neutrophils are replaced by macrophages with deposition of fibrin, the exudates are demarcated from the alveolar wall by a clear space
Resolution 8–14 days	The firmer areas revert back to the crepitant areas gradually	Macrophages are predominant in the alveolar spaces, with degenerated cell debri and liquefaction of the exudates which is coughed out or absorbed.

Complete resolution of the infective process occurs by 1–3 weeks after the initial infection. The lung parenchyma returns back to its normal condition. Generally, no residual deformity is seen.

Clinical profile: Lobar pneumonia is characterized by sudden onset of fever with rigor, pleuritic pain, shallow and rapid breathing with productive cough. The sputum is rusty in color.

Complications: Complications of lobar pneumonia are rarer compared to bronchopneumonia.

The common complications include:

- *Pleural effusion and empyema:* Seen in 5% of the individuals due to accumulation of inflammatory exudates within the pleural space.
- *Lung abscess:* Very rare complication, seen in infection with highly virulent organism and in immunocompromised states.
- *Dissemination of infection:* Spread of infections into other distant sites is a very rare complication.

Primary Atypical Pneumonia (Syn Interstitial Pneumonia) (Fig. 7.7)

This is a special form of inflammatory disorder of lung in which there is a patchy inflammatory reaction confined to the interstitial space between the alveoli. The alveolar spaces are clear without any inflammatory exudates.

Causative organisms: Most common organisms responsible for interstitial pneumonia are the viruses, such as respiratory syncytial virus (RSV), influenza virus, adenovirus, rhinovirus, cytomegalovirus and a bacterial organism, such as *Mycoplasma pneumoniae.*

Predisposing factors: The common predisposing factors include malnutrition, chronic alcoholism and any chronic debilitating illness.

Pathology: On gross examination, there is an irregular patchy consolidation of the affected lobe with a mild pleural reaction. Microscopically, there is an intense chronic inflammatory cell infiltration in the alveolar interstitium with thickening of the alveolar wall and edema. Other associated features include necrotizing inflammation of the bronchioles.

Complications: The most common complications are superimposed bacterial infection and interstitial fibrosis.

Clinical profile: The clinical features include irregular fever with malaise and non-productive cough. Chest radiograph shows patchy consolidation.

Pulmonary Tuberculosis

It is a granulomatous inflammation caused by *Mycobacterium tuberculosis* **(Fig. 7.8)**.

Fig. 7.7: Histomicrograph of interstitial pneumonia.

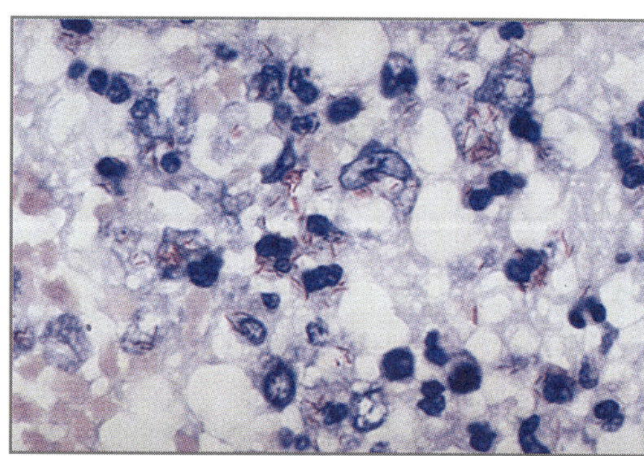

Fig. 7.8: *Mycobacterium tuberculosis*, pink rod-shaped organisms in AFB staining.

It is very common infectious disease in developing and under developed countries. Roughly around 1.7 billion people affected by this disease with an incidence of 8–10 million new cases each year and death rate of 1.7 million deaths per year. It is one of the leading infectious causes for death.

Organism: This disease is caused by slender aerobic rods which grow in straight/branching chains. The bacteria have a waxy cell wall with mycolic acid which gives the property of acid fastness. The most common causative organisms are:

- *M. tuberculosis:* Pulmonary tuberculosis
- *M. bovis:* Intestinal and oropharyngeal tuberculosis.

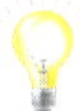

Case Scenario

A 48 year old female presented to the OPD with complaints of swelling and pain abdomen, altered bowel habits since two months. History of fever on and off seen.

On examination she was thin , anaemic .Vitals stable. There was a vague lesion palpable in the right iliac fossa.

Barium studies: Diffuse thickening and obstruction of ileum and ileo caecal junction

Endoscopy: Thickening of the ileum with mucosal ulcers.

Question:

What is your provisional diagnosis?

Answer:

Intestinal tuberculosis

Predisposing factors: The following are some of the important predisposing factors for this disease. They are:

- Poverty
- Over crowding
- Chronic debilitating illness
- AIDS/immunosuppression
- Diabetes mellitus
- Hodgkin's lymphoma
- Chronic lung disease—silicosis
- Chronic renal failure
- Malnutrition
- Alcoholism

Pathogenesis: Depends on the development of antimycobacterial cell mediated immunity which confers resistance to the bacteria and results in development of hypersensitivity reaction to tubercular antigens.

The macrophages are the primary cells that encounter the organism. The organism enters the macrophage through mannose receptors which bind to lipoarabinomannan, a bacterial cell wall glycolipid and the opsonized bacteria is internalized. Within the macrophage, the bacteria replicate within the phagosome and blocks the fusion of the phagosome with lysosome by inhibiting calcium signals which blocks the recruitment and assembly of proteins that mediate the fusion. Genetic makeup of host influences the course of the disease. Helper cell response is mounted that activates the macrophages to become microbicidal. The T lymphocytes are stimulated by the mycobacterial antigens. The activated T cells secrete Interferon-gamma, which makes the macrophages competent. IFN-γ stimulates phagolysosome fusion and exposes the bacteria to hostile acid pH and stimulates release of nitric oxide which leads to oxidative destruction of mycobacteria. Due to action of the T lymphocytes the activated macrophages secrete TNF which differentiates to epithelioid cells and forms granulomas. TH1 response critical and any deficiency leads to disease progression.

Pathology: There are usually two forms of tuberculosis. They are primary and secondary tuberculosis. Lungs are involved in both forms of tuberculosis.

Primary tuberculosis: The most common sites for primary tuberculosis are the following:

- Lung with enlarged hilar lymph node (most common)—Ghon's complex.
- Intestine (ileum) with enlarged mesenteric lymph node.

- Tonsils with enlarged jugulodigastric lymph node.

In the lungs, it usually involves distal air spaces of lower part of upper lobe and upper part of lower lobe, close to pleura (subpleural) characterized by area of grayish white consolidation of size 1–1.5 cm with the involvement of regional nodes **(Figs. 7.9 and 7.10)**. About 95% of cases undergo complete healing and about 1% of the cases develop progressive fibrosis and calcification which is referred to as Ranke complex.

Secondary tuberculosis: Secondary tuberculosis can occur due to reactivation of the primary infection or occurrence of reinfection. The initial lesion is a small focus of consolidation <2 cm occurs 1–2 cm from the apical pleura. The lesion is sharply circumscribed, grayish white areas with caseation. It heals by fibrosis and calcification.

Fibrocavitory tuberculosis (Fig. 7.11): This is mostly seen in elderly and in immunocompromised individuals. It presents as an expanded apical lesion with cavitation. The wall of the cavity is irregular and shaggy. It may erode into bronchus with the erosion of bronchial vessels resulting in hemoptysis. The cavities heal with irregular fibrous scarring and collapse.

Miliary tuberculosis (Fig. 7.12): Due to the dissemination of the infection through lymphohematogenous route to form multiple tiny lesions called the **Miliary Tuberculosis**. Expand to involve large areas. The lesions resemble millet seeds and named so. The miliary tuberculosis can confine to lungs

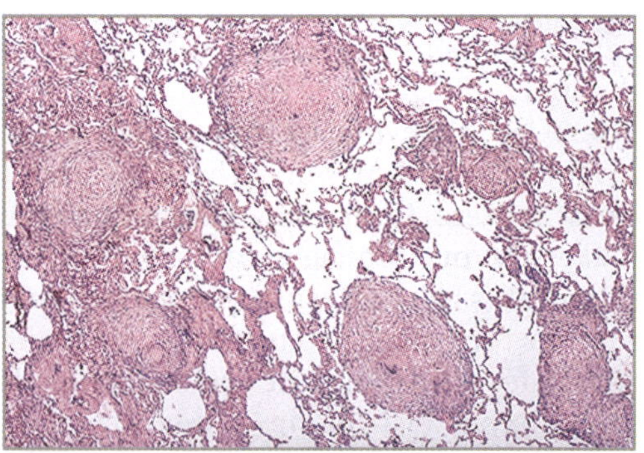

Fig. 7.9: Multiple scattered granulomas in tuberculosis of lung.

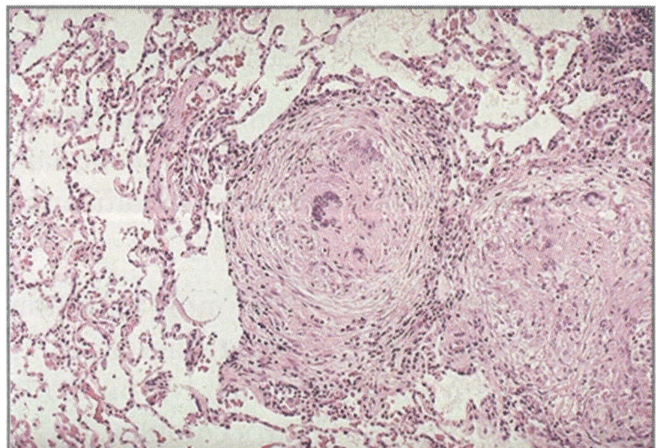

Fig. 7.10: Photomicrograph of tuberculous granuloma with prominent Langhan's type giant cells.

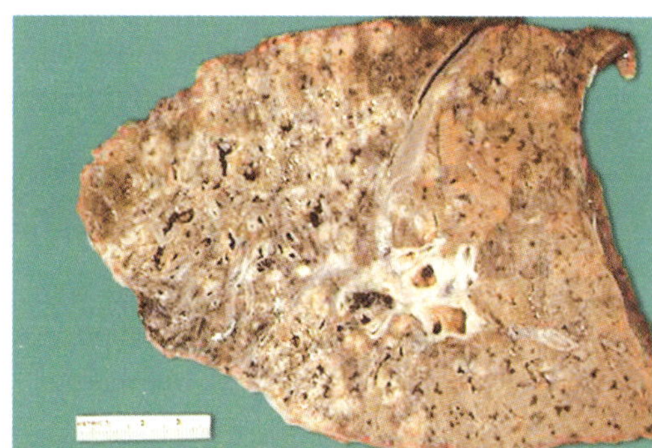

Fig. 7.11: Gross photograph of fibrocavitory tuberculosis.

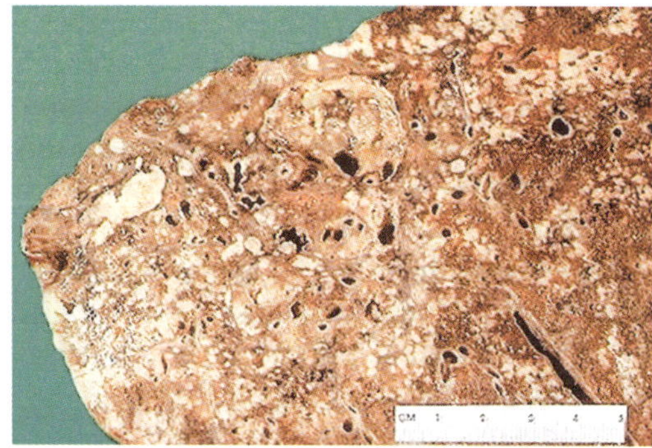

Fig. 7.12: Gross photograph of miliary tuberculosis.

or undergo extrapulmonary spread. The common organs involved are liver, bone marrow, spleen, adrenals, meninges, renal, fallopian tubes and epididymis.

Pleural involvement: Involvement of the pleura is one of the common manifestations of tuberculosis. The common pleural lesions are pleural effusion, empyema and obliterative pleural fibrosis. Other forms of pulmonary tuberculosis are endobronchial, endotracheal and laryngeal tuberculosis.

Extrapulmonary tuberculosis: Tuberculosis can involve lymph nodes (scrofula), intestine —(mostly terminal part of ileum), kidneys (renal tuberculosis), adrenals (addison's disease), bone (TB osteomyelitis), fallopian tubes (TB salpingitis), endometrium (TB endometritis) **(Fig. 7.13)**. Vertebrae (Pott's disease) and formation of cold abscess in the paraspinal region, abdomen and pelvis and meninges (TB meningitis).

Clinical features: Primary and secondary tuberculosis. The following are the common clinical symptoms associated with tuberculosis include fever—low grade—remittent, malaise, anorexia, weight loss, night sweats, productive cough, hemoptysis, pleuritic pain and extrapulmonary manifestations.

Diagnosis of tuberculosis: The diagnosis of tuberculosis is made from the following modalities of investigation. They include:

- History and physical signs
- Erythrocyte sedimentation rate
- Radiography
- Acid fast smears/culture
- Mantoux test (PPD) and ESR
- PCR amplification of *M. tuberculosis* DNA
- FNAC/tissue histopathology.

Chronic Obstructive Pulmonary Diseases (COPD)

Definition: These are group of pathological conditions of lung characterized by chronic partial or complete obstruction of airway at any level from trachea to the smallest airway resulting in functional disability. There are four important disorders categorized under this heading. They include:

1. Chronic bronchitis
2. Emphysema
3. Bronchial asthma
4. Bronchiectasis

We shall now discuss the salient features of these disorders.

Chronic bronchitis (Fig. 7.14): It is the most common form of COPD and is a common occupational respiratory disease.

Definition: Presence of persistent cough with production of sputum for a period of at least three months in two consecutive years.

Etiology: The most common etiologic agents are cigarette smoke and atmospheric pollution.

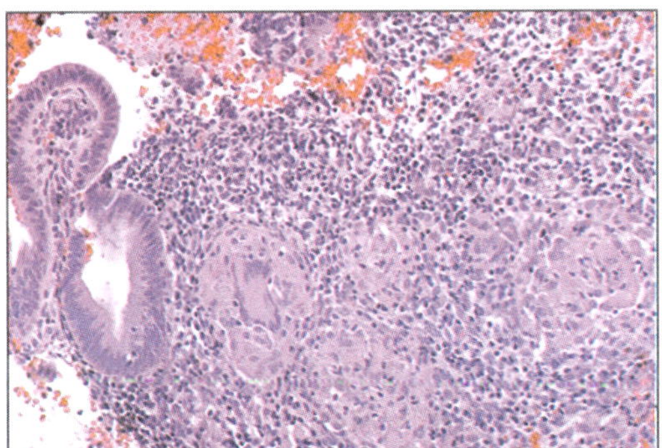

Fig. 7.13: Tuberculosis of endometrium.

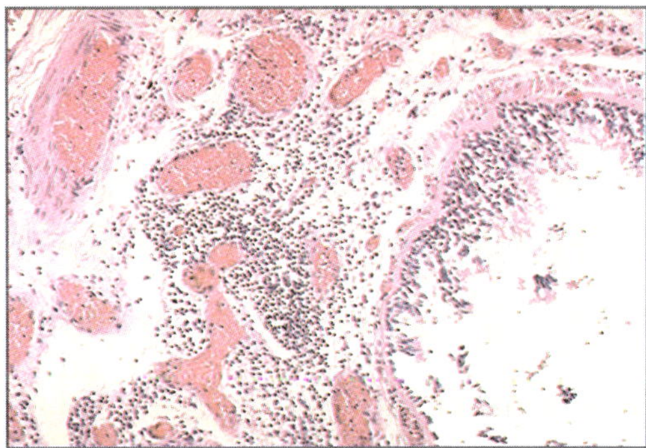

Fig. 7.14: Histomicrograph of chronic bronchitis.

This disease is more common in individuals working in cotton and plastic factories and people who are exposed to organic and inorganic dust particles.

Pathogenesis: There is marked hypertrophy and hyperplasia of the mucus secreting glands of the brochi with thickening of the bronchial wall with associated chronic inflammatory response of the bronchial wall leading to partial airway obstruction.

Pathology: On examination of the lung, the bronchial walls appear thick with the lumina showing mucus plugs. Microscopically, there is marked hypertrophy and hyperplasia of the mucus secreting glands of the bronchi with peribronchial fibrosis.

Clinical profile: This is a disease of middle-aged men characterized by persistent cough with expectoration, recurrent respiratory tract infections and difficulty in breathing. In long-standing cases, the patient may develop cyanosis and cardiac failure (cor pulmonale).

Emphysema

Definition: Abnormal permanent dilatation of the air spaces distal to the terminal bronchiole with associated destruction of the alveolar wall.

Emphysema has to be differentiated from a closely related pathology called overinflation. This is characterized by overinflated alveoli without destruction of the alveolar wall. Usually seen in senility, close to obstructive lesions, surgical complication and compensatory mechanism when a portion of lung is resected.

Etiopathogenesis: The major etiopathological factor involved in the pathogenesis of emphysema is alteration in the balance of the protease and antiprotease enzyme mechanism. The activity of the protease enzymes in naturally checked by the presence of antiprotease enzymes like the alpha-1 antitrypsin. Emphysema can occur due to increased activity of the protease enzymes or due to the deficiency of the antiprotease enzyme mechanisms.

The most common causes are smoking, air pollution and congenital deficiency of alpha-1 antitrypsin. Smoking and air pollution activates the protease enzymes mostly elastase which damages the alveolar wall. Smoking also inhibits the activity of the anti-elastase enzymes and thereby acts as a *double edged sword*.

Pathology: On gross examination, the lungs appear more voluminous with rounded edges. The air spaces appear dilated with formation of subpleural bullae. Microscopy shows dilated air spaces with destruction of the alveolar septal wall **(Fig. 7.15)**.

Classification: There are four major forms of emphysema based on the portion of the airway involved. They are:

1. *Centriacinar* **(Fig. 7.16A)**: Involves central portion of the acini of the upper lobe of lung mostly seen in smokers.
2. *Panacinar* **(Fig. 7.16B)**: Involves the entire acini and more common in the lower lobe of the lung. Seen in individuals with deficiency of alpha-1 antitrypsin.
3. *Paraseptal*: It is a localized form of emphysema involving the distal part of acini close to pleura. It is one of the most common causes for spontaneous pneumothorax.

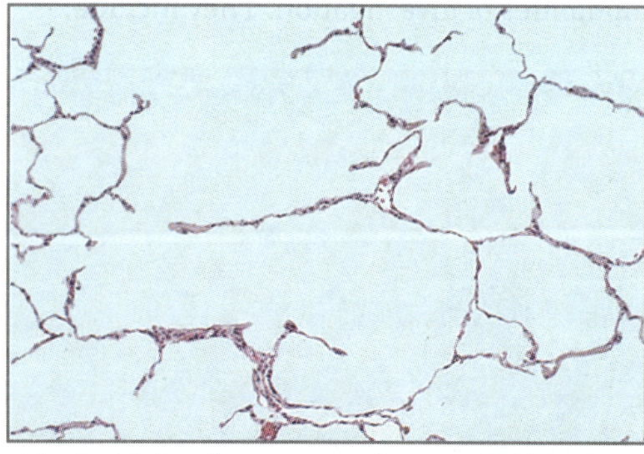

Fig. 7.15: Emphysematous lung with dilated air spaces with destruction of the alveolar wall.

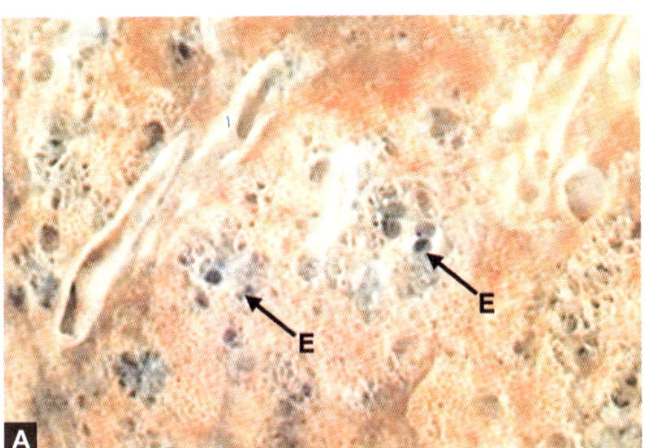

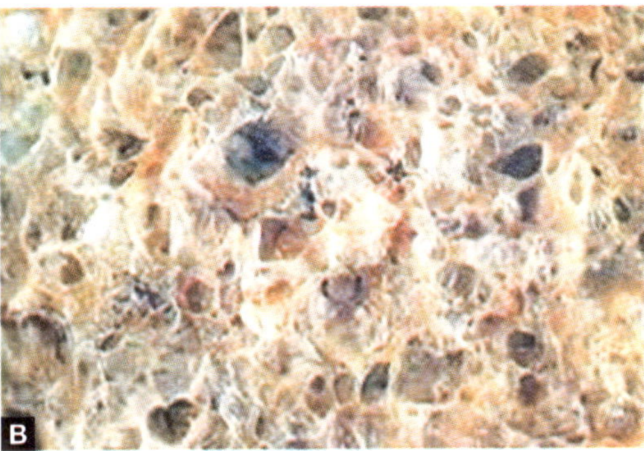

Figs. 7.16A and B: (A) Centriacinar; (B) Panacinar emphysema.

4. *Irregular and mixed pattern*: It includes more than one morphological form of emphysema and usually seen in elderly smokers.

Clinical profile: The patient usually presents with severe exertional dyspnea, tachypnea and barrel-shaped chest. Cough occurs in late stages of the disease with production of scanty mucoid sputum. Long standing case may end up with right sided cardiac failure.

Bronchiectasis (Fig. 7.17)

Definition: It is defined as an abnormal irreversible dilatation of the bronchi and bronchioles secondary to chronic necrotizing inflammatory weakening of the bronchial wall.

Etiopathogenesis: The two main etiopathogenetic factors are obstruction and infection. Obstruction may be induced by congenital defects, foreign bodies or tumors. Infection occurs secondary to obstruction.

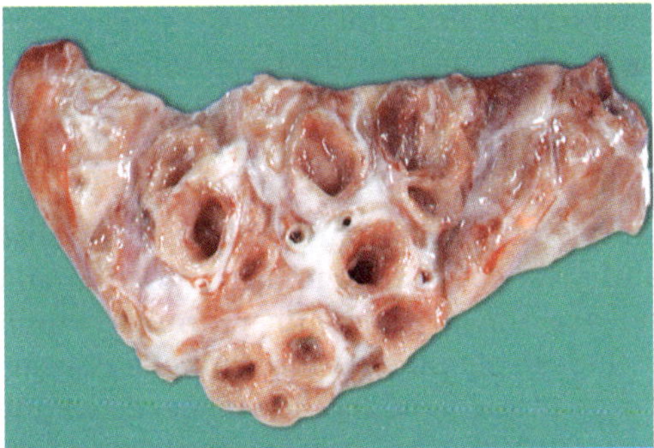

Fig. 7.17: Gross specimen of lung with bronchiectasis.

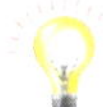

Case Scenario

A 12-year-old boy was referred to the pediatric OPD with complaints of severe cough with expectoration, fever on and off, difficulty in breathing. He had similar complaints for which he received irregular treatment. On examination, the boy was febrile, anemic, mild clubbing seen.

Question:

What is your provisional diagnosis?

Answer:

Bronchiectasis

Classification: Bronchiectasis is classified into two major types based on the etiologic agents involved and shape of the dilated airway.

Etiologic classification:

Etiologic factor	*Conditions*
Congenital	Cystic fibrosis, intralobar sequestration of lung, immotile cilia syndrome, Kartegener's syndrome
Post-obstruction	Foreign bodies, neoplasms
Post-infectious	Necrotizing pneumonia, tuberculosis, viral infections
Others	Immunodeficiency states, connective tissue disorders, graft versus host disease and others

Morphological classification

Morphological pattern	*Features*
Cylindrical	Most common form
Fusiform	Spindle-shaped dilatation
Saccular	Sac-like dilatation
Varicose	Irregular dilatation

Pathology: It involves the distal bronchi and bronchioles of the lower lobe of the lungs. It gives a honeycomb appearance to the lung with dilated airway traced up to the pleural surface. The airways are irregularly dilated with mucopurulent material within the lumina.

Microscopically, the bronchial wall is dilated with ulceration and dense peribronchial inflammatory cell infiltration with destruction of the wall **(Fig. 7.18)**. The adjacent pleura is thick and adherent.

Clinical profile: Patients usually present with irregular fever with severe cough with production of copious foul-smelling sputum or hemoptysis. The late complications include clubbing of fingers, disseminated abscess formation, amyloidosis (deposition of amyloid protein substance in the interstitium) and cardiac failure (cor pulmonale).

Bronchial asthma (Fig. 7.19)

Definition: It is defined as a hyperactive airway disease with episodic reversible bronchoconstriction, manifested as paroxysms of cough and wheezing.

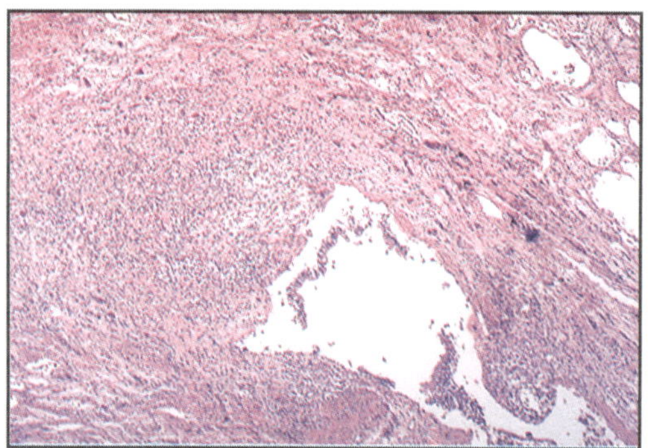

Fig. 7.18: Histomicrograph of bronchiectasis.

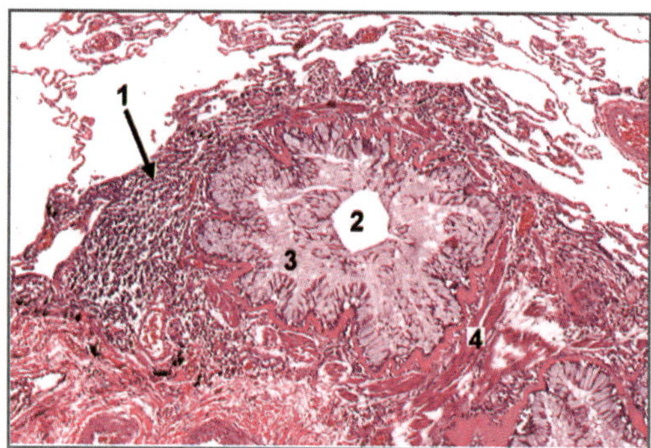

Fig. 7.19: Histomorphology of bronchial asthma: 1–inflammation, 2–lumen narrowing, 3–excess mucus, 4 –smooth muscle hyperplasia.

It is a very common respiratory illness and affects 4% of the total world population.

There are two main forms of bronchial asthma—extrinsic and intrinsic.

Extrinsic asthma	*Intrinsic asthma*
Most common	Less common
Starts in childhood	Late adult life
Family history present	No family history
Allergic response to dust, pollen, fumes and gases	No allergic response
Associated rhinitis, urticaria, eczema	Absent
Demonstrable hypersensitivity reaction	Hypersensitivity reaction to aspirin
Elevated IgE levels	Normal IgE level
Positive skin test for allergen	Skin testing negative

Pathogenesis: The disease starts with exposure of the individual to an allergen. The person becomes sensitized and results in the formation of IgE antibodies. These antibodies coat the mast cells. Re-exposure to a similar antigen triggers the immunological response and mast cells undergo degranulation and release the cytoplasmic granules which includes histamine, eosinophilic chemotactic factor, prostaglandins and platelet activating factor which causes bronchoconstriction. Repeated similar episodes lead to remodeling

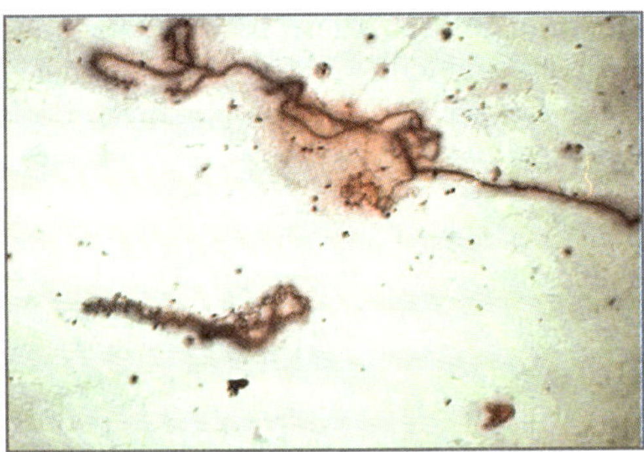

Fig. 7.20: Curschman spirals in the sputum in case of bronchial asthma.

of the bronchial wall with proliferation of the smooth muscle and fibroblasts.

Pathology: The lungs appear over distended with the bronchi showing thick viscid mucus plugs. Microscopically, the bronchial wall contains mucus plugs with degenerated respiratory epithelium called the Curschman spirals **(Fig. 7.20)**. It may also contain numerous eosinophils and diamond-shaped crystals called the Charcot-Leyden crystals **(Fig. 7.21)**. In long-standing chronic cases, the bronchial wall appears thick with thickening of the basement membrane with marked edema of the submucosal glands and infiltration by lymphocytes and plasma cells. These changes are referred to as airway remodeling.

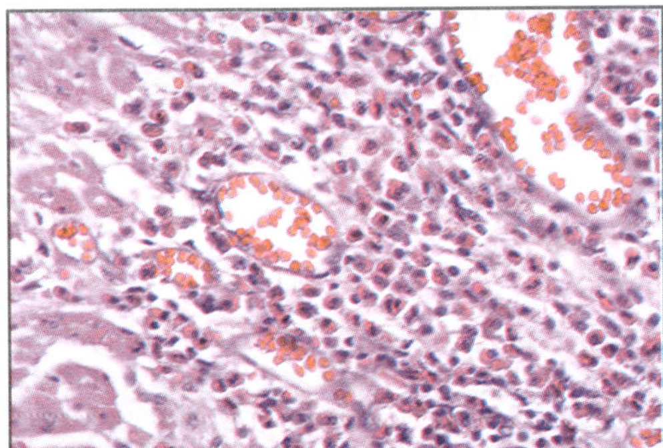

Fig. 7.21: Histomicrograph of lung in bronchial asthma, note the prominent eosinophil infiltration.

Clinical features: It is characterized by episodes to severe cough with production of thick viscid mucoid sputum and wheezing. Severe and unremitting form of asthma is called as status asthmaticus.

Case Scenario

A 35-year-old female was brought to the emergency with severe breathlessness. The bystanders gave a history of recurrent breathlessness, cough with wheeze for which the patient received treatment. On examination, patient is in shock with severe breathlessness. X-ray shows hyperinflated lung.

Question:

What is your provisional diagnosis?

Answer:

Bronchial asthma (status asthmaticus)

Lung abscess

Definition: It is defined as localized area of necrosis of lung tissue with suppurative degeneration.

Etiological agents:

- *Aspiration of foreign body:* Most common causes are aspiration of foreign bodies, food particles, decaying tooth, gastric contents, etc. This is seen in children during play, patients under general anesthesia, coma and alcoholism.
- *Spread of infection:* Patients with severe bronchopneumonia, bronchiectasis, pulmonary tuberculosis, may develop of lung abscess **(Fig. 7.22)**. It can also occur to spread of infection from empyema, suppurative pericarditis.
- Secondary to obstruction with tumors and foreign body.
- *Septic embolization:* Due to lodging of the septic emboli from cases of infective endocarditis and other causes.

Pathology: Lung abscess secondary to aspiration of foreign body is more common in the right lobe of lung because the right bronchi are in direct continuation of trachea and they

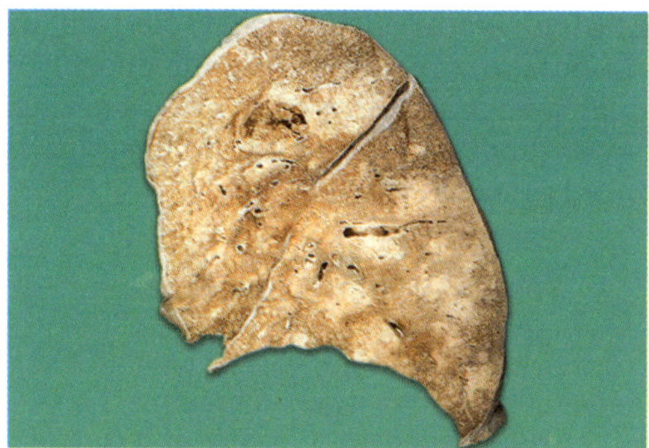

Fig. 7.22: Gross photomicrograph of abscess lung.

are often solitary whereas the abscess from other causes are usually multiple and scattered through the lung. Grossly, the abscess measures from few millimeters to 5–6 cm. The wall is usually shaggy with ragged margins. Microscopically, it shows areas of suppurative necrosis with surrounding acute and chronic inflammatory reaction.

Clinical features: The clinical manifestations include high fever with chills, malaise, cough with purulent sputum and hemoptysis. Clubbing of fingers and amyloidosis occurs in long standing cases.

Interstitial lung diseases

These are group of pathological conditions involving the delicate interstitial tissue of the lungs. They generally produce restrictive symptoms, such as tachypnea, dyspnea without any significant airway obstruction and chest radiograph shows diffuse infiltration producing a ground glass appearance.

Causes:

- *Occupational/environmental causes:* Exposure to organic and inorganic dust particles, gases and toxic fumes
- *Drugs:* Drugs, such as busulfan, bleomycin, gold, penicillamine and toxins like paraquat.
- *Other causes:* Connective tissue disorders, sarcoidosis and others.

Pneumoconiosis: These are interstitial lung disorders due to inhalation of dust particles. There are various forms of pneumoconiosis which are given below:

Disorder	*Nature of the dust particle*
Anthracosis	Carbon dust
Coal workers pneumoconiosis	Coal dust
Silicosis	Silica dust
Asbestosis	Asbestos fibers
Berylliosis	Beryllium
Siderosis	Iron dust
Stenosis	Tin dust
Baritosis	Barium dust
Bagassosis	Sugar cane dust
Byssinosis	Cotton dust

The development of the disorders depends on the amount of the dust retained in the lung, size, shaped and physiochemical property of the dust particle, concentration of the dust in the atmosphere, duration of exposure and the effectiveness of the pulmonary defense mechanisms. Normally, dust particles of size 1–5 microns induce these disorders.

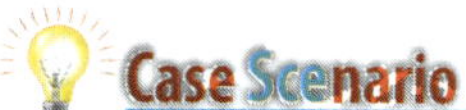

A 40-year-old chronic smoker, sand blaster by occupation died of road accident.

At autopsy gross examination of the lungs, shows discrete hard coalescent nodules and with foci of cavitation. Hilar nodes are calcified.

Question:

What is your provisional diagnosis?

Answer:

Silicosis

Spectrum of lesions: The salient pathological features induced by the common forms of pneumoconiosis are summarized below:

Type of disorder	*Pathological lesions*
Coal workers pneumoconiosis (CWP)	♦ Simple CWP ♦ Progressive Massive Fibrosis
Silicosis	♦ Fibrotic lung lesions ♦ Coexistent tuberculosis
Asbestosis	♦ Interstitial fibrosis ♦ Pleural plaque ♦ Pleural fibrosis ♦ Bronchogenic carcinoma ♦ Mesothelioma ♦ Laryngeal/colonic cancers
Berylliosis	♦ Acute pneumonitis ♦ Hilar adenopathy

Tumors of lung—bronchogenic carcinoma: It is one of the most common visceral malignancies. The incidence of tumors of lung are on a rise due to cigarette smoking and exposure to environmental pollutants. They are more common in the 5–6 decade of life and the incidence is more in men.

Etiological factors:

- *Smoking:* There is a positive relationship between smoking and occurrence of bronchogenic cancers. The risk of lung cancer is 10 times more in smokers than in non-smokers. The risk is dependent on various factors, such as amount of smoking, pattern of inhalation and duration of smoking. The cigarette smoke contains around 1200 carcinogens of which the important ones are polycyclic aromatic hydrocarbons, benzopyrene, nicotine, polonium and others. Cigarette smoking also induces cancer of other organs, such as mouth, tongue, pharynx, larynx, esophagus, pancreas, kidney and urinary bladder.
- *Industrial hazards:* Exposure to radiation, asbestos fibers, uranium, nickel, chromium, arsenic, beryllium and mustard gas also induces lung cancers.
- *Air pollution:* Exposure to radon gas has a higher risk.
- Genetic causes

Classification: The World Health Organization has classified the tumors of the lung into the following broad categories. They are:

1. Squamous cell carcinoma
2. Adenocarcinoma
3. Bronchioloalveolar carcinoma
4. Small cell carcinoma
5. Large cell carcinoma
6. *Other tumors:* Metastatic tumors, bronchial carcinoid, mesenchymal tumors
7. *Pleural tumors:* Mesothelioma-benign and malignant.

Pathological changes: Most of the tumors occur in the hilar region of lung. It appears as a localized thickening of the bronchi with piling up of the area to produce a grayish white mass lesion. The lesion usually fungates and erodes the lumina of the bronchi. There may be areas of necrosis and cavitation mostly in squamous cell carcinoma. Few of the tumors, namely adenocarcinoma present as a nodular mass in the peripheral region. The metastatic tumors are usually multiple and scattered through the lung parenchyma.

Squamous cell carcinoma—lung (Figs. 7.24 and 7.25): Most common tumor in men. Present as central hilar mass. Cavitation and necrosis are more common. Has a slow growth rate.

Adenocarcinoma: More common tumor in women and non-smokers. Present as a peripheral nodule with slow growth rate. May also be associated with old fibrous scars of lung **(Figs. 7.23 and 7.26)**.

Small cell carcinoma: Highly malignant tumor of lung, presenting as a hilar mass. Composed of small cells with scant rim of cytoplasm and round nuclei with finely granular chromatin **(Fig. 7.27)**. These tumor cells secrete various hormones and so the

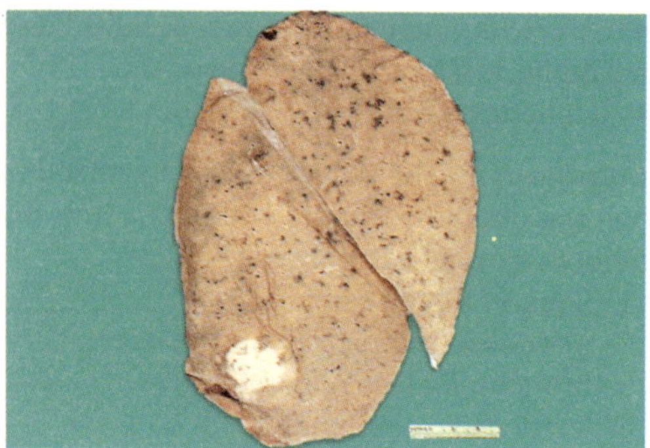

Fig. 7.23: Gross photomicrograph of adenocarcinoma lung.

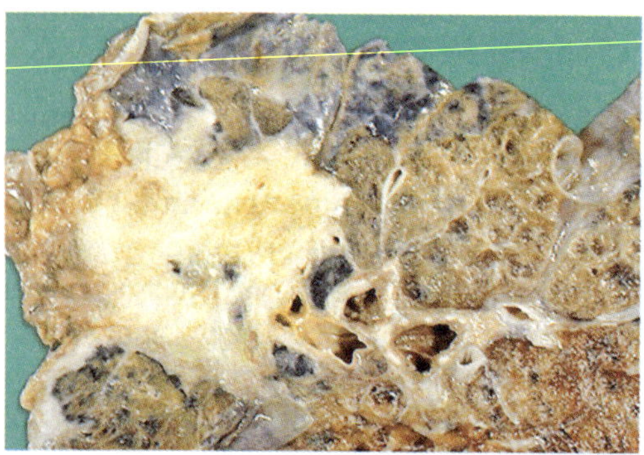

Fig. 7.24: Gross photomicrograph of squamous cell carcinoma lung.

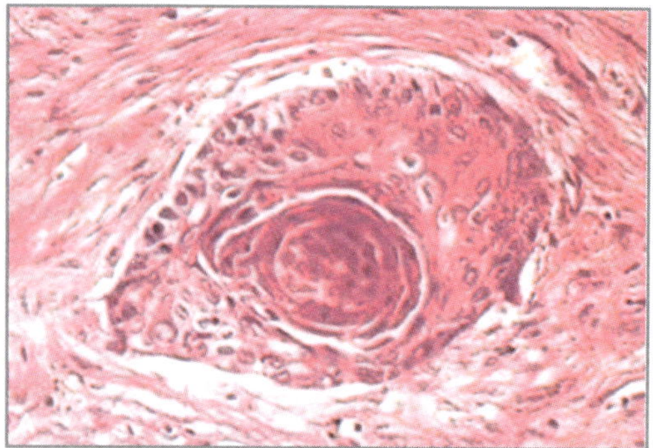

Fig. 7.25: Histomicrograph of squamous cell carcinoma of lung.

patients with this tumor present with various types of paraneoplastic syndromes.

Spread of tumors: The bronchogenic tumors can invade the adjacent structures, such as pleura, pericardium, mediastinum or undergo a spread through the lymphatics to the regional lymph nodes and hematogenous spread to distant organs, such as the liver, bones, adrenal, brain, opposite lung, and the kidneys.

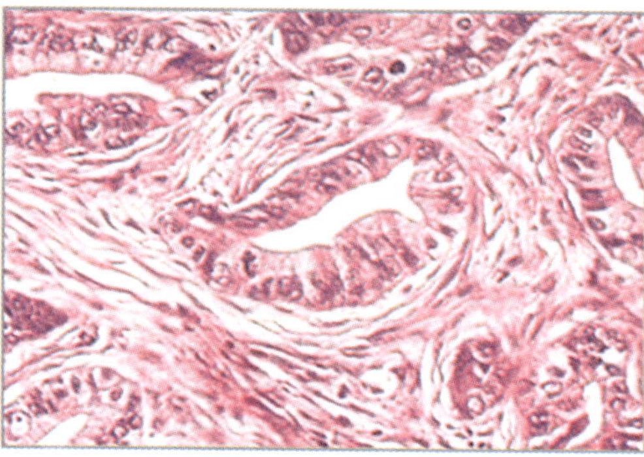

Fig. 7.26: Histomicrograph of adenocarcinoma of lung.

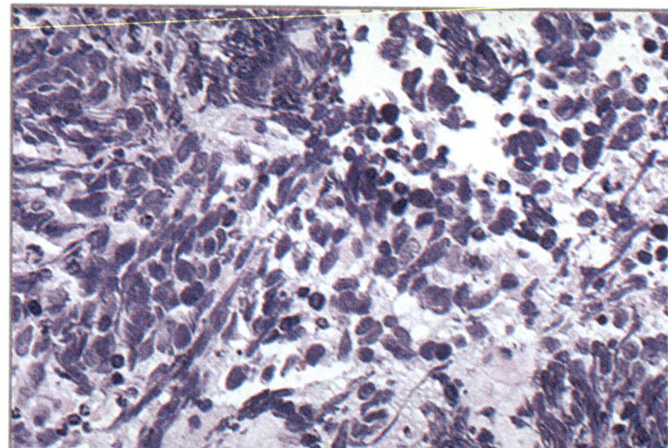

Fig. 7.27: Histomicrograph of small cell carcinoma lung.

Clinical features: The onset of the disease may be insidious or aggressive. The common clinical symptoms include cough with expectoration, hemoptysis, difficulty in breathing, chest pain, weight loss, hoarseness of voice and others.

Patient with small cell carcinoma of lung presents with a spectrum of symptoms not related to the location of the tumor due to the elaboration of hormone like substances by the tumor cells. They are called the paraneoplastic syndromes. The common features include Cushing's syndrome, hypercalcemia, carcinoid syndrome, hyponatremia, peripheral neuropathy, myasthenic syndrome, Acanthosis nigricans, leukemoid reaction and hypertrophic pulmonary osteoarthropathy (massive clubbing).

The tumors in the apical lobe of the lung (Pancoast tumor) may compress the cervical sympathetic chain of nerves which leads to Horner's syndrome characterized by enophthalmos, meiosis, ptosis and anhidrosis and erosion of the underlying rib.

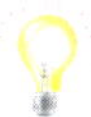

Case Scenario

A 68-year-old male patient presented with complaints of cough, weight loss, occasional hemoptysis, difficulty in breathing with chest pain.

On examination, he was thin, anemic, dyspneic, mild clubbing seen. Vitals are stable. X-ray—ill define shadow in the right upper lobe

CT scan—irregular mass lesion 3.5 × 3 cm in the right upper lobe.

Question:

What is your provisional diagnosis?

Answer:

Bronchogenic carcinoma

Diseases of pleura: The pleura is a serous membrane covering the lungs. It has two layers—the parietal and visceral pleura. The visceral pleura covers the lung and extends into the fissures of the lung. The space between the two layers contains less than 10 mL of fluid normally. Microscopically, the pleura is lined by flattened cells called the mesothelial cells.

Inflammations of pleura: The inflammatory conditions are referred to as pleuritis.

Type	*Pathological features*	*Causative factors*
Serous, serofibrinous/ fibrinous	Collection of thin serous fluid with deposition of fibrinous material	Tuberculosis, pneumonia, pulmonary infarcts, collagen diseases, rheumatic fever, uremia
Purulent	Accumulation of pus like material	Lung abscess, extension of septic abscess from nearby organs
Hemorrhagic	Accumulation of hemorrhagic fluid material	Bleeding disorders and tumors, traumatic
Hydrothorax	Accumulation of non-inflammatory watery fluid	Congestive cardiac failure, renal failure, pulmonary edema
Chylothorax	Accumulation of milky fluid	Rupture of thoracic duct, obstruction of the thoracic duct by tumors

Points to Ponder

- Pneumonia is defined as an inflammatory condition of lung caused by bacterial organisms resulting in consolidation of the lung parenchyma due to presence of an inflammatory exudate within the alveolar spaces. The two common forms are lobar pneumonia and bronchopneumonia.
- Pulmonary tuberculosis is a granulomatous inflammation caused by *mycobacterium tuberculosis*. It is very common infectious disease in developing and under developed countries.
- Chronic obstructive pulmonary diseases are group of pathological conditions of lung characterized by chronic partial or complete obstruction of airway at any level from trachea to the smallest airway resulting in functional disability. There are four important disorders categorized under this heading. They include chronic bronchitis emphysema, bronchial asthma and bronchiectasis.
- Interstitial lung diseases are group of pathological conditions involving the delicate interstitial tissue of the lungs. They generally produce restrictive symptoms, such as tachypnea, dyspnea without any significant airway obstruction and chest radiograph shows diffuse infiltration producing a ground glass appearance.
- Carcinoma of lung is one of the most common visceral malignancies The incidence of tumors of lung are on a rise due to cigarette smoking and exposure to environmental pollutants.

ASSESSMENT QUESTIONS

Essay Type Questions

1. **A 28-year-old male person came to the hospital with complaints of cough with expectoration, evening rise of temperature, difficulty in breathing, on and off chest pain. He had similar episodes before and was on irregular medications.**
   On examination, thin built, mild anemia, not jaundiced. Pulse and BP within normal limits.
   a. What is your provisional diagnosis?
   b. Substantiate your answer.
   c. Enlist the differential diagnosis in this case.
   d. Mention in brief the pathogenesis of this condition.
   e. What are the lesions you will see in the lung of this person?
   f. List the common investigations you do in this case.
   g. Enumerate the complications of this condition.
2. **A 25-year-old male already diagnosed as a case of cystic fibrosis now presents with extreme difficulty in breathing. There is progressive increase in the difficulty. He also has cough at times with no obvious sputum production.**
   a. What is your provisional diagnosis?
   b. Substantiate your answer.
   c. Enlist the differential diagnosis in this case.
   d. Mention in brief the pathogenesis of this condition.
   e. What are lesions you will see in the lung of this person?
   f. List the common investigations you do in this case.
   g. Enumerate the complication of this condition.
3. **A 25-year-old female presented to the OPD with acute difficulty in breathing. She had cough with expectoration with mucoid sputum. She had similar episodes before for which she took medical aid. She have a history of travel to her native place and visited the fields recently. There was positive family history of similar illness.**
   a. What is your provisional diagnosis?
   b. Substantiate your answer.
   c. Enlist the differential diagnosis in this case.
   d. Mention in brief the pathogenesis of this condition.
   e. What are lesions you will see in the lung of this person?
   f. List the common investigations you do in this case.
   g. Enumerate the complication of this condition.
4. **Classify tumors of lung. Enlist the common etiological factors. Describe the pathology of bronchogenic carcinoma. Add a note on the clinical features of carcinoma lung.**

Short Answer Questions

1. **Describe the composition of a pulmonary acini.**
2. **Name the common predisposing factors for bacterial pneumonia.**
3. **Define chronic obstructive pulmonary diseases (COPD).**
4. **How will you classify emphysema?**

5. Compare and contrast intrinsic and extrinsic asthma.
6. What is Caplan's syndrome?
7. What are ferruginous bodies?
8. Enumerate the common causes for atypical pneumonia.
9. Enlist the common findings in sputum in a case of bronchial asthma.
10. Classify tumors of lung.

MULTIPLE CHOICE QUESTIONS

1. Predominant lining epithelium of the respiratory tract is:
A. Squamous
B. Columnar cell
C. Pseudostratified ciliated columnar
D. Transitional

2. The most common cause for pulmonary edema is:
A. Increased hydrostatic pressure
B. Decrease in colloid oncotic pressure
C. High altitude
D. Lymphatic obstruction

3. The most common histological type of emphysema is:
A. Centriacinar
B. Panacinar
C. Paraseptal
D. Mixed

4. The earliest feature of chronic bronchitis is:
A. Dilated airways
B. Mucus hypersecretion
C. Inflammation of the bronchial wall
D. Fibrosis of the bronchial wall

5. Airway remodeling is often implicated in the pathology of:
A. Bronchial asthma
B. Emphysema
C. Chronic bronchitis
D. Bronchiectasis

6. Presence of Curschmann spirals in sputum is pathognomonic of:
A. Bronchial asthma
B. Emphysema
C. Chronic bronchitis
D. Bronchiectasis

7. Stannosis occurs due to occupational exposure to:
A. Tin
B. Coal
C. Beryllium
D. Silica

8. Presence of ferruginous bodies is pathognomonic of:
A. Anthracosis
B. Silicosis
C. Asbestosis
D. Byssinosis

9. The most common histological type of lung carcinoma is:
A. Adenocarcinoma
B. Small cell carcinoma
C. Squamous cell carcinoma
D. Large cell carcinoma

10. Egg shell calcification in chest radiograph is typical of:
A. Anthracosis
B. Silicosis
C. Asbestosis
D. Byssinosis

11. What is the purpose of the Bacillus Calmette-Guérin (BCG) vaccine in relation to tuberculosis?
A. Treatment of active tuberculosis
B. Prevention of drug-resistant tuberculosis
C. Prevention of severe lung infections
D. Prevention of disseminated tuberculosis in children

12. Which part of the respiratory system is commonly affected by pulmonary tuberculosis?
A. Upper respiratory tract
B. Trachea
C. Bronchi
D. Lungs

13. In the context of tuberculosis, what does the term "latent TB infection" refer to?
A. Active tuberculosis with severe symptoms
B. Asymptomatic infection with *Mycobacterium tuberculosis*
C. Drug-resistant tuberculosis
D. Tuberculosis affecting multiple organs

14. What is the recommended infection control measure for healthcare workers in contact with patients with pulmonary tuberculosis?
A. Wearing gloves only
B. Wearing a surgical mask
C. Wearing an N95 respirator
D. No specific precautions needed

15. Which classification system is commonly used to categorize the severity of asthma based on symptoms and lung function?
A. Mild, moderate, severe
B. Stage 1, stage 2, stage 3
C. Grade A, grade B, grade C
D. Acute, subacute, chronic

Answer Key for MCQs

1	2	3	4	5	6	7	8	9	10
C	A	A	B	A	A	A	C	C	B
11	12	13	14	15					
D	D	B	C	A					

8 CHAPTER Gastrointestinal System

Learning Objectives

At the end of reading this chapter, the student shall be able to:
- Describe the etiology, pathogenesis and pathology of common lesions of esophagus.
- Describe the etiology, pathogenesis, pathology and clinical features of peptic ulcer disease.
- Describe the etiology, pathogenesis, pathology and clinical features of gastric carcinoma.
- Describe the etiology, pathogenesis, pathology and clinical features of enteric fever, diarrhea and dysentery.
- Describe the etiology, pathogenesis, pathology and clinical features of polyps of colon, colorectal carcinoma and rare tumors like carcinoid and lymphoma.

INTRODUCTION

Gastrointestinal tract involves organs from the oral cavity and extends up to the anus. The major organs are esophagus, stomach, small intestine, large intestine and anus. This also involves other associated organs like salivary gland.

ESOPHAGUS

It is a hollow distensible muscular tube that extends from the pharynx to the gastroesophageal junction. It measures 23–25 cm. Normally, there are three physiological narrowing at the level of cricoid cartilage, left main bronchus and diaphragm. Two sphincters are present in the esophagus, upper esophageal sphincter at the level of cricopharynx and lower esophageal sphincter.

Histologically, the mucosa is lined by non-keratinizing stratified squamous epithelium with the submucosa showing blood capillaries, nerve fibers and lymphatics. The muscular layer is composed of inner circular fibers and outer longitudinal fibers. The serosa is absent.

The disorders of esophagus can be grouped into the following headings:
- *Congenital anomalies*: Atresia, tracheo-esophageal fistula
- *Motor disorders*: Achalasia cardia
- *Inflammatory*: Reflux acute esophagitis **(Fig. 8.1)**, Barrett's esophagus **(Fig. 8.2)**
- *Stenotic lesions*: Radiation, caustic injury
- Neoplasms of esophagus.

Esophagitis

This is the most common pathological condition seen in esophagus. The common causes for esophagitis are the following:

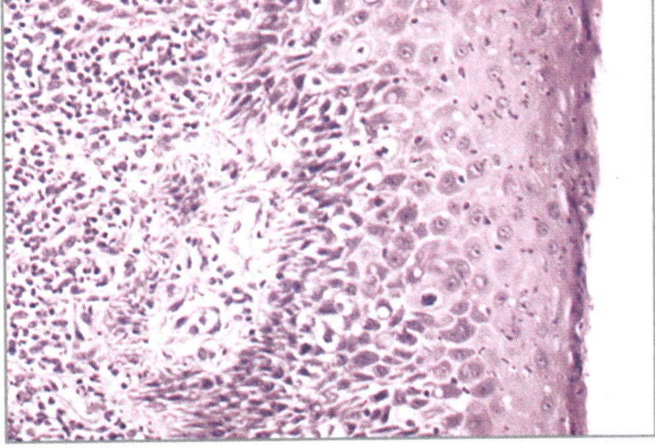

Fig. 8.1: Histomicrograph of acute esophagitis.

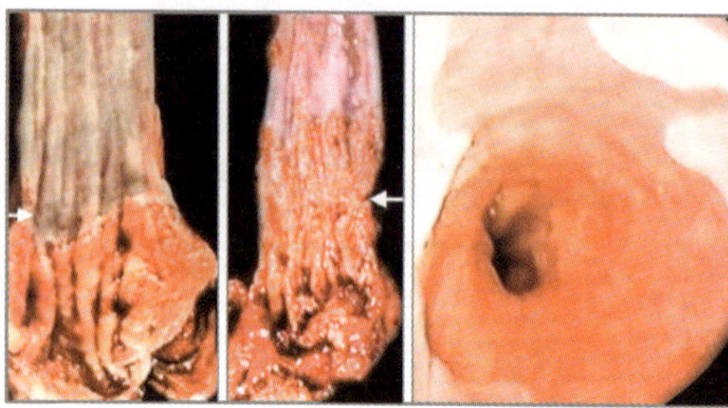

Fig. 8.2: Barrett's esophagus.

- Reflux of gastric contents (reflux esophagitis)—most common.
- Hiatal hernia
- Ingestion of corrosive acids and alkali
- Viral infections with herpes and cytomegalovirus
- Anticancer therapy
- Post-radiation
- Chronic renal disease
- Opportunistic fungal infections
- Systemic sclerosis
- Connective tissue disorders

Clinically, it presents with heartburn, regurgitation and dysphagia.

One of the common complications of long-standing reflux esophagitis is occurrence of Barrett's esophagus (**Fig. 8.3**).

In this condition, the lining squamous epithelium of the lower end of esophagus is replaced by the columnar epithelium of the stomach (metaplasia). It is a precursor for adenocarcinoma of esophagus.

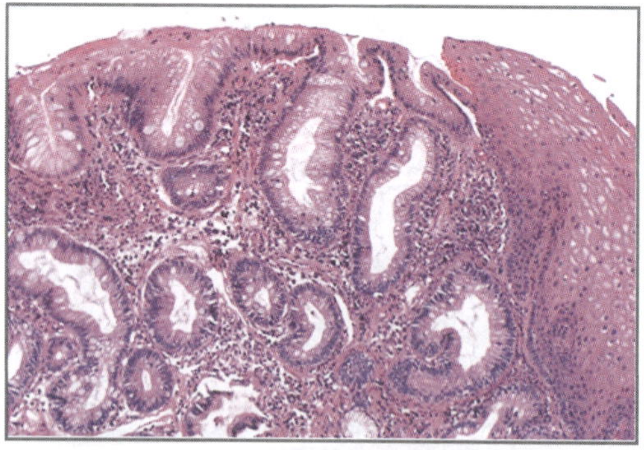

Fig. 8.3: Histomicrograph of Barrett's esophagus.

Tumors of Esophagus

It constitutes 6% of the total cancers of the gastrointestinal tract (GIT).

Etiological Factors

The common etiological factors associated with cancer of esophagus are:

- Long-standing reflux esophagitis
- Alcoholism
- Smoking
- Dietary and environmental factors
- Achalasia cardia
- Plummer-Vinson syndrome.

Site of Tumors

The tumors are more common in the middle third of esophagus followed by lower third and upper third.

Type of Tumors

The most common type of cancer is squamous cell carcinoma (**Figs. 8.4 and 8.5**) followed by adenocarcinoma (which is seen in persons with Barrett's esophagus). The tumor can occur as a polypoidal mass with obstruction of the lumen, excavated ulcerated form or a diffuse infiltrative lesion. The tumor more commonly spreads to the mediastinum and regional lymph nodes.

Clinical Profile

This is more common in men above the age of 50 years and the common clinical symptoms

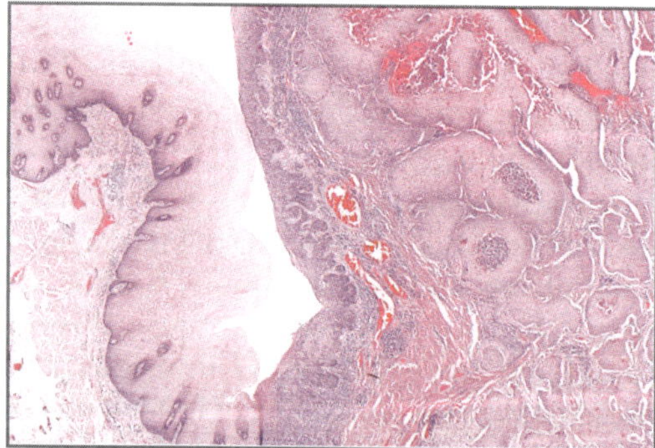

Fig. 8.4: Photomicrograph of squamous cell carcinoma of esophagus.

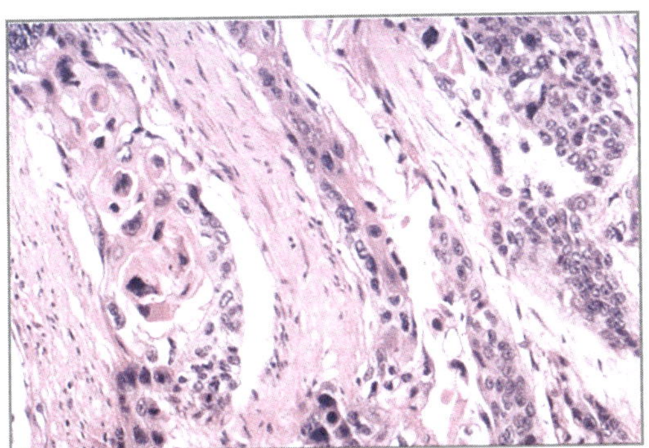

Fig. 8.5: Histomicrograph of squamous cell carcinoma of esophagus.

include progressive dysphagia. The dysphagia is initially for solid food material and gradually goes on for liquid food material also. Other symptoms include anorexia, weight loss and debilitation.

Stomach

Normal Structure

It is a saccular organ with a capacity of 1200 to 1500 mL and is divided into various regions with different functions. The part of stomach close to the esophagus is called cardia. This is followed by the fundus, the body of stomach and the pyloric antrum which extends to the first part of duodenum (**Fig. 8.6**).

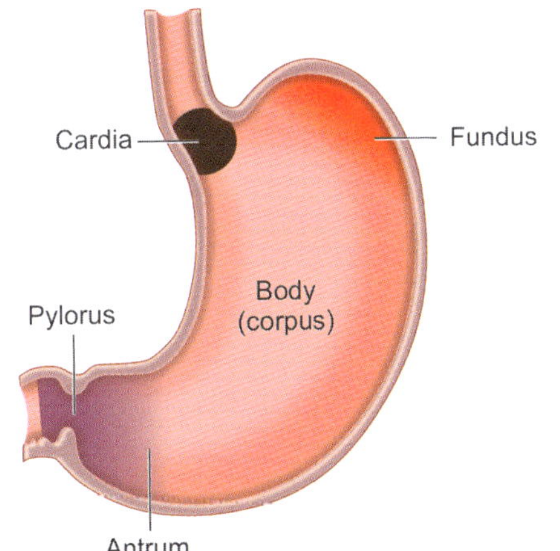

Fig. 8.6: Gross photograph of stomach, portion of esophagus is also seen.

Histology

The gastric mucosa is lined by tall columnar mucin secreting cells and is referred to as the foveolar epithelium. The fundus and the body of the stomach are rich in cells called *parietal cells,* which secrete intrinsic factor essential for the absorption of vitamin B_{12}. They also contain cells with large basophilic granules called *Chief cells* which secrete Pepsinogen. The pyloric antrum contains neuroendocrine cells called the *G cells* which secrete a hormone called gastrin.

The disorders of stomach can be grouped into the following:

- *Congenital:* Congenital pyloric stenosis
- *Inflammatory:* Acute and chronic gastritis, acid peptic disease, gastric ulcers
- *Neoplastic conditions:* Polyps and carcinoma.

Acute and Chronic Gastritis

These refer to the acute and chronic mucosal inflammatory conditions most common causes for acute gastritis include usage of drugs, such as aspirin and non-steroidal inflammatory agents, alcoholism, uremia and irradiation. Chronic gastritis is mostly due to infection with *Helicobacter pylori*. Other causes include autoimmune gastritis, pernicious anemia, biliary reflux and others.

Clinical profile: The patients usually present with epigastric pain, nausea, vomiting and rarely hematemesis.

Acid Peptic Disease (Peptic Ulcer)

Peptic ulcer is defined as a breach in the mucosa which extends through the submucosa up to the muscularis.

Most common site for peptic ulcer includes first part of duodenum (anterior wall), stomach (lesser curvature of body and pyloric antrum), ectopic gastric mucosa in Meckel's diverticulum and Barrett's esophagus.

Pathogenesis: Ulcer occurs due to imbalance between the damaging forces and gastroduodenal mucosal defense mechanisms. The most common causes include:

- Increased secretion of gastric acid (hyperacidity)
- *Helicobacter pylori* infection (**Figs. 8.7 and 8.8**)
- *Other causes*: Drugs, alcoholism, smoking, stress and psychological factors.

Morphology: The ulcers are usually solitary, circular, less than 2 cm in size, round to oval in shape. It usually appears as a punched out defect in the mucosa and the ulcer base extends lies on the muscularis.

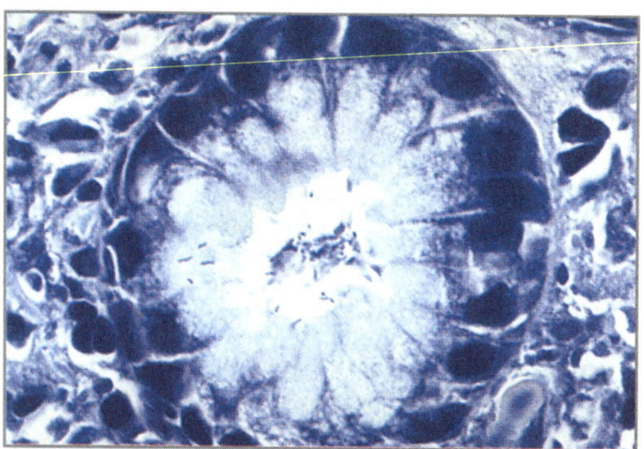

Fig. 8.7: Histomicrograph showing *Helicobacter pylori* stained with Giemsa.

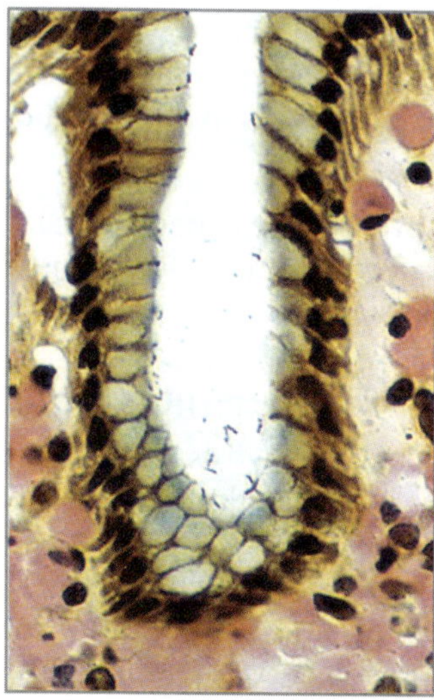

Fig. 8.8: Histomicrograph showing *Helicobacter pylori* stained with Warthin-Starry silver stain.

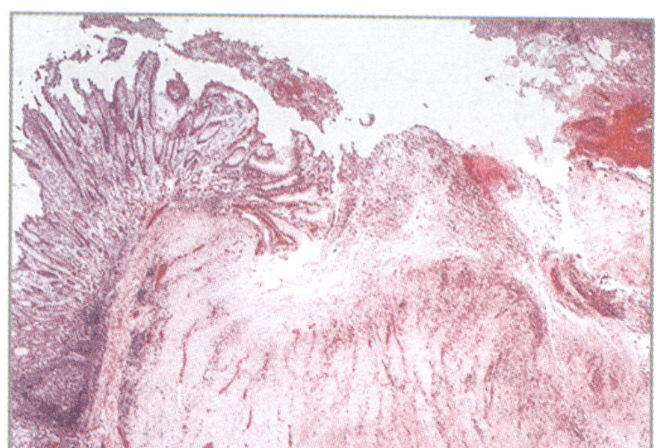

Fig. 8.9: Histomicrograph of peptic ulcer.

Microscopically, the ulcer has four layers, the superficial layer is made up of necrotic debri followed by non-specific inflammatory infiltrate, active granulation tissue and fibrous scarring in the base (**Fig. 8.9**).

Clinical profile: The common clinical symptoms include epigastric pain, vomiting. The pain is seen 1–3 hours after food.

Complications: The most common complications include bleeding, perforation, obstruction and intractable pain.

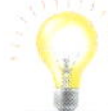

Case Scenario

A 40 year old male patient came to the OPD with complaints of epigastric pain, nausea, belching for the past one month.

The pain was very severe and knawing usually seen 1-2 hours after taking food.Worse at night few days.

Question:

What is your provisional diagnosis?

Answer:

Peptic ulcer disease

Gastric Carcinoma

General features: This is the most common form of gastrointestinal malignancies.

Etiological factors

- *Geographic factors:* It is more common in countries, such as Japan and Chile.
- *Dietary factors:* Long-term exposure to nitrites and nitrosamines, intake of salted and smoked vegetables and lack of fresh fruits and vegetables.
- *Gastric factors:* There are many predisposing factors which lead to carcinoma. They are chronic atrophic gastritis, *Helicobacter pylori* infection, intestinal metaplasia, gastric adenomatous polyps.
- *Genetic factors:* More common in persons with blood group A.
- *Location of gastric cancer:* Gastric carcinomas more common in the pyloric antrum (50–60%), cardia (25%) followed by the other portions of stomach.

Gross pathology: The gastric cancer can present as an exophytic mass protruding into the lumina, ulcerated lesion with large excavated ulcer or as a diffusely infiltrating lesion with marked thickening of the gastric wall (linitis plastica) (**Figs. 8.10 and 8.11**).

Microscopic pathology: The tumors are classified into early cancer if it is confined to the mucosa and submucosa and advanced cancer if it extends below the submucosa into the muscle wall. Most of the gastric carcinomas are adenocarcinomas (**Fig. 8.12**) made up of tumor cells arranged in glandular pattern with secretion of mucin. In few tumors, the mucin may be present within the tumor cells giving a signet ring appearance and such tumors are called as signet ring cell carcinoma (**Figs. 8.13A and B**).

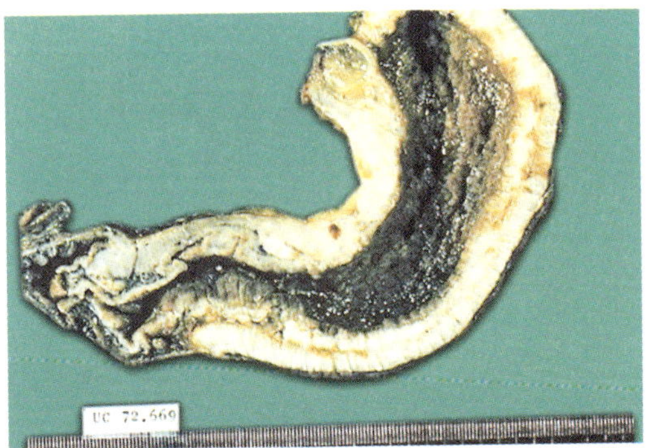

Fig. 8.10: Gross appearance of linitis plastica.

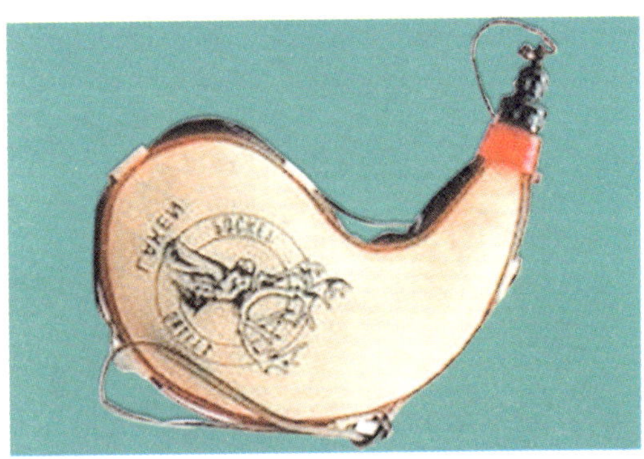

Fig. 8.11: Picture of leather bottle for comparison.

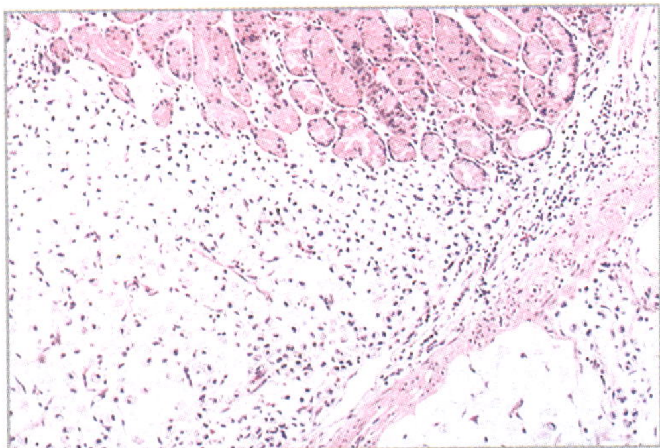

Fig. 8.12: Mucinous adenocarcinoma stomach.

Spread: The gastric carcinoma can spread to the adjacent tissue, such as duodenum and esophagus, regional lymph nodes, liver, lung, adrenals and ovary. Rarely, it can spread to the left-sided supraclavicular node (Virchow's node) (**Fig. 8.14**).

Clinical profile: The common clinical symptoms include epigastric pain, discomfort, dyspepsia, gastric outlet obstruction, anorexia, weight loss and hematemesis.

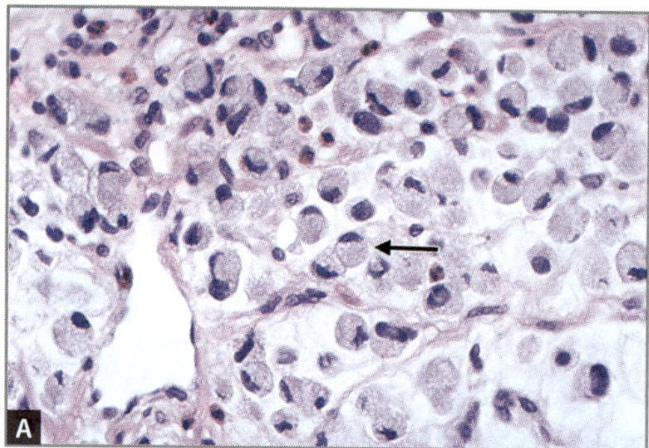

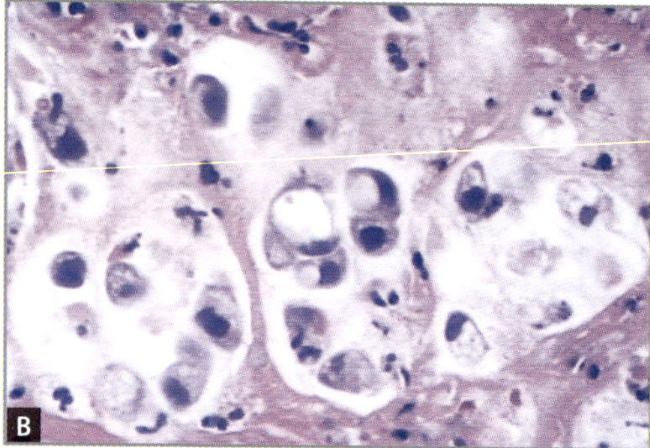

Figs. 8.13A and B: Histomicrograph showing mucin filled signet ring cell carcinoma.

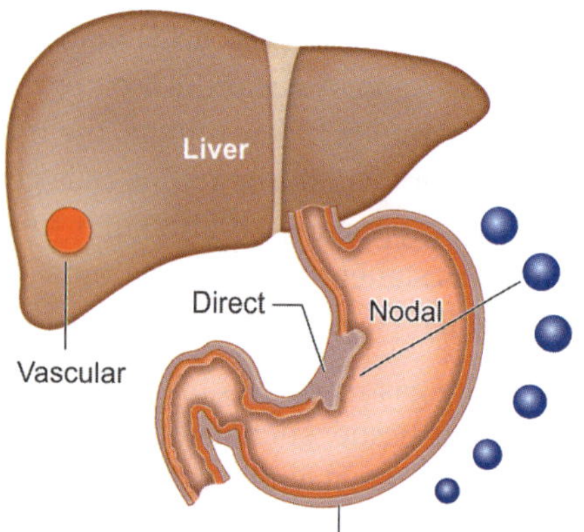

Fig. 8.14: Diaphragmatic representation of spread of gastric carcinoma.

Other rarer forms of gastric cancer include lymphoma, carcinoid tumor and gastrointestinal stromal tumors.

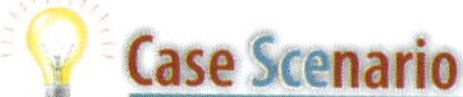

A 64 year old male patient presented to the OPD with complaints of epigastric pain , vomiting and loss of weight. He had two episodes of hematemesis last week. O/E Thin built, Anaemia present, Not jaundiced. Vitals stable. Upper GI endoscopy shows a diffuse ulceroproliferative lesion in gastric antrum with partial obstruction

Question:

What is your provisional diagnosis?

Answer:

Carcinoma stomach

Pathology of Small Intestine and Large Intestine

Normal structure: The small bowel (**Fig. 8.15**) is around 6 meters in length and divided into various portions—duodenum, jejunum and ileum. The mucosa is lined by tall columnar cells with finger-like projections called the villi. In addition to these cells, the other cells include goblet cells and neuroendocrine cells. The submucosal region is rich in lymphoid tissue mostly at the level of ileum and these lymphoid aggregates are called the Peyer's patches. The major function of small intestine is absorption of carbohydrate, fat, proteins, vitamins, minerals and electrolytes.

The large bowel (**Fig. 8.16**) is 1.5 meters in length and lined by cuboidal cells without villi. The large bowel has got various portions,

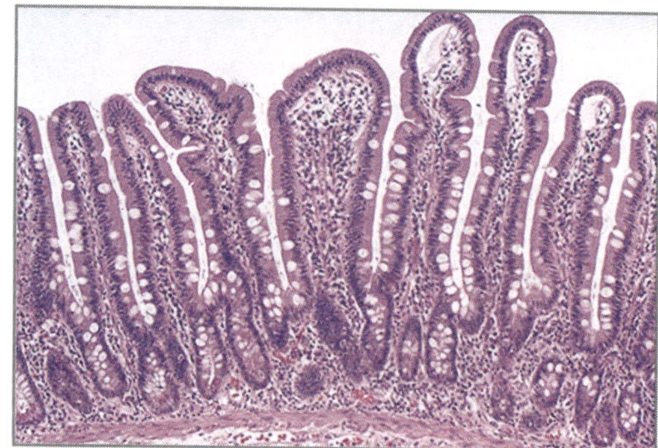

Fig. 8.15: Normal histology of small intestine.

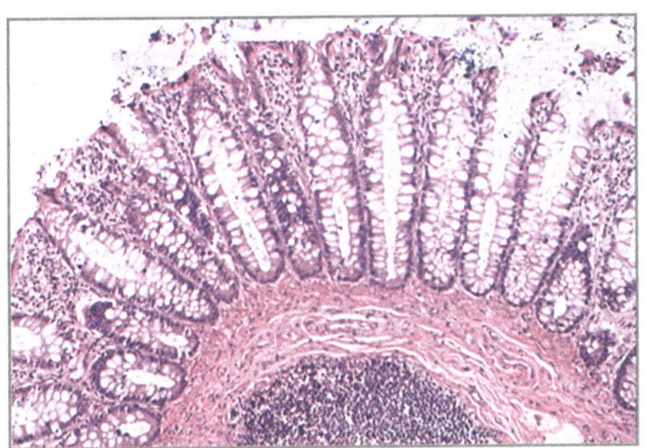

Fig. 8.16: Normal histology of large intestine.

such as the ascending colon, transverse colon, descending colon, rectum and anus.

The disorders of intestine can be grouped into the following:

- *Congenital anomalies*: Meckel's diverticulum, Hirschsprung's disease and others
- *Inflammation and infections*: Enterocolitis (diarrheal disease and dysentery)
- *Malabsorption syndrome*: Due to defective absorption
- *Immune mediated disorders*: Inflammatory bowel disease (Crohn's disease and ulcerative colitis)
- Tumors of bowel

Enteric fever

Pathogenesis: Caused by *Salmonella typhi* or paratyphi. The bacteria are ingested through contaminated water and food. The bacteria produce toxins which enters the bloodstream leading to bacteremia. The lymphoid follicles of the terminal ileum undergo enlargement which produces stretching of the overlying mucosa leading to longitudinal ulcers. These may be associated with enlargement of mesenteric nodes.

Macroscopically, the lesions are confined to the ileum. Involvement of jejunum and duodenum are rare. The ulcers are oval in shape, corresponding to the long axis of the bowel. The ulcers are usually shallow with congestion. It heals without significant fibrosis. Microscopically, the ulcer is infiltrated by phagocytic cells, lymphocytes and plasma cells. Neutrophils are significantly absent.

The main complication of typhoid ulcers are perforation of bowel wall and massive hemorrhage.

One of the major manifestations of enterocolitis is diarrhea and dysentery.

Diarrhea: It is a clinical syndrome characterized by increased frequency, fluidity and mass of the stools with sense of pain and perianal discomfort.

Dysentery: It is a clinical symptom characterized by features of diarrhea with associated pain and presence of blood and mucus in the stool.

Common causes for diarrhea and dysentery:

- *Viruses*: Vibrio cholera, rotavirus, Norwalk virus
- *Bacteria*: *E. coli*, *Clostridium*, *Salmonella*, *Shigella*
- *Others*: Use of laxatives, malabsorption syndromes, irritable bowel syndrome, inflammatory bowel diseases and others.

Tumors of intestine

The tumors of the intestine includes non-neoplastic polyps, neoplastic polyps (**Fig. 8.17**), mesenchymal lesions and lymphoid tumors.

Non-neoplastic polyps: These lesions are more common in the rectum and sigmoid colon. The polyps are grouped into the following types:

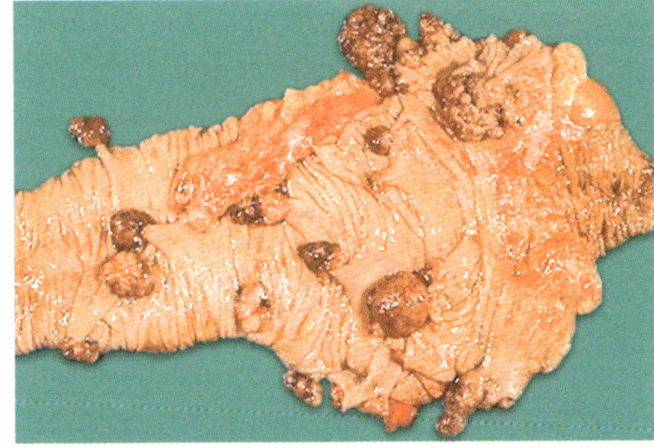

Fig. 8.17: Gross photograph of colon with multiple polyps.

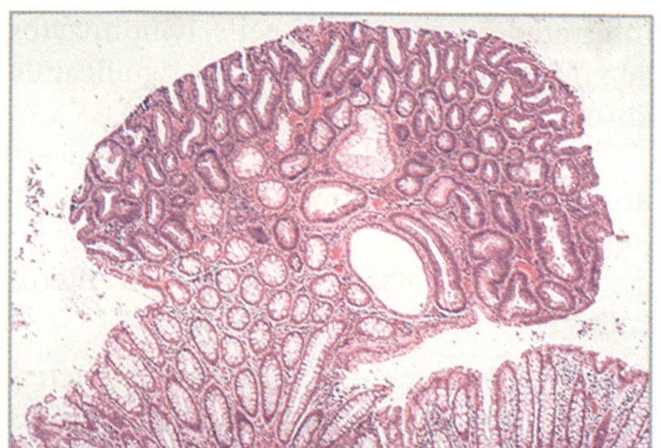

Fig. 8.18: Histomicrograph of tubular adenomatous polyp.

- *Hyperplastic polyps:* Single or multiple smaller epithelial projections composed of well-defined hyperplastic glands. They have no malignant potential.
- *Hamartomatous polyps:* These are polyps induced by deranged development. It includes:
  - Juvenile polyp: Seen in rectum in individuals < 6 years presenting as bleeding per rectum.
  - Peutz-Jeghers polyp: Characterized by multiple polyps involving stomach, colon and small bowel. Other manifestations include—pigmentation around the lips, oral cavity and face. These individuals have a risk of malignancies of pancreas, breast and lung.
- *Adenomatous polyps* (**Fig. 8.18**): These are group of benign polypoidal lesions (**Fig. 8.19**) and are classified into tubular, villous and tubulovillous adenomas based on the microscopic features.

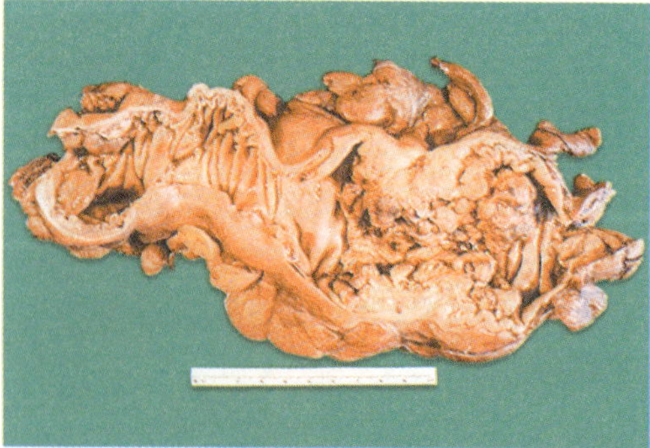

Fig. 8.19: Gross photograph of a polypoidal mass in the colon.

Tubular adenomas are usually small and pedunculated whereas the villous adenomas are large and sessile. Risk of malignant transformation is more common in villous adenoma. The most common site for these polyps is rectum and rectosigmoid.

Clinically, they present with overt rectal bleeding associated with copious secretion of mucinous material.

Familial adenomatous polyposis: This is an autosomal dominant disorder characterized by the presence of multiple tubular adenomatous polyps. The number ranging from 500 to 2000 polyps. They have a very high incidence of malignant transformation.

Colorectal Carcinoma

It is the second commonest visceral cancer after lung in men.

Etiopathogenesis:

- *Dietary factors:* Low intake of vegetable fibers, increased intake of fatty food, high intake of refined carbohydrates are some of the diet related factors.
- *Colonic factors:* Presence of familial adenomatous polyposis, villous adenomas, inflammatory bowel disease and diverticular disease.
- *Genetic factors:* Mutation of tumor suppressor gene in chromosome 5 (*APC* gene), deletion of *DCC* gene in chromosome 18 and mutation of *p53* gene.

Gross pathology: The most common site for carcinoma is rectum (60%) followed by sigmoid (25%), cecum (10%) and ascending colon (5%).The tumors of the right side of the colon often present like a cauliflower like irregular polypoidal mass projecting into the lumina whereas the tumors arising from the left side of the colon present as a diffuse infiltrative lesion which encircle the bowel wall producing obstructive manifestations.

Case Scenario

Patient X 55 years old male patient presents with complaints of persistent changes in bowel habits, including alternating constipation and diarrhea. He also reports unintentional weight loss and occasional rectal bleeding. He is having history of hypertension. During rectal examination, the nurse feels a palpable mass in the rectum. Hemoglobin level is slightly below the normal range. There is no family history of colorectal cancer in the immediate family.

Question:

Based on the presenting complaints and initial assessment, what nursing intervention should the nurse prioritize for Mr X, and why?

A. Initiate a high-fiber diet to address changes in bowel habits.
B. Schedule a colonoscopy to investigate the cause of rectal bleeding.
C. Monitor blood pressure regularly due to the history of hypertension.
D. Recommend a weight loss management program for unintentional weight loss.

Answer:

B. Schedule a colonoscopy to investigate the cause of rectal bleeding.

Microscopy: Most of the tumors are adenocarcinomas which may range from a well differentiated form to a poorly differentiated form **(Figs. 8.20 and 8.21)**.

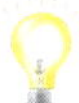

Case Scenario

A 65 year old male patient presented with complaints of altered bowel habits with pain abdomen.History of bloody diarrhoea and passing of mucus seen. He had loss of appetite and significant loss of weight. Colonoscopy shows an ulceroproliferative mass in the rectosigmoid region with partial obstruction.

Question:

What is your provisional diagnosis?

Answer:

Carcinoma colon

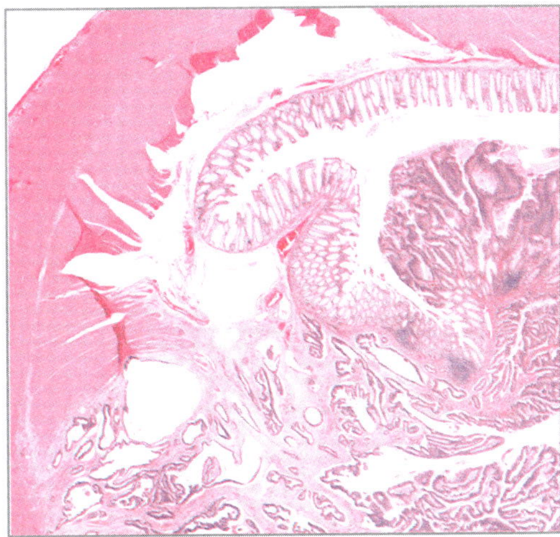

Fig. 8.20: Well differentiated adenocarcinoma with infiltration .

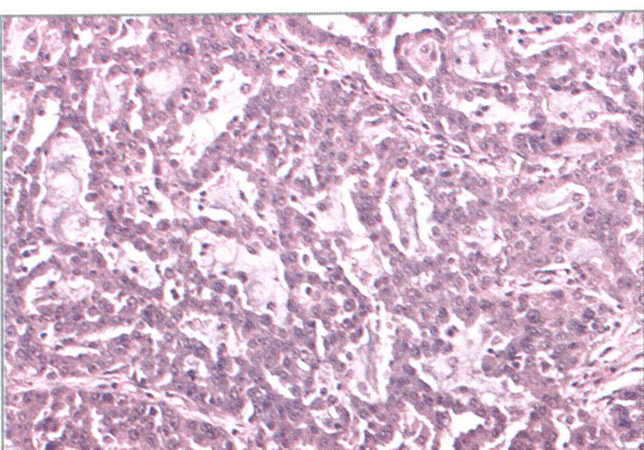

Fig. 8.21: Histomicrograph of adenocarcinoma colon.

Clinical profile: This usually occurs in men above the age of 60 years and present with fatigue, weakness, bleeding per rectum, altered bowel habits and pain abdomen. The tumor may spread locally and through the lympho-hematogenous route to liver, lung and bones.

Carcinoid Tumor (Fig. 8.22)

It is a potentially malignant neuroendocrine tumor. The common sites for the occurrence are small bowel, appendix, rectum and stomach. It presents like a submucosal nodule yellowish white in color pushing the overlying mucosa.

The tumor is made up of uniform round cells with scant pinkish granular cytoplasm

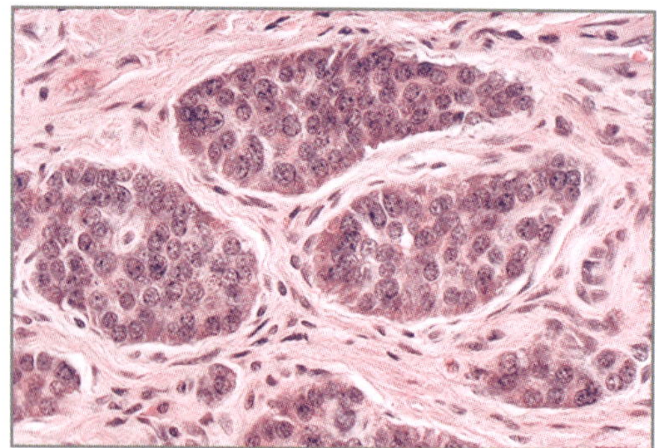

Fig. 8.22: Histomicrograph of carcinoid tumor.

and a round nuclei with stippled chromatin. These tumors may elaborate various hormonal substances which produce functional disturbances called the carcinoid syndrome. The features of this syndrome includes flushing, tachycardia, tachypnea, diarrhea, abdominal cramps, wheezing, hepatomegaly and cardiac lesions.

GIT Lymphoma (Gastrointestinal Lymphoma)

Non-Hodgkin's lymphoma (**Fig. 8.23**) is one of the tumor involving GIT. They mostly occur in stomach (60%) and small bowel (25–30%). The important predisposing factors include chronic malabsorption, immunodeficiency, HIV infection, transplantation associated and longstanding infection with *H. pylori* in stomach.

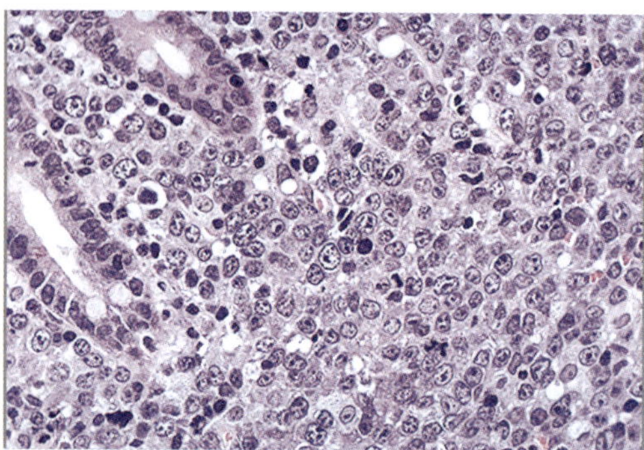

Fig. 8.23: Histomicrograph of non-Hodgkin's lymphoma of small bowel.

The lymphomas are usually of B cell origin and may be low grade or high grade. T cell lymphomas are rarer types and they occur in association with other bowel disorders. Clinically, they occur in adults and present with loss of weight, abdominal pain and other symptoms.

Points to Ponder

- Esophagitis is the most common pathological condition seen in esophagus. The common causes for esophagitis are reflux of gastric contents reflux esophagitis, hiatal hernia followed by ingestion of corrosive acids and alkali.
- The disorders of stomach can be grouped into: Congenital—congenital pyloric stenosis, inflammatory—acute and chronic gastritis, acid peptic disease, gastric ulcers and neoplastic conditions, such as polyps and carcinoma.
- Peptic ulcer is defined as a breach in the mucosa which extends through the submucosa up to the muscularis. Most common site for peptic ulcer includes first part of duodenum (anterior wall), stomach (lesser curvature of body and pyloric antrum), ectopic gastric mucosa in Meckel's diverticulum and Barrett's esophagus.
- Diarrhea is a clinical syndrome characterized by increased frequency, fluidity and mass of the stools with sense of pain and perianal discomfort.
- Dysentery is a clinical symptom characterized by features of diarrhea with associated pain and presence of blood and mucus in the stools.
- The tumors of the intestine includes non-neoplastic polyps, neoplastic polyps, mesenchymal lesions and lymphoid tumors.

ASSESSMENT QUESTIONS

Essay Type Questions

1. **Describe in detail the etiology, pathogenesis, pathology, clinical features and complications of peptic ulcer disease.**
2. **Describe the etiology, pathogenesis, pathology and clinical features of gastric carcinoma.**

Short Answer Questions

1. **Name the physiological narrowings of the esophagus.**
2. **Name the common stains used to demonstrate *Helicobacter pylori*.**
3. **Enumerate the common complications of peptic ulcers.**
4. **Define diarrhea and dysentery.**
5. **Enlist the causes for secretory diarrhea.**
6. **Enumerate the common non-neoplastic polyps of intestine.**
7. **How do you classify lymphomas of GIT?**
8. **Mention the common sites for carcinoid tumor in GIT.**
9. **What is leather bottle stomach?**
10. **Define Barrett's esophagus.**

MULTIPLE CHOICE QUESTIONS

1. **The most prevalent cause for esophagitis is:**
   A. Intake of corrosives
   B. Chronic alcoholism
   C. Gastric reflux
   D. Radiation
2. **The most common tumor that develops in a Barrett's esophagus is:**
   A. Squamous cell carcinoma
   B. Leiomyoma
   C. Adenocarcinoma
   D. Lymphoma
3. **The G cells are predominantly located in:**
   A. Cardia
   B. Body
   C. Fundus
   D. Antrum
4. **The most common malignancy of stomach is:**
   A. Carcinoid tumor
   B. MALToma
   C. Gastric adenocarcinoma
   D. Gastrointestinal stromal tumor
5. **Most common GIT site for extranodal lymphoma is:**
   A. Stomach
   B. Duodenum
   C. Ileum
   D. Rectum
6. **The most common mesenchymal tumor of stomach is:**
   A. Gastrointestinal stromal tumor
   B. Lipoma
   C. Neuroma
   D. Carcinoid tumor
7. **The hallmark of malabsorption is:**
   A. Anemia
   B. Weight loss
   C. Anorexia
   D. Steatorrhea
8. **The most common tumor of appendix is:**
   A. Adenocarcinoma
   B. Leiomyoma
   C. Neuroendocrine tumor
   D. Lymphoma

9. Most common malignancy of small intestine is:

A. Adenocarcinoma
B. Lymphoma
C. Carcinoid
D. Leiomyosarcoma

10. Which colonic polyps have the least malignant potential?

A. Turcot's syndrome
B. Gardner's syndrome
C. Juvenile polyps
D. Familial polyposis

11. What is the most common type of gastrointestinal lymphoma?

A. Hodgkin lymphoma
B. Non-Hodgkin lymphoma
C. Burkitt lymphoma
D. Mantle cell lymphoma

12. Where in the gastrointestinal tract does primary gastrointestinal lymphoma most commonly occur?

A. Stomach
B. Small intestine
C. Colon
D. Esophagus

13. Which immunoglobulin is often elevated in the serum of patients with gastrointestinal lymphoma?

A. IgA
B. IgD
C. IgE
D. IgM

14. Which of the following is a significant risk factor for the development of colorectal carcinoma?

A. Young age
B. High-fiber diet
C. Family history of colorectal cancer
D. Regular physical activity

15. What is the most common site for the development of colorectal carcinoma?

A. Ascending colon
B. Transverse colon
C. Descending colon
D. Rectum

Answer Key for MCQs

1	2	3	4	5	6	7	8	9	10
C	C	D	C	A	A	D	C	C	C
11	**12**	**13**	**14**	**15**					
B	A	C	C	A					

Chapter 9: Liver, Gallbladder and Pancreas

Learning Objectives

At the end of reading this chapter, the student shall be able to:

- Describe the steps of bilirubin metabolism. Enlist the causes for jaundice. Describe the pathology and clinical features of jaundice.
- Describe the etiology, pathogenesis, pathology and clinical features of viral hepatitis.
- Define cirrhosis. Describe the etiology, pathogenesis, pathology, clinical features and complications of cirrhosis.
- Describe the etiology, pathogenesis, pathology and clinical features of common tumors of liver.
- Describe the etiology, pathogenesis, pathology, clinical features and complications of acute and chronic pancreatitis.
- Describe the etiology, pathogenesis, pathology and clinical features of carcinoma of exocrine pancreas.

LIVER

INTRODUCTION

Normal Structure

The liver is located in the right hypochondrial region of the upper abdomen and weighs around 1400–1600 g. It is reddish-brown in color with a capsule.

Functions of Liver

The following are some of the chief functions of liver:

- Metabolism of fat, carbohydrate, proteins and vitamins
- Synthesis of serum proteins, coagulation factors and others
- Biotransformation and detoxification of drugs and chemicals
- Functions as a reticuloendothelial organ

Histology (Fig. 9.1)

The liver is made up of hexagonal units called the hepatic lobule. Each lobule has trabeculae of hepatocytes arranged around central vein with portal triad at the periphery. The hepatocytes are polygonal cells with granular cytoplasm and round nuclei. These are actively dividing cells. The space between the hepatocytes is thin-walled vascular spaces called the sinusoids lined by fenestrated endothelial cells. They also contain Kupffer cells which functions as macrophage of the liver. The space close to the sinusoid is called as space of Disse and it contains Ito cells which stores vitamin A and may transform into fibroblastic cells. The biliary canaliculi are formed at the level of the hepatocytes, they join to form interlobular and interlobar bile ducts and finally open into main bile duct.

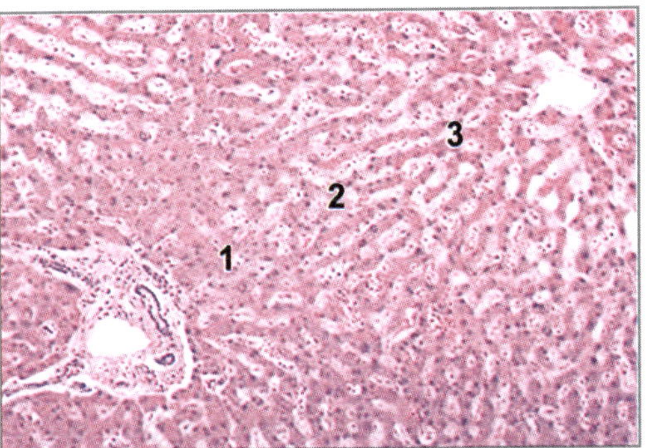

Fig. 9.1: Normal histomorphology of liver with central vein and portal triad: 1. Periportal zone, 2. Midzone, 3. Centrilobular zone.

PATHOLOGY OF LIVER

Jaundice

This is a clinical term used to denote an increase in the concentration of serum bilirubin more than 2.0 mg/dL. The normal range in less than 1 mg/dL.

Pathophysiology

Liver is the major organ involved in bilirubin metabolism. It is an end product of heme degradation.

The metabolic pathway is as follows:

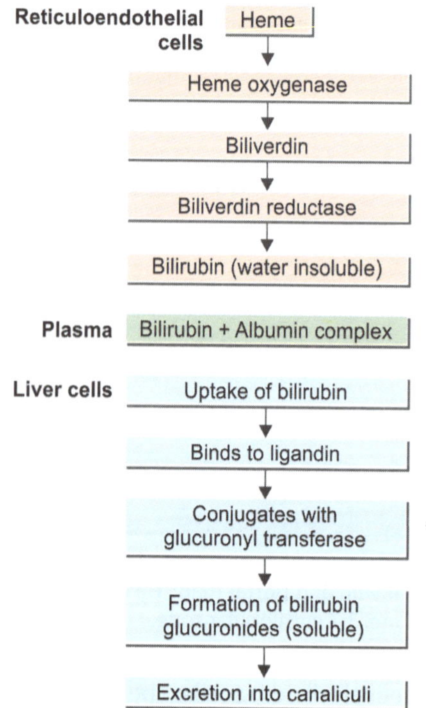

Causes for Jaundice

It can occur at any level of this pathway. The common causes include the following:

Precipitating cause	*Conditions*
Increased production	♦ Hemolytic anemia ♦ Ineffective erythropoiesis
Reduced uptake	♦ Drug induced
Impaired conjugation	♦ Physiologic—newborn ♦ Genetic defects of conjugation ♦ Diffuse hepatic disease, Hepatitis
Impaired excretion	♦ Impaired canalicular transport ♦ Drugs—oral pills ♦ Intrahepatic obstruction
Extrahepatic obstruction	♦ Gallstones ♦ Carcinoma head of pancreas ♦ Biliary strictures ♦ Fluke infestation

Contd...

Clinical Features

There is yellow coloration of the sclera **(Fig. 9.2)**, skin and other tissue. Other symptoms include fever, malaise, nausea, vomiting, loss of appetite, pruritus, abdominal pain and features of malabsorption. The histology of the liver shows marked bile stasis within the biliary canaliculi **(Fig. 9.3)**.

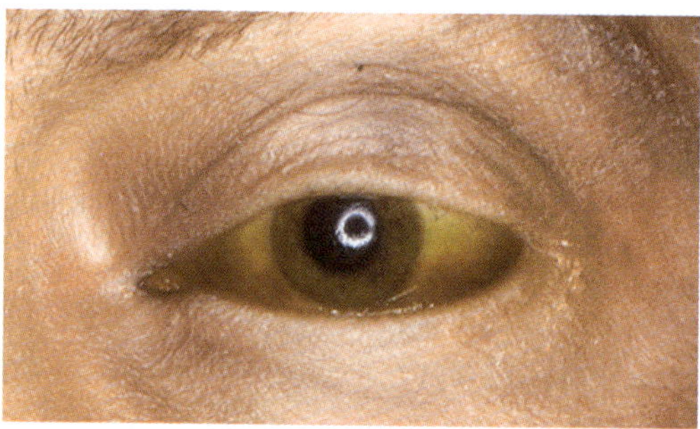

Fig. 9.2: Yellowish coloration of sclera in jaundice.

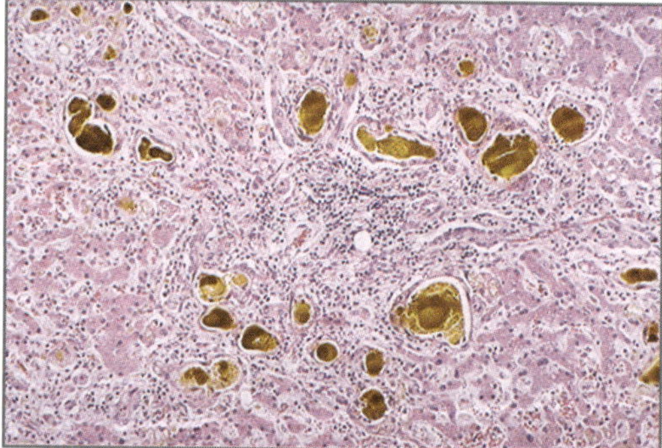

Fig. 9.3: Liver biopsy showing cholestasis in a case of jaundice.

The laboratory findings include elevated serum bilirubin, serum alkaline phosphatase, alterations in the liver function tests. Urine analysis shows presence of bile salts and bile pigments.

HEPATITIS

This term refers to the inflammatory conditions of the liver induced by various organisms and toxins. The most common cause includes viral infection and the term hepatitis is generally used to indicate viral hepatitis.

Common agents implicated in hepatitis are viruses, such as hepatitis viruses, Epstein-Barr virus, adenovirus, cytomegalovirus, yellow fever virus, rubella and enteroviruses. Many bacterial organisms like the leptospirosis, *Pseudomonas* is also associated with hepatitis. We shall now discuss the role played by the various hepatitis viruses in causing a liver injury.

Hepatitis Viruses

This is a family of viruses having a tropism for the liver. They are labeled as hepatitis A, B, C, D, E, G and other types. The **Table 9.1** summarizes the spectrum of lesions induced by these various types of viruses.

Clinicopathological Syndromes

Acute Hepatitis

It is characterized by non-specific constitutional symptoms, such as fever, malaise, loss of appetite, fatiguability, headache, myalgia followed by features of jaundice with pruritus and defects in liver function.

The liver may be enlarged and microscopy shows isolated cell necrosis with features of bile stasis and fatty change. The Kupffer cells look prominent and the portal triad is expanded with non-specific inflammatory cell infiltration.

TABLE 9.1: Spectrum of lesions induced by the various types of viruses.

Virus	*Type of virus*	*Route of spread*	*Incubation period*	*Spectrum of Lesions*
HAV	RNA	Feco-oral	2–6 weeks	♦ Acute hepatitis ♦ Fulminant hepatitis ♦ No carrier/chronic state
HBV	DNA	Blood, blood products, sexual, drug abuse, transplacental (vertical)	4–26 weeks	♦ Acute hepatitis ♦ Chronic hepatitis ♦ Carrier state ♦ Cirrhosis ♦ Hepatocellular Ca
HCV	RNA	Transfusion associated	2–26 weeks	♦ Acute hepatitis ♦ Chronic hepatitis ♦ Carrier state ♦ Cirrhosis ♦ Hepatocellular Ca
HDV	RNA—incomplete virus	Co-infection/ superinfection with HBV	2–20 weeks	♦ Acute hepatitis ♦ Chronic hepatitis ♦ Carrier state ♦ Cirrhosis ♦ Hepatocellular Ca
HEV	RNA	Waterborne	2–6 week	♦ Acute hepatitis ♦ Fulminant hepatitis ♦ No carrier/chronic state

Chronic Hepatitis

Definition: It is a term used to refer to the presence of symptomatic, biochemical or serological evidence of hepatic disease for more than 6 months after an acute hepatitis.

Causes: The common causes include the following:

- *Viral hepatitis*: Due to HBV, HCV and HDV
- Wilson's disease
- Autoimmune hepatitis
- *Drug induced*: Isoniazid, alpha-methyldopa, methotrexate
- Idiopathic

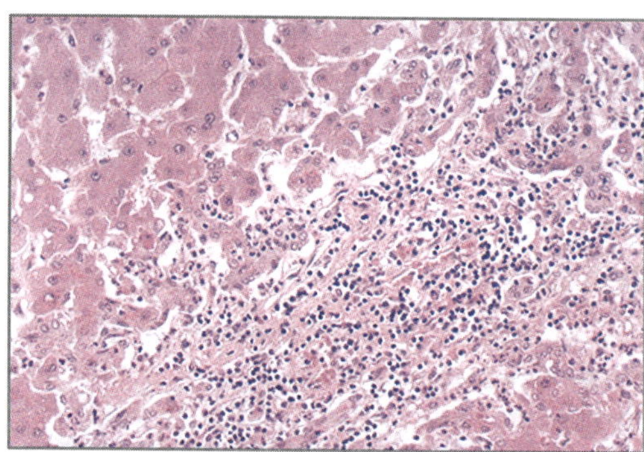

Fig. 9.4: Histomicrograph of chronic active hepatitis showing piecemeal necrosis.

Classification and types: The chronic hepatitis is classified into four main types based on the histomorphological alterations. They include:

1. Chronic persistent hepatitis
2. Chronic active hepatitis
3. Chronic lobular hepatitis
4. *Non-specific reactive hepatitis*: Do not have specific histomorphological features.

The common histological features are summarized below:

Type of chronic hepatitis	*Histological features*
Chronic persistent hepatitis	Milder form—enlarge portal tract—infiltration by chronic inflammatory mononuclear cells. No parenchymal spillover
Chronic active hepatitis	Severe form—presence of piecemeal necrosis **(Fig. 9.4)** and bridging necrosis with spill over of inflammation from the portal tract associated with variable fibrosis and bile duct lesions
Chronic lobular hepatitis	Confined to the hepatic lobule with major changes seen in the periportal area

Hepatitis—Carrier state: This refers to individuals who harbor the organisms without any overt clinical manifestation. This is more common with HBV infection. Carrier state is more commonly seen in infants who receive the infection through transplacental route and in immunocompromised individuals.

The histological findings of a carrier state include presence of ground glass hepatocytes with finely granular cytoplasm and sanded nuclei. They represent the surface antigen and core antigen of the hepatitis B virus.

Diagnosis of hepatitis: The diagnosis of hepatitis is made on the clinical grounds and detection of the various serological markers. Most common of them include the detection of HBsAg and antibodies to HBsAg. They indicate the severity of the infection.

Cirrhosis

Definition: It is defined as an end stage liver disease characterized by distorted parenchymal architecture of liver with many regenerative nodules rimmed by fibrosis along with altered vasculature. The fibrosis can extend from central vein to portal tract or central vein to other central vein and portal tract to other portal tract. The gross image of the liver in cirrhosis is shown in **Figure 9.5.** The histomicrograph of liver in cirrhosis in both higher and lower power is depicted in **Figures 9.6A and B**.

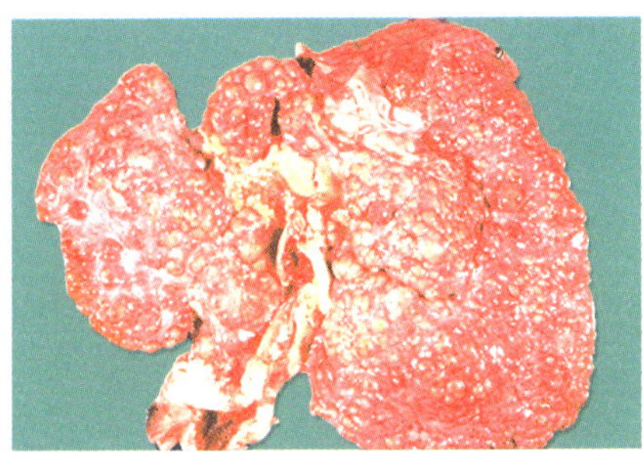

Fig. 9.5: Gross photograph of liver in cirrhosis.

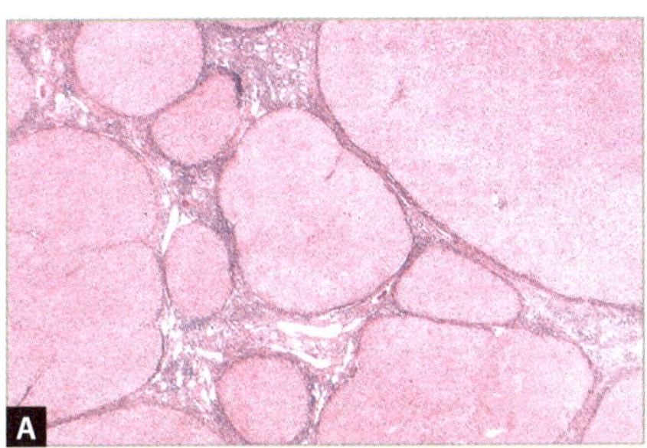

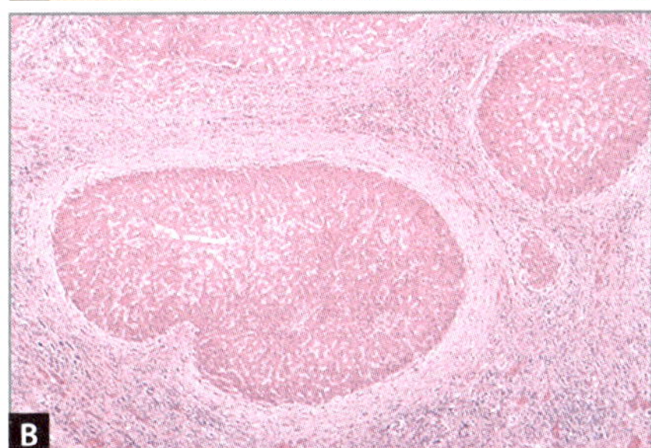

Figs. 9.6A and B: (A) Histomicrograph of liver in cirrhosis (lower power); (B) Histomicrograph of liver in cirrhosis (higher power).

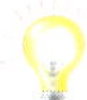

Case Scenario

A 58-year-old male patient was brought to the casualty in a state of shock. He had two bouts of massive hematemesis. He was a chronic alcoholic for the past 25 years. On examination, he was drowsy, PR 102/ mt—feeble and thready, BP 80/60 mm of Hg. His limbs were cool. There was protuberant abdomen with free fluid.
Spleen was palpable.

Question:

What is your provisional diagnosis?

Answer:

Cirrhosis liver with portal hypertension.

Classification: Cirrhosis can be classified according to the size of the nodules (morphological classification) and on the precipitating cause (etiological classification).

Morphological classification:

- *Micronodular:* Nodules less than 3 mm
- *Macronodular:* Nodules more than 3 mm
- *Mixed:* Combination of both

Etiological classification:

- Alcoholic cirrhosis
- Biliary cirrhosis
- Postnecrotic cirrhosis
- *Metabolic cirrhosis:*
  - Hemochromatosis
  - Wilson's disease
  - Alpha-1 antitrypsin deficiency
- Indian childhood cirrhosis
- Cardiac cirrhosis
- Idiopathic

Case Scenario

Mrs Nina, a 50-year-old woman, is admitted to the hospital with a diagnosis of cirrhosis of the liver. She has a history of non-alcoholic fatty liver disease (NAFLD) and recently presented with jaundice, ascites, and confusion. As the attending physician, you are responsible for her care.

Question:

Which of the following risk factors is most likely associated with Mrs Thompson's non-alcoholic fatty liver disease (NAFLD) leading to cirrhosis?

A. Chronic alcohol consumption
B. Viral hepatitis infection
C. Obesity and metabolic syndrome
D. Autoimmune liver disease

Answer:

C. Obesity and metabolic syndrome.

Pathogenesis: Progressive deposition of collagen fibrosis is the main pathological change. The major source of collagen comes from the Ito cells which transform into fibroblastic cells due to chronic liver cell injury and secrete many inflammatory cytokines which stimulate the synthesis of collagen proteins which are deposited in the liver.

We shall now discuss the salient features of some of the important forms of cirrhosis.

- *Alcoholic liver disease:* Alcohol is rapidly absorbed in the stomach and get transformed into acetaldehyde and acetate. Acetaldehyde is a hepatotoxic substance and it induces hepatocytic injury. The spectrum of lesions induced by alcohol includes alcoholic fatty liver, alcoholic hepatitis and cirrhosis.

  Alcoholic fatty liver: It is a reversible lesion characterized by the presence of fat vacuoles within the hepatocytes with minor degree of fibrosis.

  Alcoholic hepatitis: This occurs following alcoholic fatty liver and is characterized by malaise, anorexia, weight loss, jaundice and pain abdomen with tender hepatomegaly. Microscopically, it shows ballooning degeneration of the cytoplasmic body located close to the nuclei. Other features include infiltration by neutrophils and presence of perivenular fibrosis.

  Alcoholic cirrhosis: It is a micronodular form of cirrhosis. The size of the liver is reduced and it looks brownish and shrunken with visible nodules giving a hob nail appearance **(Fig. 9.7)**.

  Microscopically, it shows regenerative nodules with variable fibrosis with features of alcoholic hepatitis **(Fig. 9.8)**. The major manifestations are that of portal hypertension.

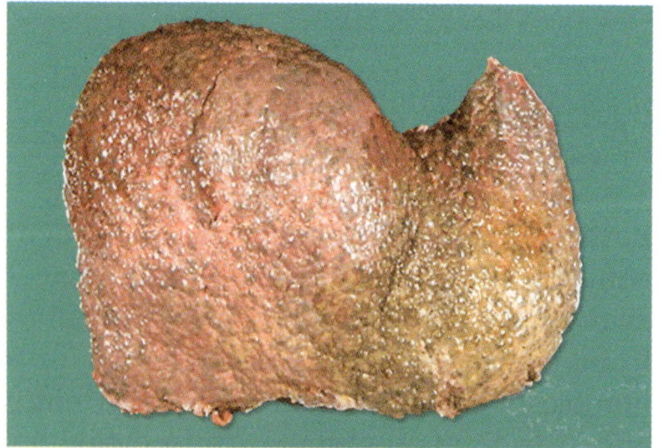

Fig. 9.7: Gross photograph of micronodular cirrhosis in alcoholism.

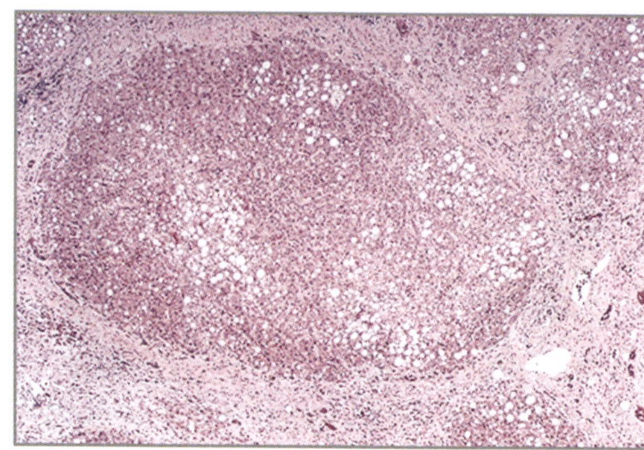

Fig. 9.8: Histomicrograph of micronodular alcoholic cirrhosis with fatty change.

- *Postnecrotic cirrhosis:* This is a form of cirrhosis that occurs following viral hepatitis, toxic liver injury due to carbon tetrachloride, acetaminophen and phosphorus. It is a macronodular form of cirrhosis with wide areas of necrosis and fibrosis.
- *Biliary cirrhosis:* This is a chronic progressive cholestatic liver disease induced by immune mediated destruction of the intrahepatic bile ducts with fibrosis. This occurs mostly in women and clinically presents with pain abdomen, jaundice and hepatomegaly. The bile ducts are damaged by the generation of the antimitochondrial antibodies. Microscopically, it is characterized by significant destruction of bile ducts with lymphoplasmacytic cells with formation of granuloma. Other features include presence of Mallory bodies and piecemeal necrosis.
- *Hemochromatosis:* This is a term used to indicate excessive deposition of iron in the reticuloendothelial cells and in the parenchyma cells. Liver is one of the major organs involved in hemochromatosis. Other organs involved are heart, exocrine pancreas, skin, joints, testis, adrenals and thyroid.

  The liver looks golden yellow in color with prominent micronodules. The iron accumulates within the Kupffer cells and

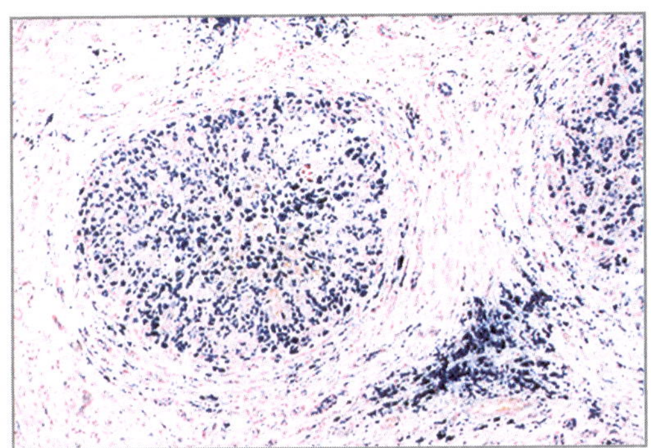

Fig. 9.9: Histomicrograph of liver in hemochromatosis stained with Perls Prussian blue.

also in the hepatic parenchyma around the portal tracts. There is gradual development of fibrosis. Perls Prussian blue stain is used to demonstrate the iron within the hepatocytes **(Fig. 9.9)**.

Clinically, it presents with hepatomegaly, abdominal pain, diabetes mellitus and skin pigmentation. The symptom complex is called Bronze diabetes (Micronodular cirrhosis + Diabetes + Skin pigmentation).

- *Wilson's disease:* This is an autosomal recessive disorder of copper metabolism with excessive accumulation of copper within the liver, brain and cornea of eye. There is progressive accumulation of copper within the hepatocytes. The spectrum of lesions includes fatty change of liver, acute hepatitis, chronic hepatitis and cirrhosis. Other manifestations include deposition of copper in the basal ganglia and in the Descemet's membrane of the cornea producing Kayser-Fleischer ring. The stains used to demonstrate copper are rhodanine and rubeanic acid.
- *Alpha-1 antitrypsin deficiency:* Deficiency produces features of neonatal hepatitis, cholestasis and cirrhosis. It is a micronodular form of cirrhosis with irregular fibrosis.

One of the most common clinical complications of cirrhosis is the development of portal hypertension. Due to cirrhosis, there is increased resistance to the blood flow within the sinusoids. The major manifestations of portal hypertension include splenomegaly, ascites and abnormal portosystemic shunts at the lower end of esophagus (esophageal varices) presenting as hematemesis, rectum (hemorrhoids), retroperitoneum and abdominal wall. It may progress to hepatic encephalopathy or hepatic coma.

Tumors of Liver

Hepatocellular carcinoma: Carcinoma of liver is one of the common visceral malignancies seen more in men with a mean age of 50 years.

Etiological factors: The following are some of the common etiological agents associated with hepatocellular carcinoma. They are:

- Hepatitis B virus infection
- End stage cirrhosis
- *Aflatoxin:* It is a toxin produced by *Aspergillus flavus*, which grows on wet cereals and pulses.
- Alcoholic liver disease
- Hemochromatosis
- Metabolic liver diseases

Macroscopically, it is characterized by the presence of irregular grayish-yellow mass with infiltrative margins and areas of hemorrhage and necrosis **(Fig. 9.10)**.

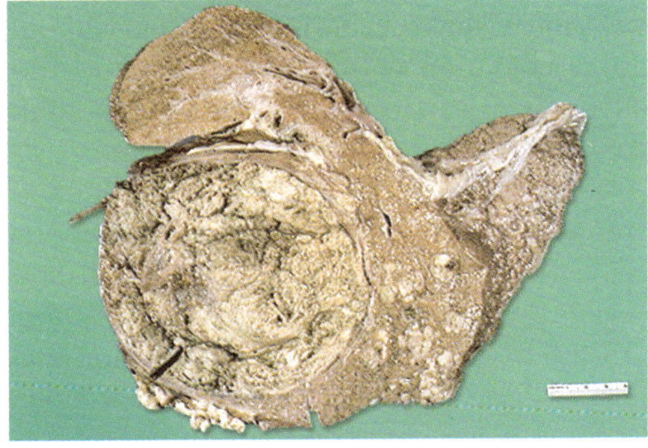

Fig. 9.10: Gross photograph of hepatocellular carcinoma.

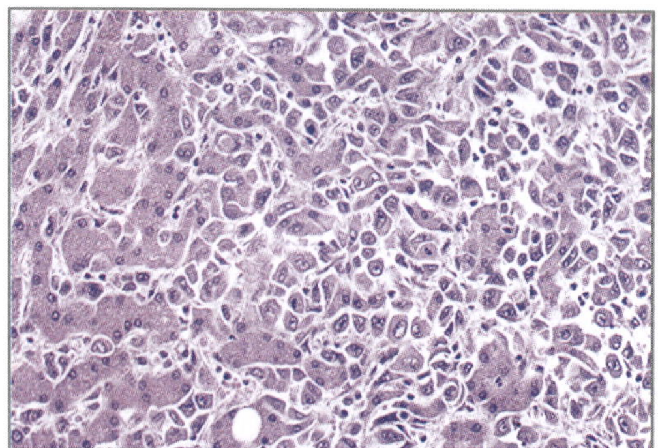

Fig. 9.11: Histomicrograph of hepatocellular carcinoma.

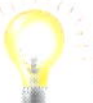

Case Scenario

A 54-year-old male patient presented to the surgical OPD with complaints of pain and swelling abdomen. Loss of appetite and weight. On examination, there was fullness in the right hypochondrium. USG reveled a huge mass in the left lobe of liver 8 x 6 cm.

Question:

What is your provisional diagnosis?

Answer:

Hepatocellular carcinoma.

Microscopically, it is composed of neoplastic hepatocytes with trabecular, acinar and glandular pattern in a richly vascular stroma **(Fig. 9.11)**. The tumor is capable of invading the blood vessels. There is a variant of hepatocellular carcinoma called fibrolamellar carcinoma which occurs in young men without any association with hepatitis B virus and cirrhosis. It carries a better prognosis than conventional hepatocellular carcinoma.

The tumor is a highly aggressive in nature and spreads through the lymphohematogenous route to the regional lymph nodes and distant organs, such as lung, brain and bones.

Clinical features include upper abdominal pain, malaise, fatigue, fever and jaundice. Alpha fetoprotein is a very important tumor marker for the diagnosis of hepatocellular carcinoma.

Cholangiocarcinoma: It is a rarer form of liver malignancy. The etiological agents include infusion of radiocontrast media like thorotrast, infestation with liver fluke *Opisthorchis sinensis*. It presents as a firm to hard gritty small nodule. Microscopically, it is an adenocarcinoma seen within a markedly desmoplastic stroma. The tumor spreads to the regional lymph nodes and generally carry a worser prognosis.

Hepatoblastoma: It is a pediatric malignant liver tumor presenting as a mass abdomen. The tumor is composed of small round undifferentiated cells with the stroma showing presence of mesenchymal elements, such as cartilage and bony tissue. The prognosis of hepatoblastoma is poor.

Points to Ponder

- **Jaundice** is a clinical term used to denote an increase in the concentration of serum bilirubin more than 2.0 mg/dL. The normal range is less than 1 mg/dL.
- **Hepatitis** refers to the inflammatory conditions of the liver induced by various organisms and toxins. The most common cause includes viral infection and the term hepatitis is generally used to indicate viral hepatitis. Common agents implicated in hepatitis are viruses, such as hepatitis viruses, Epstein-Barr virus, adenovirus, cytomegalovirus, yellow fever virus, rubella and enteroviruses.
- **Chronic hepatitis** is a term used to refer to the presence of symptomatic, biochemical or serological evidence of hepatic disease for more than 6 months after an acute hepatitis.
- **Cirrhosis** is defined as an end stage liver disease characterized by distorted parenchymal architecture of liver with many regenerative nodules rimmed by fibrosis along with altered vasculature. It is classified according to the size of the nodules (morphological classification) and on the precipitating cause (etiological classification).
- **Carcinoma** of liver is one of the common visceral malignancies seen more in men with a mean age of 50 years. The common etiological factors are hepatitis B virus infection.

GALLBLADDER

INTRODUCTION

The most common pathological conditions involving gallbladder are formation of gallstones (cholelithiasis) **(Fig. 9.12)** with subsequent inflammatory changes and tumors. We shall now discuss the salient pathological features.

PATHOLOGY OF GALLBLADDER

Cholelithiasis (Gallstones)

These are concretions formed from normal or abnormal constituents of bile. The most common chemical components are cholesterol, calcium bilirubinate and calcium carbonate. The stones are grouped into three classes: **Mixed stones (80%), pure stones (10%) and compound stones (10%)**.

Risk Factors and Etiological Agents

Cholesterol stones: Obesity, familial, geographic, high calorie diet, Crohn's disease, cystic fibrosis, pancreatic insufficiency, increased estrogen, pregnancy, multiparity and diabetes mellitus.

Pigment stones: Geographic, chronic hemolysis, alcoholic cirrhosis, biliary infection.

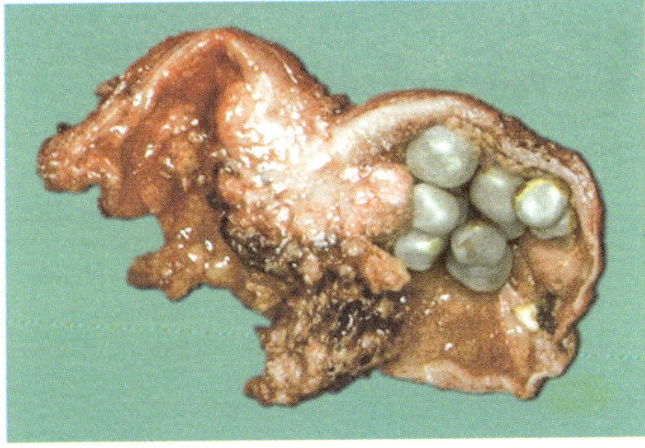

Fig. 9.12: Gallbladder with calculi.

Pathogenesis

The formation of calculi occurs either due to supersaturation of the bile or stasis of the bile with superadded infection.

Morphology

Cholesterol stones: They are solitary yellowish stones with granular external surface. The size may go up to 5 cm. These stones are radiolucent and float in bile.

Pigment stones: They are small and multiple stones brownish or black in color.

Clinical Implications of Calculi

The gallstones may induce the following pathological changes:

- Obstruction and biliary colic
- Gallbladder dysfunction—malabsorption
- Cholecystitis
- Malignancy

Of the above clinical syndromes, the most common is cholecystitis.

There are two forms of cholecystitis—acute and chronic.

Common causes include—calculi (90%), other causes include bacteremia, diabetes mellitus, arteritis and others.

Acute cholecystitis: Grossly, the gallbladder is enlarged and tense. The surface appears grayish-red. Cut section usually reveals a calculi in the neck of the gallbladder.

Microscopically, there is evidence of mucosal erosion or ulceration with dense acute inflammatory cell infiltration **(Figs. 9.13A and B)**.

Chronic cholecystitis: The gallbladder may be slightly enlarged or normal in size. It appears opaque grayish-white.

Microscopically, it shows mucosal injury with chronic mononuclear inflammatory cell infiltration with invagination of the mucosa into the muscularis layer forming Rokitansky-Aschoff sinuses and a thick fibrotic serosa **(Fig. 9.14)**.

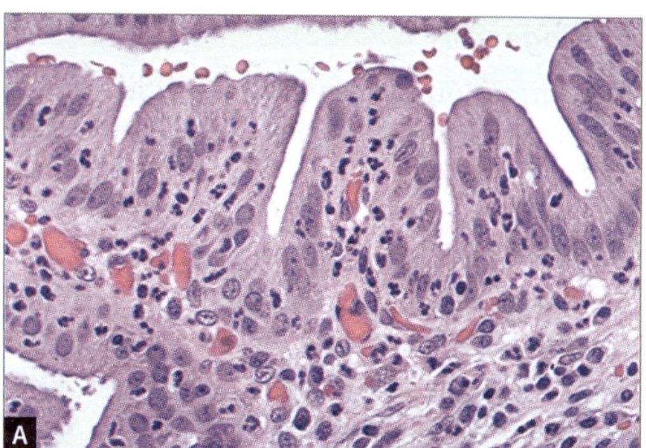

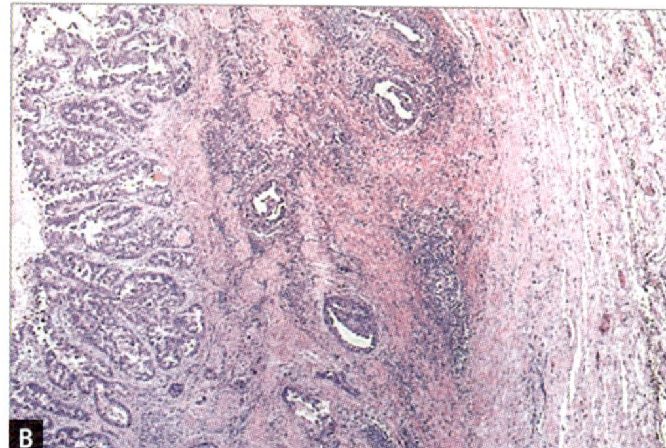

Figs. 9.13A and B: (A) Histomicrograph of acute cholecystitis; (B) Photomicrograph.

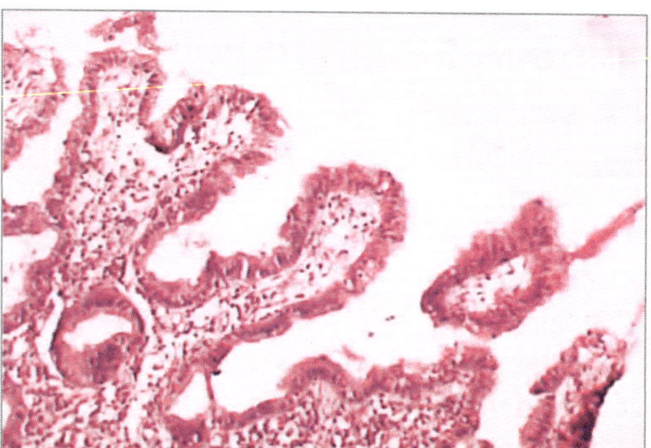

Fig. 9.14: Histomicrograph of chronic cholecystitis.

Carcinoma Gallbladder

It is the fifth common site for occurrence of tumor in gastrointestinal tract (GIT). The common etiological agents include long standing calculi, chemical carcinogens like nitrosamines, patients with chronic ulcerative colitis, chronic typhoid carriers and history of previous surgeries in the biliary tract.

Gallbladder carcinoma is more common in women with a mean age of 65. It is generally a slow growing tumor. Grossly, it presents as a polypoidal fungating mass or a diffusely infiltrating ulcerative form.

Microscopically, it is usually an adenocarcinoma. The tumor undergoes lymphohematogenous spread to the pancreaticoduodenal and para-aortic lymph nodes.

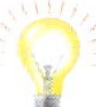

Case Scenario

Mrs X 55-year-old female, presents to the emergency department with severe right upper quadrant abdominal pain, nausea, and vomiting. She describes the pain as colicky and radiating to her back. On examination, Murphy's sign is positive, and laboratory tests reveal elevated liver enzymes. Imaging studies confirm the diagnosis of cholelithiasis.

Question:

What is the primary pathophysiological process underlying the development of cholelithiasis in Mrs X?

A. Chronic alcohol consumption
B. Excessive dietary fat intake
C. Gallbladder inflammation
D. Formation of gallstones in the biliary system

Answer:

D. Formation of gallstones in the biliary system.

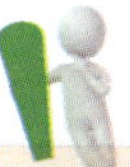

Points to Ponder

- **Gallstones** are concretions formed from normal or abnormal constituents of bile. The most common chemical components are **cholesterol, calcium bilirubinate and calcium carbonate**. The stones are grouped into three classes—mixed stones (80%), pure stones (10%) and compound stones (10%).

Contd...

Contd...

- The most common clinical implications of calculi are obstruction and biliary colic, gallbladder dysfunction—malabsorption, cholecystitis and malignancy.
- Carcinoma gallbladder is the fifth common site for occurrence of tumor in GIT. The common etiological agents include long-standing calculi, chemical carcinogens like nitrosamines, patients with chronic ulcerative colitis, chronic typhoid carriers and history of previous surgeries in the biliary tract. It is more common in women with a mean age of 65.

PANCREAS

NORMAL STRUCTURE

The exocrine pancreas is made up of numerous acinar structures separated by a delicate fibrovascular septa **(Fig. 9.15)**. The lining cells are rich in cytoplasmic enzymes. The pancreas secrets around 22 enzymes, such as protease, amylase, elastase, lipase and others. These enzymes aid in digestion of the food substances by breaking them into simple molecules. All these enzymes are stored in an inactive precursor form within the cells and they are activated when released into the second part of duodenum.

PATHOLOGY OF EXOCRINE PANCREAS

Pancreatitis

It is defined as an inflammatory degeneration of the exocrine pancreas. There are two forms of pancreatitis—acute and chronic.

Acute Pancreatitis

It is characterized by sudden onset of acute abdominal pain with increased release of pancreatic enzymes into the circulation due to inflammatory necrosis of the pancreatic tissue.

This is more common in men with a mean age of 40 years.

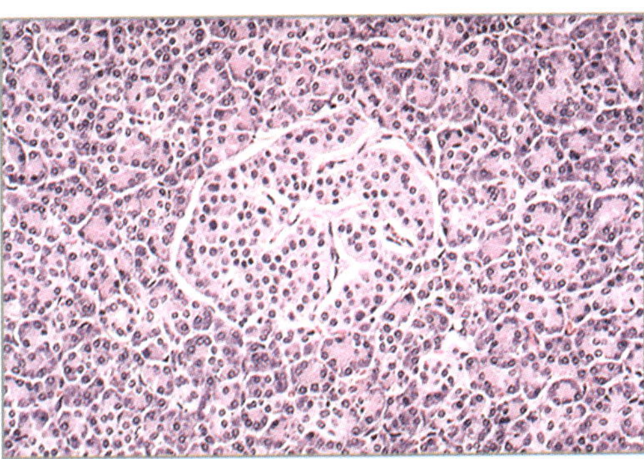

Fig. 9.15: Normal exocrine pancreas with many acinar structures.

Etiological factors: The following are some of the common etiological agents associated with acute pancreatitis. They include:

- *Obstructive biliary tract disease*: Gallstones
- Alcoholism
- *Infections*: Mumps virus
- *Toxins*: Alpha methyldopa, diuretics
- *Metabolic causes*: Uremia, hyperlipidemia
- *Endocrine causes*: Hyperparathyroidism
- *Vascular*: Ischemia, shock
- *Congenital*: Duct anomalies
- Traumatic
- Idiopathic

Pathogenesis: The major pathogenetic changes are injury to the acinar cells and release of the enzymes, such as amylase, proteinase, lipase and elastase. The acinar cells may be injured directly or due to the release of the duodenal enzymes, such as lecithin into the pancreas (duodenal reflux) or due to deranged transport of enzymes from the acinar cells.

Pathology: The organ is enlarged and edematous. The gross image of pancreas in acute pancreatitis is shown in **Figure 9.16**. Cut section shows chalky white areas admixed with congested areas. Microscopically there is destruction and necrosis of the acinar epithelial cells with areas of edema **(Fig. 9.17)**. In severe cases the whole pancreatic tissue may be converted into a large blood clot.

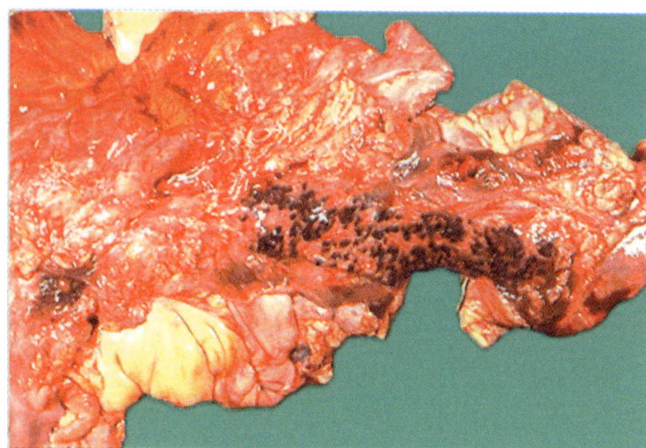

Fig. 9.16: Gross photograph of pancreas in acute pancreatitis.

The peritoneal cavity shows presence of fatty turbid and brownish oil tinged fluid (chicken broth fluid) due to extensive fat necrosis of the omentum.

Clinical features: It is a medical emergency. There is sudden onset of severe abdominal pain with radiation to the back and the patient develops peripheral vascular collapse (shock).

Diagnosis: Laboratory estimation of serum amylase and lipase levels are useful in confirming the diagnosis. There is marked elevation of these enzymes in cases of acute pancreatitis.

Chronic Pancreatitis

It is a persistent progressive inflammatory pathology of the pancreas characterized by irregular fibrosis and sclerosis of the gland which leads to sever functional impairment.

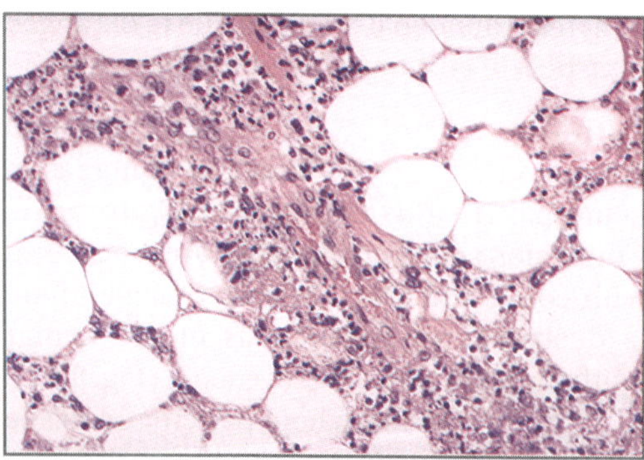

Fig. 9.17: Histomicrograph of acute pancreatitis.

The common etiological agents include the following:

- Chronic alcoholism
- Protein malnutrition
- Obstructive conditions
- Idiopathic

Pathology: The organ is shrunken grayish white and firm to hard with areas of calcification. Microscopically, there is diffuse acinar cell damage with fibrosis and hyalinization. Few of the pancreatic ducts may be dilated **(Fig. 9.18)**.

Clinical features: It usually presents with recurrent attacks of abdominal pain usually after a bout of alcohol intake or a fatty meal. Patients may also present with diabetes mellitus due to the fibrotic compression of the endocrine portion of pancreas (secondary diabetes mellitus).

CARCINOMA PANCREAS

It is one of the common visceral malignancies seen in association with smoking. Carcinoma pancreas is common in men with a mean age of 60 years. The common etiological agents include smoking, chemical carcinogens, such as beta naphthylamines, nitrosamines and chronic pancreatitis.

Pathology: The carcinoma is more common in the head of pancreas (670%) followed by the body (20%) and tail (10%). It presents as

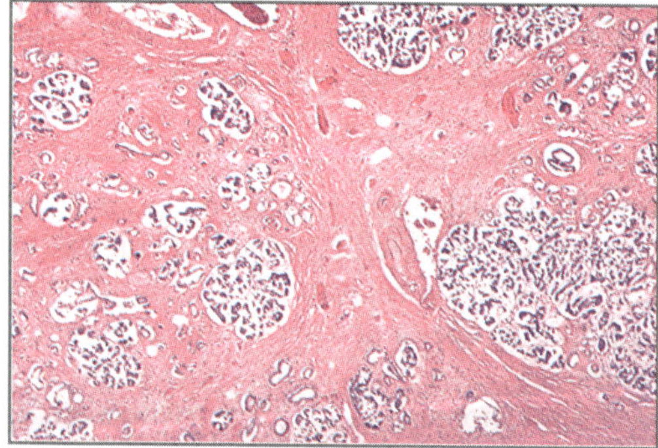

Fig. 9.18: Histomicrograph of chronic pancreatitis.

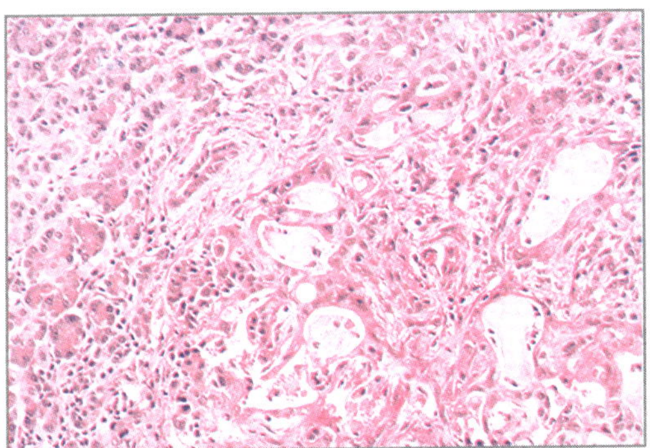

Fig. 9.19: Histomicrograph of adenocarcinoma pancreas.

Case Scenario

Dr Patel, a 35-year-old physician, presents with recurrent acute pancreatitis episodes despite abstinence from alcohol. Imaging studies reveal chronic pancreatitis.

Question:

What additional investigations would you consider identifying the underlying etiology of Dr Patel's chronic pancreatitis, and how would you approach the management of this condition?

A. Genetic testing for cystic fibrosis and supportive care with pancreatic enzyme replacement
B. Endoscopic ultrasound (EUS) and sphincterotomy for biliary stones
C. Serial imaging to monitor disease progression and symptomatic relief with pain management
D. Liver biopsy and initiation of corticosteroids for autoimmune pancreatitis

Answer:

A. Genetic testing for cystic fibrosis and supportive care with pancreatic enzyme replacement.

an irregular grayish white firm to hard mass with infiltrative margins.

Microscopically, it is an adenocarcinoma with variable differentiation **(Fig. 9.19)**. Other microscopic forms include acinar type, cystadenocarcinoma type, adenosquamous type and others.

Clinical features: It presents with abdominal pain jaundice, weight loss, malaise and venous thrombosis. Occurrence of venous thrombosis in pancreatic carcinoma is due to release of thromboplastin, such as substances by the tumor cells into the circulation—Trousseau's sign.

Points to Ponder

- The **exocrine pancreas** is made up of numerous acinar structures separated by a delicate fibrovascular septa. The lining cells are rich in cytoplasmic enzymes.
- **Pancreatitis** is defined as an inflammatory degeneration of the exocrine pancreas. There are two forms of pancreatitis—acute and chronic.
- **Acute pancreatitis** is characterized by sudden onset of acute abdominal pain with increased release of pancreatic enzymes into the circulation due to inflammatory necrosis of the pancreatic tissue.
- **Carcinoma pancreas** is one of the common visceral malignancies seen in association with smoking. It is common in men with a mean age of 60 years. The common etiological agents include smoking, chemical carcinogens, such as beta-naphthylamine, nitrosamines and chronic pancreatitis.

ASSESSMENT QUESTIONS

Essay Type Questions

1. **Describe the etiology, pathogenesis, pathology and clinical features of viral hepatitis.**
2. **A 64-year-old male patient presented to the hospital with complaints of hematemesis for the past 2 days. He had similar episodes for which he took some native treatment. He is a chronic alcoholic and is consuming alcohol for the past 20 years.**

On examination, the patient is conscious, oriented, anemic, not jaundiced, vitals within normal limits. Abdomen appears bloated with free fluid. Spleen palpable. Liver not palpable.

a. What is your provisional diagnosis?
b. Substantiate your answer.
c. Enlist the differential diagnosis in this case.
d. Mention in brief the pathogenesis of this condition.
e. Describe the pathology of liver in this condition.
f. List the common investigations you do in this case.
g. Enumerate the complications of this condition.

3. **Define a gallstone.**
4. **Name the predisposing factors for cholesterol stone.**
5. **Describe the microscopic pathology of chronic cholecystitis.**
6. **Enumerate the clinical complications of gallstones.**
7. **Enlist the causes for pigmented gallstones.**
8. **Enlist the common causes for acute pancreatitis.**
9. **Name the various enzymes released due to pancreatic acinar injury.**
10. **Define chronic pancreatitis.**
11. **What are the common causes for chronic pancreatitis?**
12. **Mention the common sites of occurrence of carcinoma pancreas.**

Short Answer Questions

1. **Mention the major functions of the liver.**
2. **Enumerate the common causes for chronic hepatitis.**
3. **Define cirrhosis.**
4. **How will you classify cirrhosis morphologically?**
5. **Name the common complications of portal hypertension.**
6. **Name the common tumor markers associated with hepatocellular carcinoma.**
7. **Enlist the common clinical signs in a case of jaundice.**
8. **Enumerate the common etiological factors for hepatocellular carcinoma.**
9. **What is Wilson's disease?**
10. **What are the common causes for postnecrotic cirrhosis?**

MULTIPLE CHOICE QUESTIONS

1. **The most common cause for cirrhosis is:**
   A. Chronic alcoholism
   B. Biliary obstruction
   C. Metabolic disorders
   D. Viral hepatitis
2. **The most common cause for portal hypertension is:**
   A. Portal vein thrombosis
   B. Cirrhosis
   C. Constrictive pericarditis
   D. Splenic vein embolism
3. **One of the following hepatotropic virus is a DNA virus:**
   A. Hepatitis A virus
   B. Hepatitis B virus
   C. Hepatitis C virus
   D. Hepatitis E virus

4. Necrosis of the limiting plate of hepatocytes is referred to as:
A. Bridging necrosis
B. Piecemeal necrosis
C. Spotty necrosis
D. Dropout necrosis

5. In hemochromatosis deposition of iron occurs in:
A. Hepatocytes
B. Macrophages
C. Both A and B
D. Ito cell

6. The gene of Wilson's disease is located in chromosome:
A. 6
B. 14
C. 18
D. 13

7. Fibrolamellar type HCC is characterized by all, *except*:
A. Occurs in young male
B. History of cirrhosis
C. Good prognosis
D. Solitary mass

8. Hepar lobatum is due to:
A. Hepatitis A
B. Syphilis
C. Hepatitis B
D. Biliary atresia

9. HBV is not associated with:
A. Chronic active hepatitis
B. Chronic persistent hepatitis
C. Postnecrotic necrosis
D Cholangiocarcinoma

10. One of the following is hepatitis virus is feco-orally transmitted:
A. Hepatitis A
B. Hepatitis B
C. Hepatitis C
D. Hepatitis D

11. Most common type of gallstone is:
A. Pigment
B. Cholesterol
C. Mixed
D. Brown stone

12. Strawberry gallbladder refers to:
A. Cholesterolosis
B. Empyema
C. Acute cholecystitis
D. Chronic cholecystitis

13. Presence of Rokitansky-Aschoff sinuses are pathognomonic of:
A. Cholesterolosis
B. Empyema
C. Acute cholecystitis
D. Chronic cholecystitis

14. Porcelain gallbladder is due to:
A. Gangrenous cholecystitis
B. Xanthogranulomatous cholecystitis
C. Dystrophic calcification
D. Cholesterolosis

15. Most favored location of carcinoma gallbladder is:
A. Lateral wall
B. Neck
C. Ducts of Luschka
D. Fundus

16. One of the following infection causes acute pancreatitis:
A. *Mycoplasma*
B. Mumps
C. *Salmonella*
D. *Pseudomonas*

17. Elevation of one of the following enzymes occurs in the early phase of acute pancreatitis:
A. Lipase
B. Elastase
C. Amylase
D. Protease

18. Chicken broth ascitic fluid is pathognomonic of:
A. Chronic pancreatitis
B. Acute pancreatitis
C. Pseudocyst of pancreas
D. Pancreatic abscess

19. Most common cause for chronic pancreatitis is:
- A. Alcoholism
- B. Gallstones
- C. Mumps
- D. Malnutrition

20. Most favored location of carcinoma pancreas is:
- A. Body
- B. Tail
- C. Head
- D. Ampulla of Vater

21. The paraneoplastic syndrome associated with carcinoma pancreas is:
- A. Migratory thrombophlebitis
- B. Hypercalcemia
- C. Polycythemia
- D. Acanthosis nigricans

Answer Key for MCQs

1	2	3	4	5	6	7	8	9	10	11
A	B	B	B	C	D	B	B	D	A	C
12	**13**	**14**	**15**	**16**	**17**	**18**	**19**	**20**	**21**	
A	D	C	B	B	C	B	A	C	A	

10

CHAPTER

Kidney and Urinary Tract

Learning Objectives

At the end of reading this chapter, the student shall be able to:

- Describe the normal anatomy and histology of kidney.
- Define and classify glomerular diseases. Enumerate the etiology, pathogenesis, mechanisms of glomerular injury and clinical features of common type of glomerulonephritis.
- Enumerate and describe the glomerular manifestations in diabetes and systemic lupus erythematosus.
- Describe the etiology, pathogenesis, pathology and clinical features of tubulointerstitial nephritis.
- Define, classify, describe the clinical syndromes and laboratory features of acute and chronic renal failure.
- Describe the etiology, pathogenesis, pathology and clinical features of urolithiasis.
- Classify and describe the etiology, genetics, pathogenesis, pathology and clinical features of tumors of kidney.
- Describe the etiology, pathogenesis, pathology and clinical features of cystitis.

INTRODUCTION

Kidneys are paired organ weighing 150 g. The major functions of kidney are excretion of metabolic waste products, maintenance of the acid-base balance and secretion of rennin, erythropoietin and other substances (endocrine function). Kidneys are richly vascular organ receiving 25% of the total cardiac output.

FUNCTIONS OF THE KIDNEY

The kidney has various functions which include:

- Excretion of end products of metabolism and excess substance from the diet
- Regulation of water and electrolyte balance
- Maintenance of the acid-base balance
- Reabsorption of essential substances
- Secretion of hormones—erythropoietin and renin

ANATOMY OF THE KIDNEY

The kidneys are encased by a thin capsule which could be peeled of easily. Gross examination of kidney shows an outer cortex and inner medulla (**Fig. 10.1**). The cortex is 1.5 cm thick and is granular in texture. It is mostly composed of the glomeruli and proximal convoluted tubules. The cortex is richly vascular in nature. The inner medulla is made up of a series of pyramidal structures with striped appearance. The apex of the pyramid points to the collecting system. The collecting system of kidney is called as the renal pelvis. It is a funnel shaped and drains the major and minor calyces and opens into ureter.

Nephron is the basic structural and functional unit of kidney. Each nephron is made up of glomeruli, which is a collection of capillaries covered by a thin membrane called the Bowman's membrane. The space is called Bowman's space. This is continuous with the

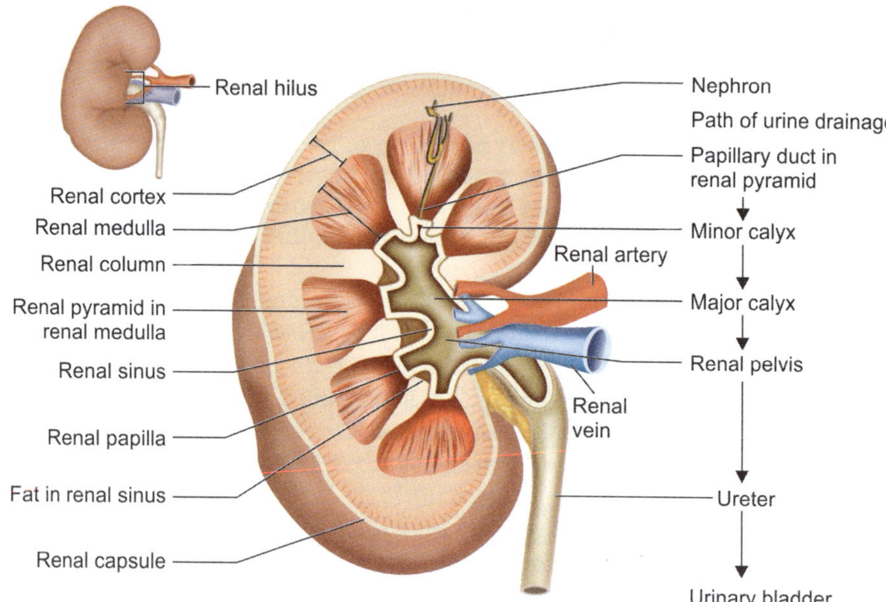

Fig. 10.1: Frontal view of normal right kidney.

orifice of the proximal convoluted tubules through which the glomerular filtrate is drained.

The kidney is made up of a cortex and medulla. The medulla consists of renal pyramids, the apices of which are called papillae, and each is related to a calyx. As the ureter enters the kidney at the hilus, it dilates into a funnel-shaped cavity called the pelvis, from which derive two or three main branches, the major calyces; the latter subdivides again into three of four minor calyces.

The functional unit of the kidney is called the nephron. There are approximately 1 million nephrons in the kidney. Each nephron consists of a glomerulus which filters the urine, and a tubule, through which the filtered urine passes. As the filtered urine passes through the tubules, certain constituents are reabsorbed by the cells lining the tubules, and other substances are secreted in the lumen for eventual excretion.

Each glomerulus consists of a network of capillaries surrounded by a membrane called the Bowman's capsule. This continues to form the Bowman's space and the beginning of the renal tubule. The uppermost portion of the tubular portion of the nephron is called the proximal convoluted tubule and is continuous with the glomerulus. The distal portion is called as the distal convoluted tubule. The descending limb of the proximal tubule and the ascending limb of the distal tubule form the loop of Henle. The distal convoluted tubules from several nephrons drain into the collecting tubule. A number of these coalesce to form the collecting duct. The collecting ducts then join together to form papillary ducts. These then empty at the tips of the papillae into the calyces which in turn drain into the bladder, where it remains until voided.

GLOMERULI

The glomeruli are an important structural component of the nephron. It is made up of an afferent arteriole, tuft of capillaries and an efferent arteriole. When the glomeruli are studied under electron microscope (**Fig. 10.2**) it shows the following structures.

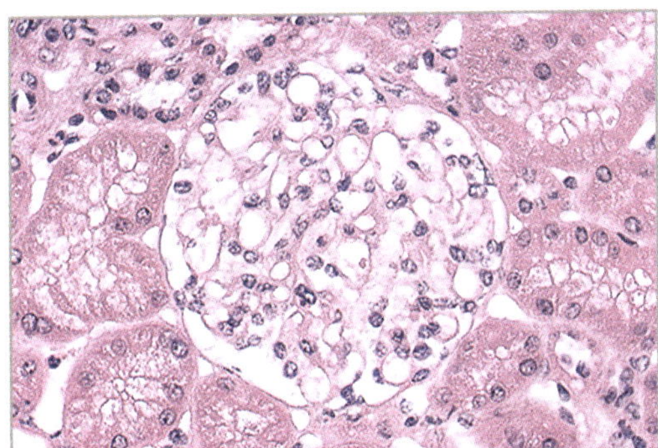

Fig. 10.2: Histomicrograph of normal glomeruli.

The inner side of the glomerular capillary wall is lined by endothelial cells with fixed gaps between the cells. It is called **fenestrated endothelium**. The length of the gaps is 70–100 nm.

The endothelial cells rest on a basement membrane called the glomerular basement membrane (GBM), which is a three-layered structure. The central portion is called as **lamina densa**, as it is electron dense. The inner portion is called **lamina rara interna** and the external portion is called **lamina rara externa**.

The GBM is made up of collagen and other non-collagenous proteins such as **laminin, polyanionic proteoglycans, fibronectin, entactin and glycoproteins**.

The outer side of the capillary wall is called the **epithelial layer**. It is made up of cells called the visceral cells. These cells have interdigitating cytoplasmic processes which are referred to as foot processes and they rest on the lamina rara externa. Since this cell is having foot such as extensions it is called **podocyte (podo-foot, cyte-cell)**. The space between the foot processes is referred to as the filtration slit and the width is 20–30 nm.

The Bowman's space is lined by flattened cells called the **parietal epithelial cells**.

The glomerular structures are supported by a supporting tissue called the **mesangium**. It comprises of mesangial matrix and mesangial cell. The mesangial cells have got a wide range of functions and they act as macrophage of the kidney.

GLOMERULAR FILTRATION

The major function of the kidney is excretion of the urine, which is an ultrafiltrate of plasma. The substances are filtered from the circulation and allowed to pass through the renal tubules and excreted into the collecting system. This filtration function is dependent on two major factors:

1. *Size dependent filtration:* The glomeruli can allow only substances with a molecular size less than 3.5 nm and molecular weight less than 70,000 Daltons to pass through it. Any particle which is large than this is less permeable through the GBM.
2. *Charge dependent filtration:* The GBM is normally an ionically charged due to the presence of polyanionic proteoglycans. If the substance is cationic it easily passes through it and if it is anionic it is impermeable. Neutral charged particles are retained in the mesangium.

In addition to the glomeruli the kidneys also contain renal tubules, renal blood vessels, juxtaglomerular apparatus and the renal interstitium.

PATHOLOGY OF RENAL SYSTEM

The renal diseases can be grouped into the following headings:

- Diseases of glomeruli (glomerulonephritis),
- Diseases of tubules and interstitium (tubulointerstitial diseases),
- Diseases of blood vessels (renovascular diseases) and
- Tumors of kidney

Clinical Profile of Renal Diseases

Patients with renal disease will have varied clinical presentations which are generally grouped into the following headings:

- *Acute nephritic syndrome* (*acute GN*): This is characterized by mild-to-moderate proteinuria, hematuria (gross or microscopic) and hypertension.

- *Nephrotic syndrome:* This is characterized by massive proteinuria, edema, hypoalbuminemia and hyperlipidemia.
- Asymptomatic proteinuria/hematuria
- *Acute renal failure:* Acute onset renal shut down with oliguria and azotemia.
- *Chronic renal failure:* (Syn: Uremia) end stage renal disease with multiorgan dysfunction.
- *Others:* Urinary tract infection, obstructive uropathy—calculi and renal tumors.

GLOMERULAR DISEASES

The glomerular disease can be generally classified into primary and secondary glomerular diseases. The exact etiological mechanism is unclear in primary form and the secondary form is a form of glomerular damage secondary to an existing primary disease such as diabetes mellitus, systemic lupus erythematosus (SLE) and others.

Pathogenesis

As we have already discussed, the glomeruli are a tuft of capillary encased within a thin membranous Bowman's capsule. Injury to the glomeruli is mostly mediated by immunological reactions. These reactions can be mediated by the antibodies, cytotoxic T lymphocytes or the complement system components.

Antibody mediated glomerular damage is the most common form. The damage can be induced by the following type of antibodies:

- Formation of antigen and antibody complexes at the level of the GBM. The antibodies may be directed against fixed intrinsic antigens or against planted antigens.
- *Entrapment of the circulating immune complexes*: In this category, the immune complexes are not formed at the level of the glomeruli. They are formed elsewhere in the circulation and they get trapped at the level of the GBM due to the physiochemical properties. This type of glomerular injury is seen in many immune complex disorders, such as SLE and others.
- Glomerular injury may also be induced by the activation of the alternate pathway of the complement system and by the cytotoxic lymphocytes.

Mechanism of Glomerular Damage

Following deposition of the immune complexes in GBM, there will be infiltration of the inflammatory cells due to the release of cytokines and various chemical mediators of inflammation which damage the glomeruli.

Common Histological Alterations of Glomeruli in Glomerulonephritis

The following are the common histological alterations:

- *Hypercellularity:* There will be proliferation of the endothelial cells or epithelial cells or mesangial cells.
- *Thickening of the basement membrane:* Due to the deposition of the immune complexes.
- *Leukocytic infiltration:* The glomeruli may be infiltrated by acute and chronic inflammatory cells.
- *Others:* Crescents—these are hemispherical cellular structures seen in the Bowman's space due to the proliferation of the parietal epithelial cells, hyalinization and sclerosis—seen in the end stage glomerular disease.

Histomorphological Profile of Various Forms of Glomerulonephritis

Acute Poststreptococcal Proliferative Glomerulonephritis

It is one of the most common causes for acute GN in children.

Etiopathogenesis: It is a glomerular disease that occurs following a streptococcal skin infection, due to deposition of immune complexes against the streptococcal antigens.

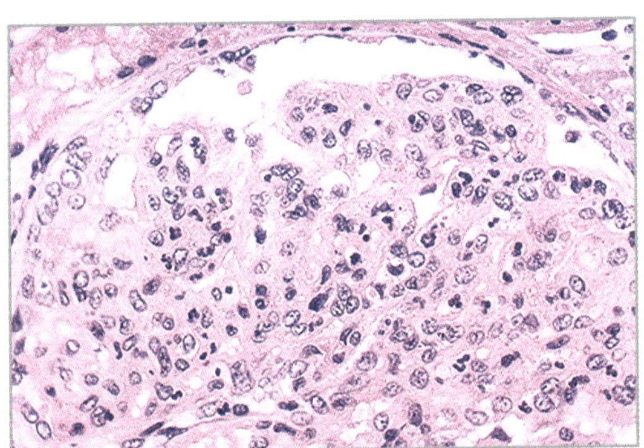

Fig. 10.3: Histomicrograph of acute poststreptococcal glomerulonephritis.

Microscopy: The glomeruli are hypercellular with infiltration by neutrophils (**Fig. 10.3**).

Immunofluorescence: Shows deposition of granular immune complexes in the mesangium and subepithelium. Electron microscopy (EM) also shows electron dense deposits in the same site.

Clinical profile: Seen in children of age 6–10 years. It follows a streptococcal skin infection mostly an impetigo. The clinical features include fever, malaise, oliguria with features of acute GN. There is complete recovery in 95% of the cases.

Membranous GN

It is the most common cause for nephrotic syndrome in adults.

Etiopathogenesis: It is an immune mediated glomerular damage induced by antibodies formed against glomerular antigens. This may also occur secondarily to drug reaction, malignancies, viral infections and in diabetes mellitus.

Microscopy: There is uniform diffuse thickening of the glomerular basement membrane (GBM). If shows granular deposits of immune complexes in the epithelial side of the GBM (**Fig. 10.4**). EM shows deposition of electron dense complexes in the epithelial side.

Clinical profile: It is characterized by the features of nephrotic syndrome.

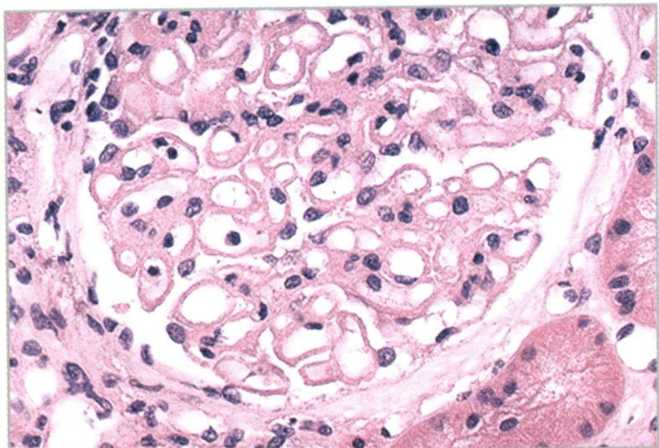

Fig. 10.4: Histomicrograph of membranous glomerulonephritis.

Minimal Change Disease (Lipoid Nephrosis)

It is the most common cause for nephrotic syndrome in children.

Etiopathogenesis: In this disorder, the glomerular damage is induced by the loss of polyanionic proteoglycans and damage to the foot processes of the visceral epithelial cells. There is no deposition of immune complexes.

Microscopy: The glomeruli look normal without any immune deposits. EM is diagnostic which demonstrates the loss of the foot processes and damage of the podocytes.

Clinical profile: It involves children of age 2–6 years characterized by the features of nephrotic syndrome.

Rapidly Progressive GN

It is characterized by severe immune mediated glomerular damage leading to acute renal failure.

Etiopathogenesis: It is an immune complex mediated disease due to deposition of immune complexes at the level of the GBM. The antibodies are directed against certain fixed antigens of the GBM. It may also be induced by deposition of circulating immune complexes or activation of anti neutrophilic cytoplasmic antibodies (ANCA).

Microscopy: The glomeruli are enlarged and pale with proliferation of the endothelial and mesangial cells. The hall mark of this lesion is the presence of crescents within the Bowman's space. If shows linear deposition of the immune complexes in the GBM in most of the cases. In few cases, the deposits are granular and interrupted (**Fig. 10.5**). EM shows similar electron dense deposits.

Clinical profile: The patients present with moderate proteinuria, hematuria, hypertension, edema and features of acute renal failure. In few cases, the patient may have hemoptysis due to similar damage to the alveolar basement membrane of the lung, this is called the Goodpasture's syndrome.

Membranoproliferative GN

It is an immune mediated glomerular disease presenting with nephrotic syndrome.

Etiopathogenesis: The damage to the GBM may be induced by the entrapment of the immune complexes or due to the abnormal activation of the alternate pathway of the complement system.

Pathology: The glomeruli are large and hypercellular with marked thickening of the GBM. It shows a double contour and referred to as the tram track basement membrane. If shows granular deposition of the immune complexes in the subendothelial aspect of GBM. Electron microscope (EM) shows marked thickening of the GBM with the deposition of the electron dense immune deposits and the change is referred to as the dense deposit disease (**Fig. 10.6**).

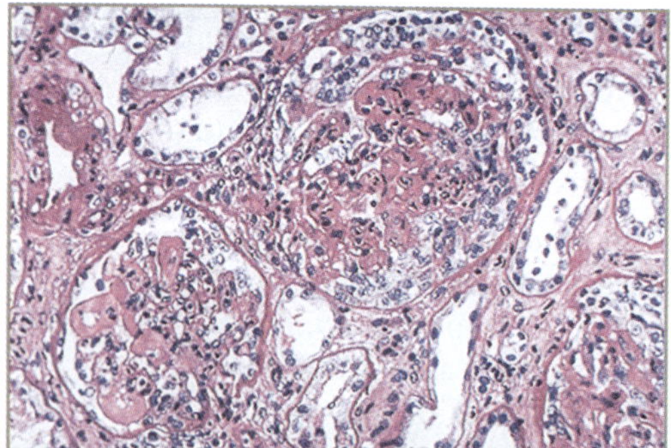

Fig. 10.5: Histomicrograph of rapidly progressive GN with crescents.

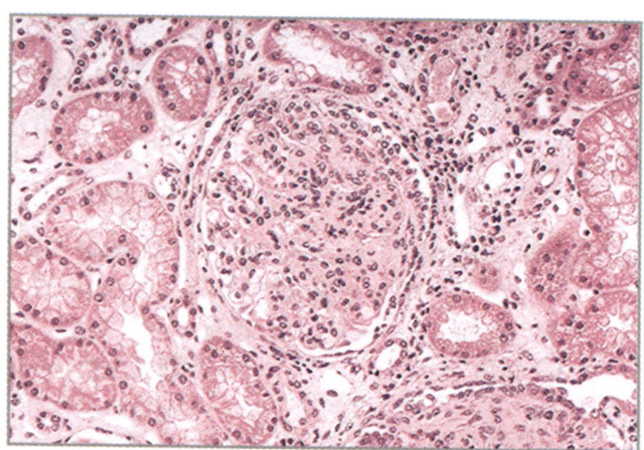

Fig. 10.6: Histomicrograph of membranoproliferative GN.

Clinical profile: It is characterized by the features of nephrotic syndrome.

IgA Nephropathy (Berger's Disease)

This is a form of glomerular disease induced by the deposition of IgA within the mesangium. Patients with this disease have higher serum levels of IgA which gets trapped in the mesangium and induces an inflammatory response by activating the alternate pathway of the complement.

Pathology: There is marked widening of the mesangium with proliferation of the mesangial cells. If is diagnostic and it shows characteristic deposition of IgA within the mesangium. EM shows electron dense deposits in the mesangium (**Fig. 10.7**).

Clinical profile: It often presents with recurrent gross hematuria.

Secondary GN

There are many primary causes which may lead to GN. They include diabetes mellitus, SLE, amyloidosis, hypertension.

Drug-induced damage, preeclampsia and in transplant rejection.

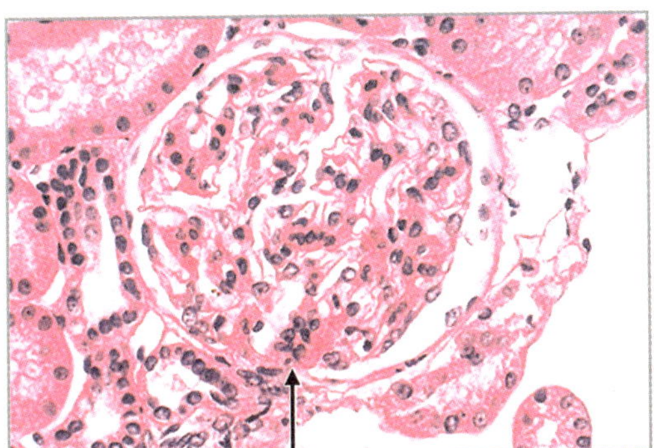

Fig. 10.7: Histomicrograph of IgA nephropathy deposition of IgA indicated by arrow.

Diabetic Nephropathy

This is more common with type I insulin dependent DM than type II form and one of the major causes for renal morbidity. The common glomerular lesion seen are:

- *Thickening of the GBM:* It is a very common finding. There is progressive widening of the GBM. This is due to diabetic microangiopathy.
- *Nodular glomerulosclerosis:* It is a pathognomonic lesion of diabetic nephropathy and is characterized by the formation of nodular sclerotic lesions in the glomeruli (**Fig. 10.8**). It is also referred to as Kimmelstiel-Wilson lesion.
- *Diffuse glomerulosclerosis*: This is seen in end stage of the disease with complete obliteration of the glomeruli.

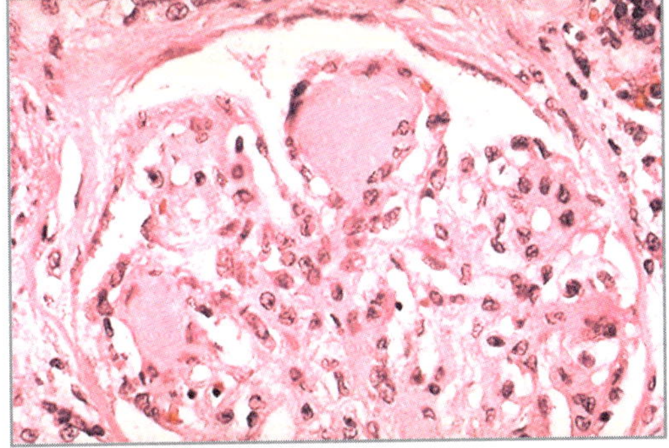

Fig. 10.8: Histomicrograph of nodular glomerulosclerosis of diabetic nephropathy.

- *Fibrin cap and capsular drop*: These are minor lesions seen in the Bowman's space.

Other changes seen in the kidney includes accumulation of glycogen within the tubules, recurrent urinary tract infection leading to pyelonephritis and renal papillary necrosis.

The clinical features include non-nephrotic proteinuria, nephrotic proteinuria, chronic renal failure and without any symptoms.

Lupus Nephritis

Kidney is one of the important organs involved in the pathology of systemic lupus erythematosus (SLE). There are various lesions seen in the kidney. The renal glomeruli gets damaged due to the trapping of the circulating immune complexes and subsequent immune mediated damage. The lesion includes mesangial lupus nephritis, focal proliferative glomerulonephritis (GN), diffuse proliferative GN and membranous GN. The patient presents with nephritic and nephritic range of proteinuria.

Chronic Glomerulonephritis

This is a chronic end stage renal disease following acute glomerular damage. The most common causes include rapidly progressive GN, focal segmental glomerulosclerosis, membranous GN, membranoproliferative GN and IgA nephropathy.

Grossly, the kidneys are symmetrically contracted with diffuse fine granularity on the surface. The cortex is markedly thinned out. Microscopically, it shows features of the primary glomerular disease with hyaline degeneration and obliteration of the glomerular capillary loops. These changes are associated with interstitial fibrosis.

TUBULOINTERSTITIAL DISEASES

Pyelonephritis

It is an inflammatory disorder affecting the tubules and the interstitium. There are two forms of pyelonephritis—acute and chronic.

Etiopathogenesis

Mostly due to gram negative bacilli, such as *E. coli*, *Streptococci*, *Proteus*, *Klebsiella* and *Enterobacter*.

Source of Infection

The bacteria usually originate from the patients fecal flora.

Route of Spread

The most common route of spread is ascending infection and rarely hematogenous spread.

Ascending infection is the most common route by which the organism colonizes the renal pelvis. Some of the **common predisposing factors** include:

- Urethral catheterization and instrumentation
- *Female gender:* Due to short urethra, increased risk of urethral trauma, absence of the antibacterial prostatic secretions and increased adherence of the bacteria to the distal urethra.
- Defects in bladder function.
- *Vesicoureteral reflux:* This condition occurs due to incompetence of the vesicoureteral valve. During micturition, a small amount of urine is flushed back into the ureter and then into the renal pelvis. This may be due to congenital incompetence of the valve or abnormal shortening of the intravesical portion of the ureter. Diagnosis of this condition can be made by voiding cystourethrogram.

Pathology

Acute pyelonephritis: It is characterized by acute suppurative inflammation of tubules and the intersititum with formation of abscesses. **Figure 10.9** shows histomicrograph of acute tubulointerstitial inflammation. The glomeruli remain normal.

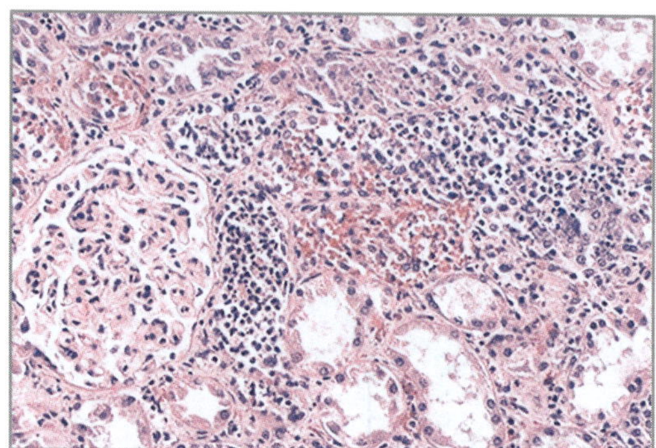

Fig. 10.9: Histomicrograph of acute tubulointerstitial inflammation.

Complications of acute pyelonephritis: The most common complications are:

- *Renal papillary necrosis*: Necrosis of the apex of the renal pyramid, mostly seen in patients with diabetes mellitus.
- *Pyonephrosis*: Severe form of suppuration, where the kidney is converted to a bag of pus.
- *Perinephric abscess*: Due to spillover of inflammation into the perinephric tissues.

Clinical Features

It is characterized by fever, pain and tenderness in the renal angle, frequency and urgency of urination and painful micturition. Examination of urine shows many leucocyte casts. Diagnosis can be made by doing a urine culture.

Chronic pyelonephritis: This is a chronic form of tubulointerstitial damage. Grossly, the kidneys are asymmetrically contracted with large irregular pitted scars. The pelvicalyceal system is markedly distorted.

Histologically, it shows predominant tubulointerstitial inflammation with lymphoplasmacytic infiltration (**Fig. 10.10**). The tubules are dilated and filled with colloid cast like material. This change is called **thyroidization (as the renal tubules mimic thyroid follicles)**. The interstitial vessels show thickening and there will be periglomerular fibrosis.

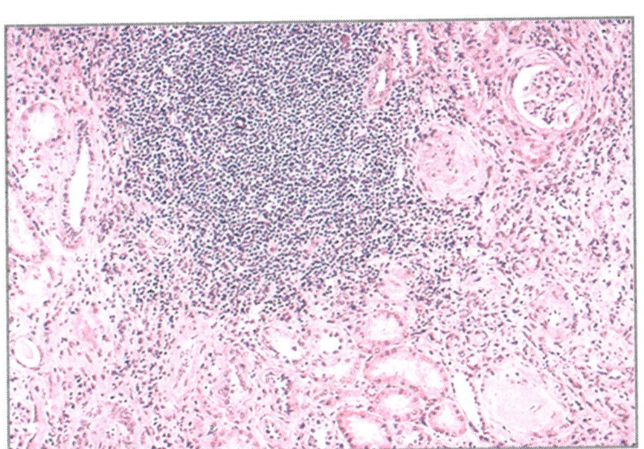

Fig. 10.10: Histomicrograph of chronic pyelonephritis.

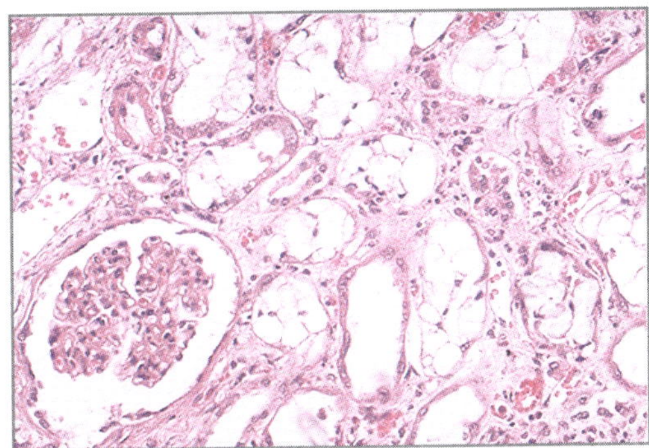

Fig. 10.11: Histomicrograph of toxic acute tubular necrosis.

Renal Failure

This is a form of severe renal dysfunction. It may be acute and chronic.

Acute Renal Failure

Most common cause for acute renal failure is acute tubular necrosis. It is a reversible lesion with severe damage to the tubular epithelium. There are two forms of acute tubular necrosis: ischemic and toxic.

Ischemic acute tubular necrosis: It is caused by severe ischemia to the renal circulation as in case of shock, following transfusion reaction, severe sepsis, massive hemorrhage and disseminated intravascular coagulation.

Toxic acute tubular necrosis: It is induced by various toxins and drugs which include heavy metals, such as mercury, chromium, bismuth, gold and arsenic, chemical, such as carbon tetrachloride, ethylene glycol, drugs such as sulfonamides, non-steroidal anti-inflammatory agents, anesthetic agents, such as halothane, radiocontrast material and chemotherapeutic agents.

These disorders are characterized by marked tubular dysfunction mostly involving the proximal convoluted tubules as they are very sensitive for ischemia. **Figure 10.11** shows histomicrograph of toxic acute tubular necrosis.

Clinical features: It is characterized by sudden reduction in the urinary output with rise in the levels of blood urea nitrogen. It progresses to severe form of oliguria, with metabolic acidosis and hyperkalemia. If the disease is recognized and treated at this phase the disease reverts back to normal. The recovery is indicated by a steady increase in the volume of urine.

Chronic Renal Failure

It is an end stage renal disease characterized by increase in the blood levels of urea and creatinine with marked reduction in the glomerular filtration. **Figure 10.12** shows histomicrograph of end stage renal disease. It is a multisystem disease and the common clinical manifestations include the following.

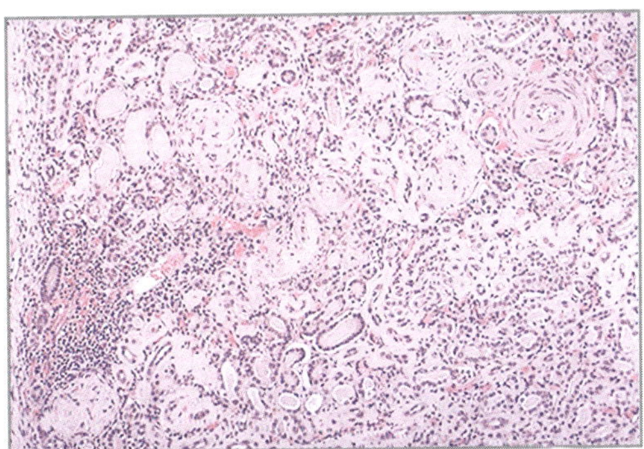

Fig. 10.12: Histomicrograph of end stage renal disease.

System involved	Manifestations
Fluid and electrolyte	♦ Dehydration ♦ Edema ♦ Hyperkalemia ♦ Metabolic acidosis
Calcium metabolism	♦ Hypocalcemia ♦ Hyperphosphatemia
Skeletal system	♦ Renal osteodystrophy ♦ Spontaneous fractures ♦ Impaired bone growth
Cardiovascular	♦ Congestive cardiac failure ♦ Uremic pericarditis
Respiratory	♦ Pulmonary edema ♦ Uremic pneumonia
GIT	♦ Uremic gastroenteritis ♦ Superficial ulcerations
Hematologic	♦ Anemia ♦ Bleeding disorders
Neuromuscular	♦ Myopathy ♦ Peripheral neuropathy
Dermatologic	♦ Dermatitis ♦ Sallow colored skin

Urolithiasis

It is one of the common causes that causes obstructive uropathy. The common types of renal calculi include the following:

- Calcium phosphate and calcium oxalate (75–80%)
- Magnesium ammonium phosphate (15%)
- Uric acid stones (6%)
- Cystine stones (1–2%)

Etiological Factors

- Increased concentration of crystalloids, e.g., hypercalciuria, hyperuricemia, hyperparathyroidism and other metabolic diseases.
- Highly concentrated urine
- Infection with bacteria such as proteus
- Lack of substances that inhibit crystallization.

Morphology

The calculi are mostly unilateral in location (80%). They are located in the renal calyces, pelvis and urinary bladder. **Figure 10.13** shows the gross image of kidney with calculi. Most of the calculi are small 2–3 mm in size except the triple phosphate stones which are very large and the assume the shape of the pelvicalyceal system. These are called the **stag horn calculi**.

Clinical Features

Small calculi generally induces sever renal colic, whereas large calculi induced hematuria. Most of the calculi induces obstruction which predisposes to urinary tract infection.

Case Scenario

Mr Kumar, a 40-year-old male, presents to the emergency department with severe colicky right lower abdominal pain and hematuria. He describes the pain as intermittent and radiating to the groin. On examination, he is restless and has tenderness over the right costovertebral angle. Laboratory tests show microscopic hematuria. A non-contrast CT scan of the abdomen reveals a 6 mm stone in the right renal pelvis.

Question:

What is the most likely diagnosis for Mr Kumar's condition based on the clinical presentation and imaging findings?

A. Acute appendicitis
B. Diverticulitis
C. Urolithiasis
D. Acute pancreatitis

Answer:

C. Urolithiasis

Tumors of Kidney

Kidneys and urinary tract are one of the common sites for the occurrence of the tumors. The tumors of the kidney are classified as follows:

- *Epithelial tumors:*
  - Renal cell adenoma

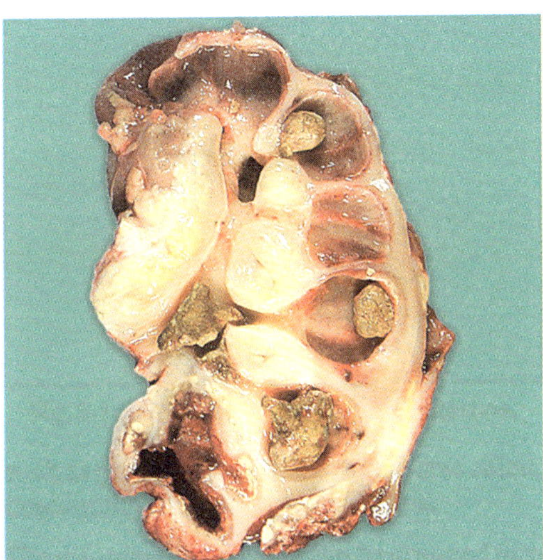

Fig. 10.13: Gross photograph of kidney with calculi.

- Oncocytoma
- Renal cell carcinoma (RCC)

❖ *Nephroblastic tumors (embryonal tumors):*
- Nephroblastoma (Wilms', tumor)
- Mesoblastic nephroma

❖ *Non-epithelial tumors:*
- Angiomyolipoma
- Fibroma
- Hemangioma

❖ *Miscellaneous:*
- Reninoma
- Clear cell sarcoma
- Renomedullary interstitial tumor
- Malignant rhabdoid tumor
- Teratoma

Metastatic Tumors

Common primary sites include—breast, lung and opposite kidney.

We shall now discuss the salient pathological features of the common forms of renal tumors.

Renal Cell Carcinoma

They constitute 1–3% of all visceral tumors. It is the most common form of malignant renal tumor. This is more common in men in age of 6–7 decade of life.

Etiological factors: The common etiological agents associated with RCC include:

❖ Cigarette smoking
❖ Obesity
❖ Hypertension
❖ Estrogen therapy
❖ Asbestosis
❖ Chronic renal failure
❖ Acquired cystic disease of kidney
❖ Tuberous sclerosis
❖ Familial conditions, such as von Hippel-Lindau syndrome, hereditary form of clear cell carcinoma, hereditary papillary carcinoma and others.

Gross: It presents with a solitary mass in the upper pole of kidney. The size varies from 3–15 cm. The cut section shows bright yellowish areas with areas of hemorrhage and cystic change (**Fig. 10.14**).

Histologically, it is an adenocarcinoma made up of cells with clear cytoplasm arranged in trabecular, tubular, solid pattern with irregular nuclei (clear cell adenocarcinoma) (**Fig. 10.15**).

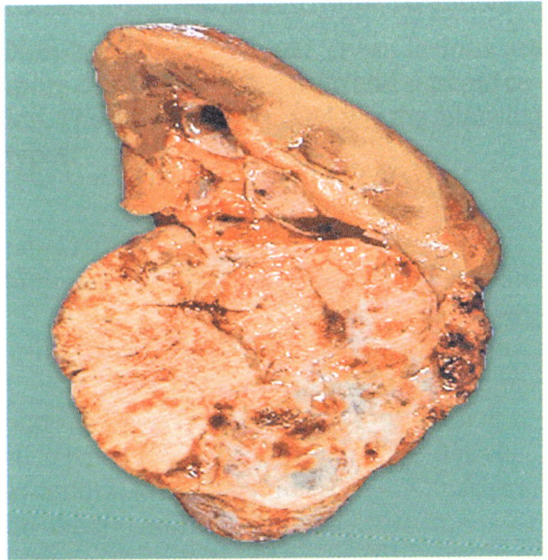

Fig. 10.14: Gross photograph of renal cell carcinoma.

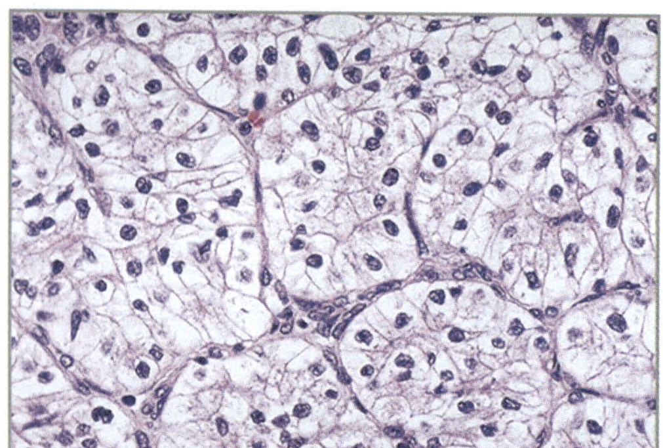

Fig. 10.15: Histomicrograph of renal cell carcinoma with lobules of clear cells.

Clinical features: Renal cell carcinoma typically presents with a diagnostic triad of costovertebral pain, palpable mass with hematuria. The patient is also prone for many paraneoplastic syndromes, such as polycythemia, hypercalcemia, hypertension, feminization and leukemoid reaction.

Spread: The tumor undergoes a direct spread to the renal pelvis and it has an angioinvasive property. The tumor cells invade the renal veins and spread through the veins. The various sites for metastasis includes lung, bones, adrenal, brain and opposite kidney.

Nephroblastoma (Wilms' Tumor)

It is one of the most common pediatric renal tumor seen in children of age 2–6 years. It is associated with other congenital anomalies, such as Denys-Drash syndrome, Beckwith Wiedemann syndrome and others.

Grossly, it presents like a large irregular mass with wide areas of hemorrhage and fleshy areas in cut section (**Fig. 10.16**).

Histologically, the tumor has a triphasic pattern.

It is composed of blastemal cells, stromal cells and epithelial cells. The blastemal cells are primitive cells with scant rim of cytoplasm and round nuclei. The epithelium is made up of abortive tubules. The stroma shows myxoid areas and other heterologous elements (**Fig. 10.17**).

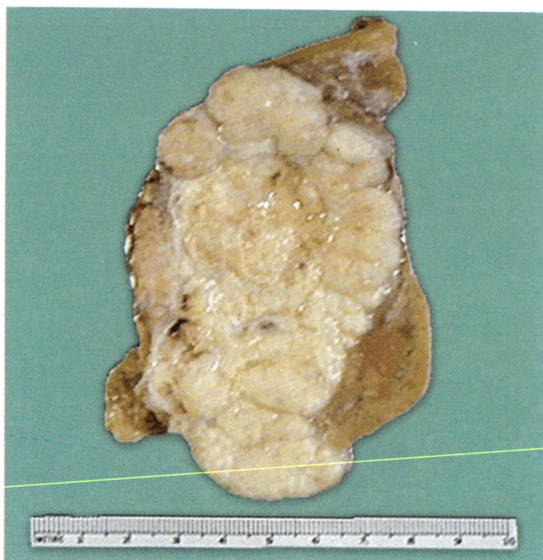

Fig. 10.16: Gross photograph of nephroblastoma.

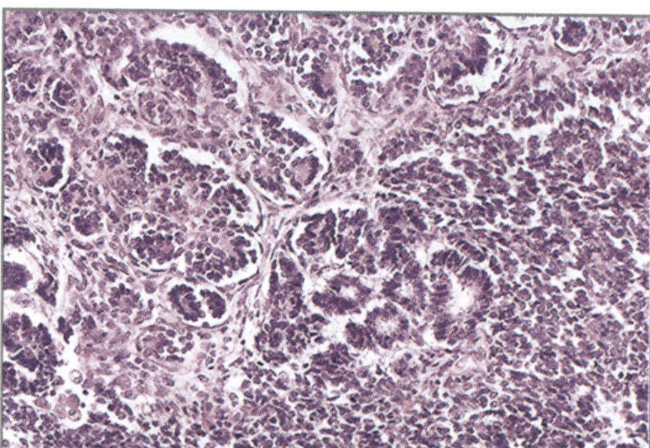

Fig. 10.17: Histomicrogrpah of nephroblastoma with epithelial and blastemal elements.

Clinically, it presents with large abdominal mass with pain abdomen and hematuria. The tumor spreads to the perirenal tissue, adrenals, liver, lung and vertebrae.

Cystitis

It is defined as an inflammatory degeneration of the urinary bladder mucosa. There are two forms—acute or chronic. Common causative factors such as *E. coli*, *Proteus*, *Klebsiella*, *Enterobacter*, *Candida*, Schistosomiasis, and drugs, such as cyclophosphamide..

Special Forms of Cystitis

Ulcerative interstitial cystitis: It is also referred to as Hunner's ulcer. This is more common in women with superficial ulceration and underlying fibrosis.

Emphysematous cystitis: This form is characterized by the presence of bullae, seen in diabetic individuals.

Malakoplakia: It is a peculiar form of chronic cystitis with formation of yellowish raised lesions within a pink mucosa. Histologically, it typically shows the presence of foamy macrophages (von Hansemann cells) and laminated mineralized concretions with targetoid appearance (Michaelis-Gutmann bodies). This occurs in infection with *E. coli*, *Proteus* and in immunocompromised patients.

Points to Ponder

- The glomeruli is an important structural component of the nephron. It is made up of an afferent arteriole, tuft of capillaries and an efferent arteriole.
- The glomerular disease can be generally classified into primary and secondary glomerular diseases. The exact etiological mechanism in primary form is an immune mediated glomerular damage and the secondary form is secondary to an existing primary diseases, such as diabetes mellitus, systemic lupus erythematosus.
- The common histological alterations of glomeruli in glomerulonephritis are hypercellularity, thickening of the basement membrane—due to the deposition of the immune complexes, leucocytic infiltration and others.
- Pyelonephritis is an inflammatory disorder affecting the tubules and the interstitium. There are two forms of pyelonephritis—acute and chronic. Mostly due to gram negative bacilli, such as *E. coli*, streptococci, *Proteus*, *Klebsiella* and *Enterobacter*.
- Renal failure is a form of severe renal dysfunction. It may be acute and chronic.
- Most common cause for acute renal failure is acute tubular necrosis.
- Urolithiasis is one of the common cause for obstructive uropathy.
- Renal cell carcinoma constitute 1–3% of all visceral tumors. It is the most common form of malignant renal tumor. This is seen in men in age of 6–7 decade of life. The most common clinical presentation is costovertebral pain, palpable mass with hematuria.
- Cystitis is defined as an inflammatory degeneration of the urinary bladder mucosa. There are two forms—acute or chronic.

ASSESSMENT QUESTIONS

Essay Type Questions

1. **An 8-year-old boy was brought to the pediatric OPD with complaints of swelling of the face and leg with reduction in the urinary output. The boy had taken treatment for a skin infection of the hands recently.**
   On examination, periorbital edema is seen, pulse rate within normal limits, blood pressure is elevated.

Examination of the urine: Cola-colored urine, positive for proteins [+++]. Urine microscopy shows red blood cells and RBC casts.

a. What is your provisional diagnosis?
b. Substantiate your answer.
c. Enlist the differential diagnosis in this case.
d. Mention in brief the pathogenesis of this condition.
e. What are lesions you will see in the glomeruli?
f. Enumerate the complication of this condition?

2. **A 38-year-old person was admitted to the medical ward with complaints of swelling of the face and leg with reduction in the urinary output.**
   On examination, massive edema is seen. Pulse rate within normal limits, blood pressure is normal.
   Examination of the urine: Positive for proteins [++++]. He has elevated levels of cholesterol, triglycerides and low density lipoproteins.
   a. What is your provisional diagnosis?
   b. Substantiate your answer.
   c. Enlist the differential diagnosis in this case.
   d. Mention in brief the pathogenesis of this condition.
   e. What are lesions you will see in the glomeruli?
   f. Enumerate the complication of this condition.
3. **Classify tumors of kidney. Discuss in detail the etiology, genetics, pathology and clinical features of renal cell carcinoma.**

Short Answer Questions

1. **Enlist the biochemical composition of the glomerular basement membrane.**
2. **Define nephrotic syndrome.**
3. **Enlist the causes for secondary glomerulonephritis.**
4. **What are the glomerular changes in diabetic nephropathy?**
5. **What are the causes for anemia in chronic renal failure?**
6. **What are the reasons that make women more prone for urinary tract infections?**
7. **Name the common types of renal calculi.**
8. **Enumerate the common malignant tumors of kidney.**
9. **What is malakoplakia?**
10. **Enlist the common predisposing factors for carcinoma urinary bladder.**

MULTIPLE CHOICE QUESTIONS

1. **The anionic nature of the glomerular basement membrane is due to:**
   A. Collagen
   B. Proteoglycans
   C. Fibronectin
   D. Entactin
2. **Nephrotic syndrome is characterized by all, *except*:**
   A. Hypertension
   B. Hypoalbuminemia
   C. Massive edema
   D. Proteinuria
3. **The most common cause for nephrotic syndrome in adults is:**
   A. Membranous GN
   B. Membranoproliferative GN
   C. IgA nephropathy
   D. Minimal change disease

4. **Presence of oval fat bodies in urine is commonly seen in:**
   A. Acute renal failure
   B. Nephrotic syndrome
   C. Nephritic syndrome
   D. Chronic renal failure
5. **The most common clinical presentation of IgA nephropathy is:**
   A. Acute renal failure
   B. Nephrotic syndrome
   C. Nephritic syndrome
   D. Recurrent hematuria
6. **Kimmelstiel-Wilson lesion is pathognomonic of:**
   A. Lupus nephritis
   B. Amyloid kidney
   C. Diabetic nephropathy
   D. Benign nephrosclerosis
7. **Most common type of renal calculi is:**
   A. Triple phosphate
   B. Uric acid
   C. Cystine
   D. Calcium oxalate
8. **One of the following is a radiolucent calculi:**
   A. Triple phosphate
   B. Uric acid
   C. Cystine
   D. Calcium oxalate
9. **The clear cytoplasm in renal cell carcinoma is due to accumulation of:**
   A. Proteins
   B. Glycogen
   C. Mucin
   D. Hyaline
10. **Hemorrhagic cystitis is commonly due to:**
    A. Tuberculosis
    B. Cyclophosphamide
    C. Candidiasis
    D. Mycoplasma
11. **The most common clinical presentation of carcinoma of urinary bladder is:**
    A. Dysuria
    B. Painless hematuria
    C. Palpable mass
    D. Intractable pain
12. **Vesicoureteric reflux is usually diagnosed by:**
    A. Intravenous pyelogram
    B. Cystoscopy
    C. Voiding cystourethrogram
    D. Ultrasonography

Answer Key for MCQs

1	2	3	4	5	6	7	8	9	10	11	12
B	A	D	B	D	C	D	B	B	B	B	C

CHAPTER 11 Male Genital System

Learning Objectives

At the end of reading this chapter, the student shall be able to:
- Define cryptorchidism and enlist the common causes with complications.
- Enumerate the common causes for infection of testis and epididymis.
- Classify tumors of testis. Describe the pathogenesis, pathology and clinical features of common testicular tumors.
- Describe the pathogenesis, pathology of prostatic hyperplasia and prostatic carcinoma.
- Describe the preneoplastic conditions, pathology and clinical features of carcinoma of penis.

NORMAL STRUCTURE

The male genital system comprises of testis, epididymis, cord structures, prostate and penis. The testis is composed of seminiferous tubules lined by spermatogenic cells which mature to form spermatozoa and larger Sertoli cells which support the germ cells. The fibrovascular stroma between the tubules is called the interstitium and it contains Leydig cells which secrete male hormones, such as testosterone and androgen **(Fig. 11.1)**.

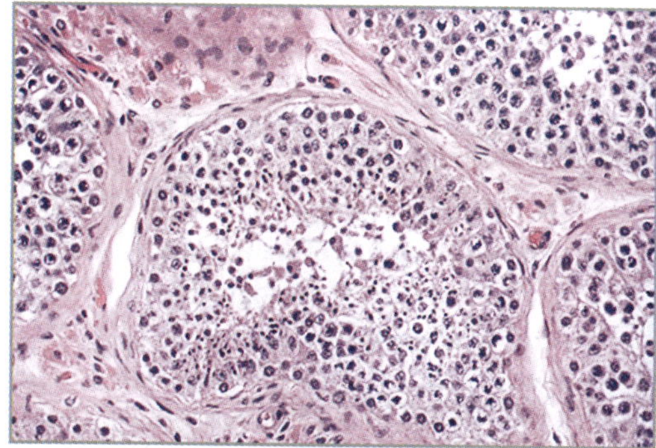

Fig. 11.1: Normal histology of testis with seminiferous tubules.

PATHOLOGY OF MALE GENITAL SYSTEM

The common pathological conditions include the following:
- *Congenital anomalies:* Cryptorchidism
- *Inflammatory conditions:* Tuberculous, filarial
- *Vascular:* Varicocele, torsion of testis, hematocele
- Tumors of testis and epididymis

CRYPTORCHIDISM

(Syn-Undescended Testis)

It is a condition in which the testis is arrested in some point of it descend from the inguinal canal. In 70% of the cases, the testis is seen in the inguinal region, in 25% in the abdomen and the rest 5% in pathway of descend.

Causes for Cryptorchidism

- Genetic factors—Trisomy 13
- Hormonal—deficiency of androgenic hormones
- Mechanical—short spermatic cord, narrow inguinal canal.

It may be unilateral or bilateral. The testis is very small and fibrotic.

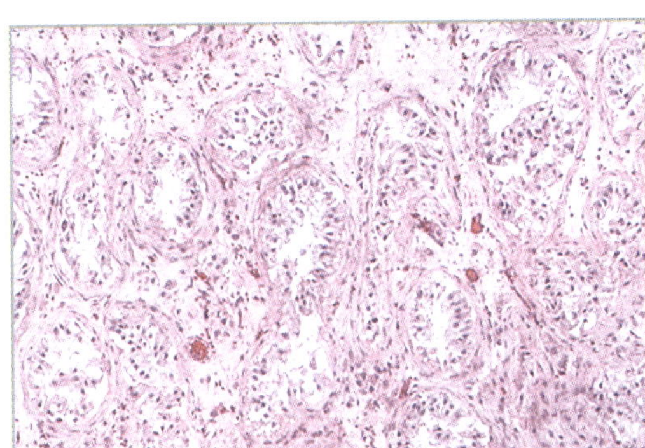

Fig. 11.2: Histomorphology of cryptorchid testis.

Histologically, the seminiferous tubules are lined by very few spermatogenic cells with markedly thickened tubular basement membrane **(Fig. 11.2)**. There is marked interstitial fibrosis. Common clinical manifestations include sterility or infertility. There is an increased incidence of developing malignant germ cell tumors of testis.

EPIDIDYMO-ORCHITIS

Inflammation of testis is called orchitis and of the epididymis is referred to as epididymitis. The common causes for these inflammatory conditions include organisms, such as *Neisseria gonorrhoeae*, *Chlamydia trachomatis*, *Escherichia coli*, *Pseudomonas* and Tuberculous epididymo-orchitis.

Tuberculous infection reaches the epididymis and testis from kidney, prostate and the lungs. The lesions heal with fibrosis and calcification.

TUMORS OF TESTIS

Testicular tumors are one of the common visceral tumors in men. The World Health Organization have classified the tumors according to the cell of origin.

They include:

I. *Germ cell tumors (95%):*
   1. Seminoma
   2. Spermatocytic seminoma
   3. Teratoma
   4. Embryonal carcinoma
   5. Yolk sac tumor
   6. Choriocarcinoma

II. *Sex cord stromal cell tumors (4%):*
   1. Leydig cell tumor
   2. Sertoli cell tumor
   3. Mixed tumors

III. Mixed tumors and others (1%)

Etiopathogenesis

Some of the common predisposing factors include cryptorchidism, dysgenetic cords, mumps orchitis, history of trauma, exposure to carcinogens and radiation.

Pathology

Seminoma is the most common germ cell tumor of testis. The tumor has a peak incidence in fourth decade. It causes uniform diffuse enlargement of the testis. Cut section shows homogenous grayish white mass without necrosis **(Fig. 11.3)**.

Histologically, the tumor is composed of lobules of round to polygonal cells with clear cytoplasm and round to oval nuclei within a fibrovascular stroma with lymphocytic infiltration. They are extremely radiosensitive tumors **(Fig. 11.4)**.

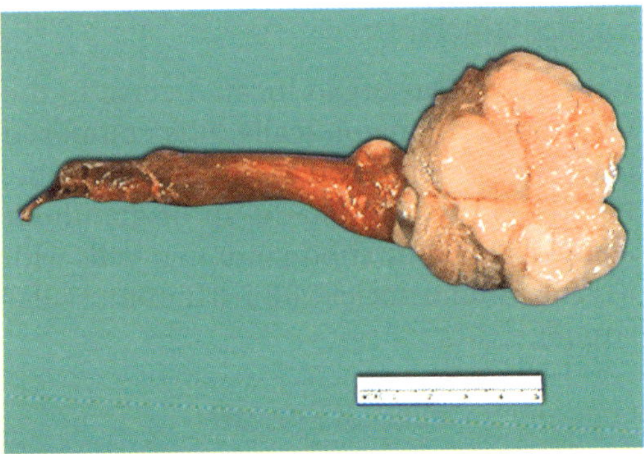

Fig. 11.3: Gross photograph of seminoma testis.

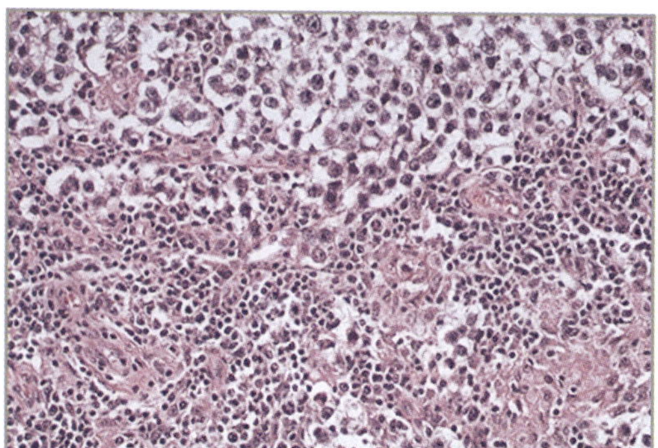

Fig. 11.4: Histomicrograph of seminoma testis.

Clinical Features

The testicular tumors usually present with gradual enlargement of testis with loss of testicular sensation. The tumors spread through the lymphatics to the paraaortic nodes and other nodes and through the blood stream to the lungs, liver, bones and brain.

Diagnosis

Diagnosis of the testicular tumors is made based on clinical and histopathological examination. In addition to the above modalities, there are a number of tumor markers, such as alpha fetoprotein, human placental lactogen and human chorionic gonadotropin are elevated in testicular tumors.

PROSTATE

Normal Structure

It is a glandular organ located close to the male urethra. Anatomically, it is composed of two lateral lobes and a small median lobe. Histologically, it is made up of glandular elements lined by cubo-columnar cells with a regular round nuclei within a fibromuscular stroma.

Common Disorders of Prostate

- *Inflammation:* Acute, chronic and granulomatous prostatitis
- Nodular hyperplasia
- *Tumors:* Adenocarcinoma of prostate

Nodular Hyperplasia of Prostate

It is the most common cause for non-neoplastic enlargement of prostate presenting with difficulty in micturition in elderly men above the age of 60.

Etiology

A number of etiologic causes have been implicated in the pathogenesis. As age advances, there is decline in the level of androgen with a compensatory increase in the level of estrogen which leads to hyperplasia of the glandular elements. Other causes include inflammatory conditions and arteriosclerosis of prostate.

Pathologically, it presents with smooth, firm, nodular enlargement of prostate **(Fig. 11.5)**.

Histologically, there is marked hyperplasia of the glandular elements in the inner periurethral region and hyperplasia of the fibromuscular supporting stroma **(Fig. 11.6)**.

Clinical Features

The person presents with symptoms, such as increased frequency of micturition, nocturia, difficulty in initiation, pain and hematuria

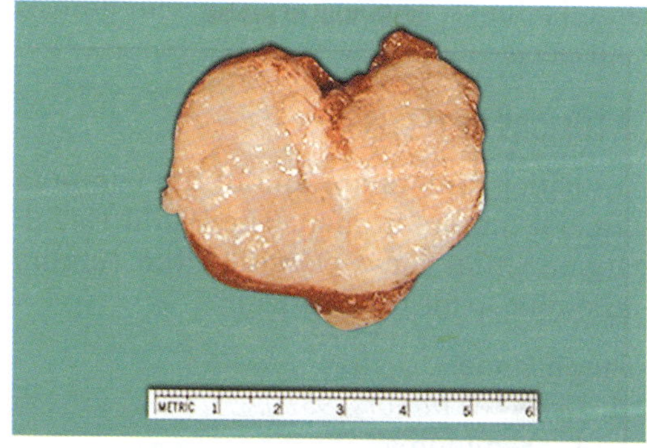

Fig. 11.5: Gross photograph of nodular hyperplasia of prostate.

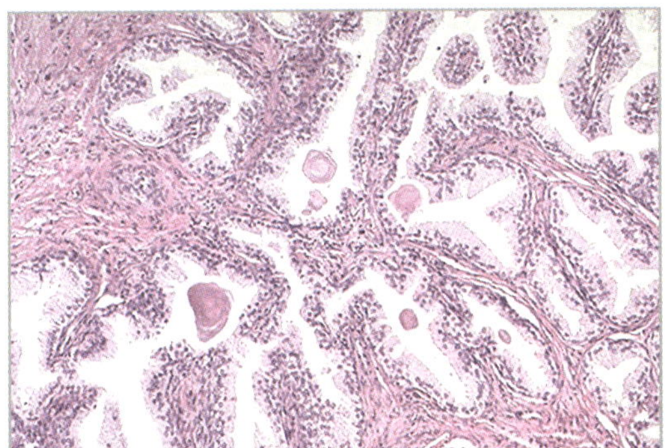

Fig. 11.6: Histomicrograph of benign adenomyomatous hyperplasia of prostate.

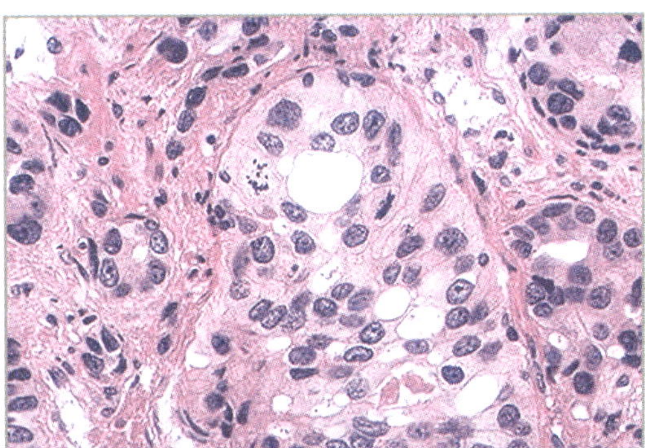

Fig. 11.7: Histomicrograph of adenocarcinoma prostate.

due to urethral obstruction or with symptoms of acute urinary retention and secondary effects, such as bladder hypertrophy, cystitis, hydroureter and hydronephrosis.

CARCINOMA PROSTATE

It is the second most common malignant tumor in men. The prevalence increases with increasing age and the peak incidence occurs between 6 and 8 decade.

Etiological Factors

There are various etiological factors implicated in the pathogenesis of carcinoma prostate. They include increased level of androgens, nodular prostatic hyperplasia of prostate and genetic factors.

Pathology

Grossly, the prostate is enlarged and the tumor is located in the peripheral zone of the prostate. The consistency of the tumor is firm to hard.

Adenocarcinoma is the most common histological pattern of tumor. The tumor is composed of irregular glands lined by cubo-columnar cells with hyperchromatic nuclei infiltrating the fibromuscular stroma **(Fig. 11.7)**.

Spread

The tumor spreads directly to the urinary bladder, seminal vesicle and urethra or spread through the lymphohematogenous route to the regional lymph nodes, pelvic and vertebral bone producing osteoblastic metastasis and to lungs, kidney and brain.

Clinical Features

It presents with urinary obstruction, dysuria, increased frequency, retention of urine and hematuria. In few, the patient presents with severe bone pain due to vertebral metastasis. Diagnosis of prostatic cancer is made from rectal examination of a hard prostate, needle biopsy showing adenocarcinoma and tumor markers, such as prostatic acid phosphatase and prostate specific antigen.

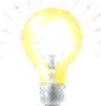

Case Scenario

Mr Z male 65-year-old, visits his primary care physician with complaints of increased frequency of urination, hesitancy, and a sensation of incomplete emptying. He has no significant medical history, but his father was diagnosed with prostate cancer. Digital rectal examination reveals a firm and enlarged prostate, and the prostate-specific antigen (PSA) level is found to be elevated.

Contd...

Contd...

Question:

Considering family history of Mr Z prostate cancer, what additional diagnostic test would be crucial in assessing the likelihood of malignancy?

A. Transrectal ultrasound (TRUS)
B. Magnetic resonance imaging (MRI) of the prostate
C. Urinalysis
D. Uroflowmetry

Answer:

B. Magnetic resonance imaging (MRI) of the prostate

TUMORS OF PENIS

Condyloma acuminatum: It is most common benign tumor of penis caused by human papillomavirus. It presents like an exophytic warty mass in the coronal sulcus of penis. The lesions are histologically made up markedly hyperplastic stratified squamous epithelium with thin walled fibrovascular core.

Squamous cell carcinoma is the most common type of penile carcinoma **(Fig. 11.8)**. There is a wide variation in the incidence of penile cancer in various nations. There are many premalignant lesions of penis which include Bowen's disease, Bowenoid Papulosis and Erythroplasia of Queyrat.

Circumcision provides protection against carcinoma of penis. It occurs in age group of 40–60 years and presents grossly as an exophytic mass with/without ulceration. The tumor spreads along the lymphatic channels to the regional lymph nodes. Hematogenous spread is very rare.

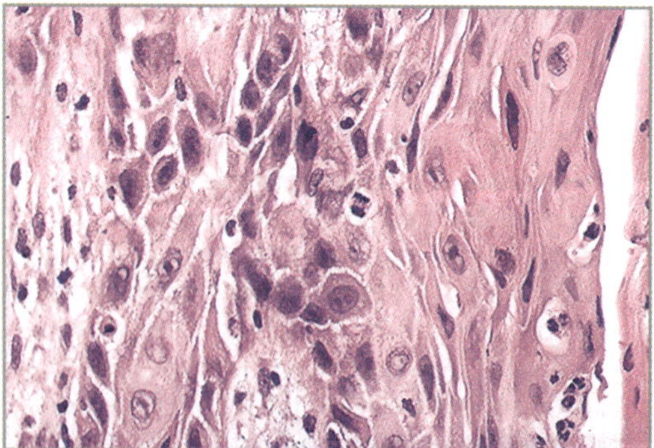

Fig. 11.8: Histomicrograph of squamous cell carcinoma penis.

Points to Ponder

- The male genital system comprises of testis, epididymis, cord structures, prostate and penis.
- Cryptorchidism is a condition in which the testis is arrested in some point of its descend from the inguinal canal.
- Inflammation of testis is called orchitis and of the epididymis is referred to as epididymitis. The common causes for these inflammatory conditions include organisms, such as *Neisseria gonorrhoeae*, *Chlamydia trachomatis*, *Escherichia coli*, *Pseudomonas* and tuberculous epididymo-orchitis.
- Testicular tumors are one of the common visceral tumors in men. The World Health Organization have classified the tumors according to the cell of origin. Seminoma is the most common germ cell tumor of testis. The tumor has a peak incidence in fourth decade.
- Nodular hyperplasia of prostate is the most common cause for non-neoplastic enlargement of prostate presenting with difficulty in micturition in elderly men above the age of 60.
- Carcinoma prostate is the second most common malignant tumor in men. The prevalence increases with increasing age and the peak incidence occurs between 6–8 decade.
- Condyloma accuminatum is most common benign tumor of penis caused by human papillomavirus.
- Squamous cell carcinoma is the most common type of penile carcinoma. There is a wide variation in the incidence of penile cancer in various nations. There are many premalignant lesion of penis which include Bowen's disease, Bowenoid papulosis and erythroplasia of Queyrat.

ASSESSMENT QUESTIONS

Short Answer Questions

1. **Enumerate the common causes for cryptorchidism.**
2. **What are the common microorganisms associated with epididymo-orchitis?**
3. **Classify tumors of testis.**
4. **Describe the gross and microscopic features of seminoma testis.**
5. **Enlist the common premalignant lesions of carcinoma penis.**
6. **What are the common risk factors for carcinoma prostate?**
7. **Name the common testicular tumors seen in prepubertal boys.**
8. **Describe the mode of spread of carcinoma prostate.**

MULTIPLE CHOICE QUESTIONS

1. **All of the following are precancerous lesions of penis, *except*:**
   A. Condyloma accuminatum
   B. Bowen's disease
   C. Bowenoid papulosis
   D. Erythroplasia of Queyrat
2. **Most common germ cell tumor of testis is:**
   A. Embryonal carcinoma
   B. Yolk sac tumor
   C. Seminoma
   D. Teratoma
3. **Condyloma accuminata is caused by:**
   A. HSV-1
   B. HSV-11
   C. HPV 6,11
   D. HIV 1
4. **The most common testicular tumor in young children is:**
   A. Seminoma
   B. Embryonal carcinoma
   C. Teratoma
   D. Yolk sac tumor
5. **Prostatic carcinoma involves________lobe of prostate.**
   A. Anterior
   B. Middle
   C. Posterior
   D. Lateral
6. **Gleason's grading system is used in grading cancer of:**
   A. Prostate
   B. Urinary bladder
   C. Seminal vesicle
   D. Testis

Answer Key for MCQs

1	2	3	4	5	6
A	C	C	D	D	A

CHAPTER 12 Female Genital System

Learning Objectives

At the end of reading this chapter, the student shall be able to:
- Describe the epidemiology, etiology, pathogenesis, pathology, precancerous lesions screening and diagnosis of carcinoma uterine cervix.
- Describe the normal pattern of endometrium.
- Describe the etiopathogenesis, pathology and clinical features of endometrial carcinoma.
- Describe the etiopathogenesis, pathology and clinical features of leiomyoma and adenomyosis.
- Enlist the common types of non-neoplastic cysts of ovary.
- Classify ovarian tumors and describe the etiopathogenesis, pathology and clinical features of carcinoma ovary.
- Classify and describe the lesions of trophoblastic tissue.

ANATOMY OF FEMALE GENITAL TRACT

The normal anatomical structures of the female genital tract include the vulva, vagina, uterine cervix, uterus, ovaries and fallopian tubes with supporting tissues **(Fig. 12.1)**.

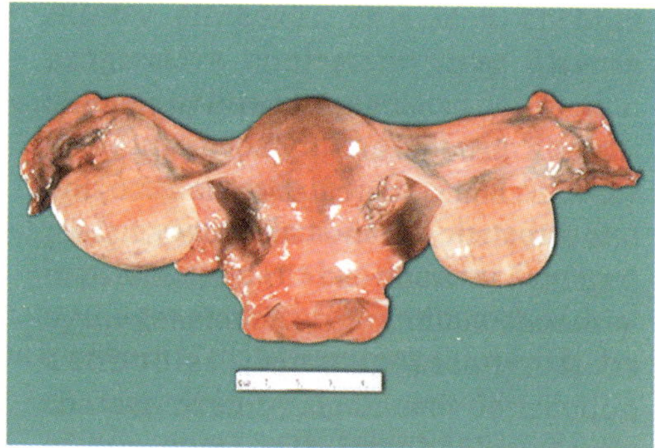

Fig. 12.1: Normal anatomical structures of the female genital tract.

CERVIX

Normal Structure

The cervix is a specialized organ that communicates with the endometrial cavity through the internal os and with that of the vagina through the external os.

It has two histological components, the ectocervix which is the portion of cervix that is exposed to the vagina and it is lined by stratified squamous epithelium. The endocervix is the inner part which is lined by a mucosa composed of tall columnar cells with mucus rich cytoplasm and basally placed regular nuclei. This mucosa is thrown into folds and clefts forming endocervical glands. The junction between the ectocervix and endocervix is called the junctional mucosa or the transitional zone (squamocolumnar junction) **(Fig. 12.2)**.

Pathology of Cervix

Common lesions of cervix: The common pathological lesions of cervix include the following:
- *Inflammatory conditions:* Acute and chronic cervicitis

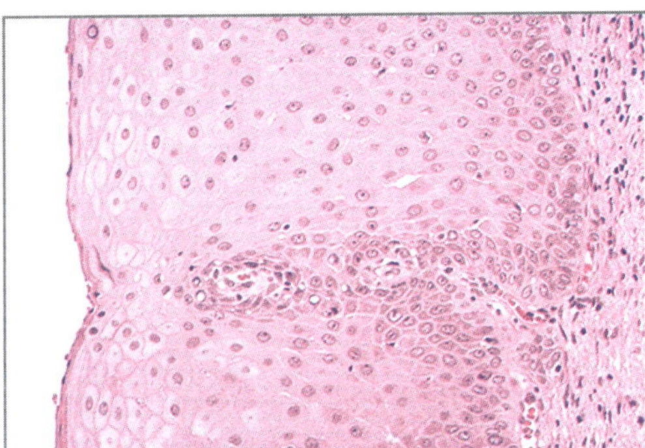

Fig. 12.2: Normal ectocervical mucosa with stratified squamous cells.

- Cervical intraepithelial neoplasia (CIN)
- Invasive carcinoma of cervix

Cervical Intraepithelial Neoplasia

It is one of the important pathological entities of the cervix. It is a lesion that develops gradually and progresses into an invasive carcinoma later. Identification and treatment of these lesions are of great importance in reducing the mortality of invasive carcinoma.

These generally refer to atypical cytological changes seen in the lining stratified squamous epithelium of cervix and they are grade according to the thickness of the mucosa involved **(Fig. 12.3)**.

- *CIN I:* Less than one-third of the thickness of the epithelium is involved (mild dysplasia).

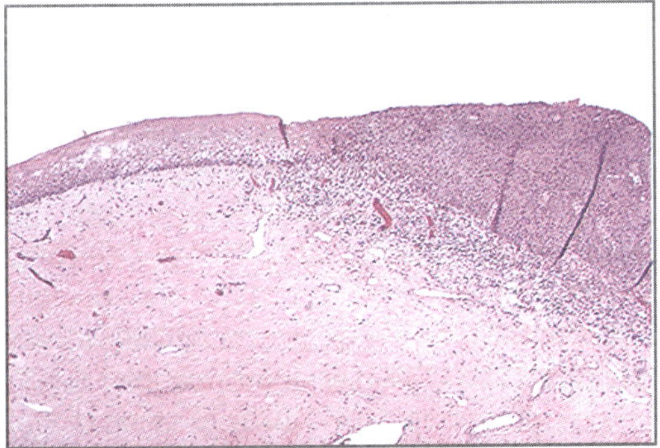

Fig. 12.3: Cervical epithelium showing dysplastic features.

- *CIN II:* More than one-third and less than two-third of the epithelium involved (moderate dysplasia).
- *CIN III:* Full thickness of the epithelium involved without any break in the basement membrane.

The new Bethesda system of classification divides these lesions into two broad categories, the low grade squamous intraepithelial lesion (it includes mild dysplasia and virus induced epithelial changes) and high grade squamous intraepithelial lesion which includes moderate dysplasia and CIN III.

Etiopathogenesis: There are several risk factors associated with the occurrence of cervical intraepithelial neoplasia and subsequent invasive carcinoma. They include:

- Multiparity
- Onset of early age of sexual activity
- Multiple sex partners
- Infection with human papillomavirus (HPV)

Human papillomavirus and cervical cancer: It is one of the well documented example of virus-induced carcinogenesis. There are various subtypes of the virus involved in cervical cancer. HPV types 6 and 11 are called the low-risk types and serotypes 16, 18, 31, 33 and 35 are termed as high-risk types.

Clinical profile: There is no well-defined clinical symptoms associated with CIN. The diagnosis can be suspected on the basis of Schiller's test. In this, Lugol's iodine (a solution of iodine and potassium iodide) is painted in the suspected area. The cancerous foci will fail to stain with this solution as it lacks glycogen. Tissue material can be taken from these sites to confirm the diagnosis. Exfoliative cytologic studies (Pap screening) are extremely useful in tracking the cases of CIN. It is a simple and cost-effective method and can be employed as a mass screening program. The cells are collected using a special Ayre. Spatula and the smears are stained with Papanicolaou stain for the detection of the cytological atypia **(Figs. 12.4A and B)**.

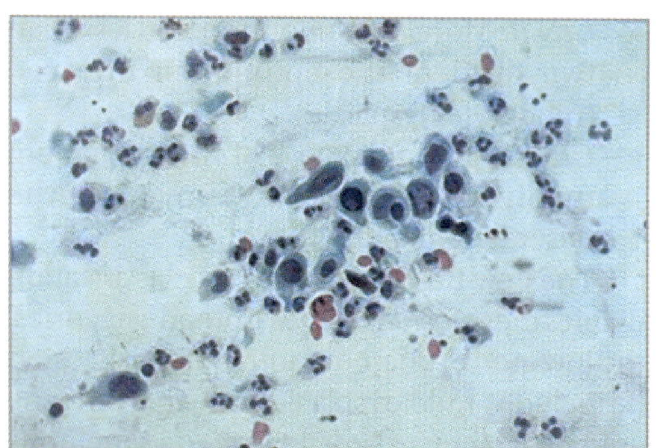

Fig. 12.4A: Exfoliative cytology smear malignancy of cervix (Papanicolaou stain).

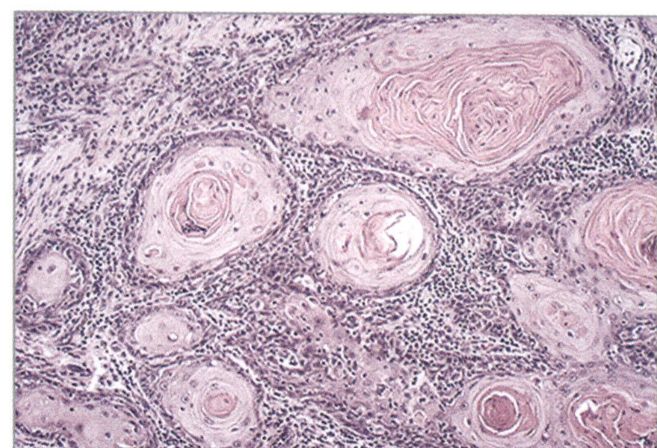

Fig. 12.5: Histomicrograph of invasive squamous cell carcinoma—keratinizing type.

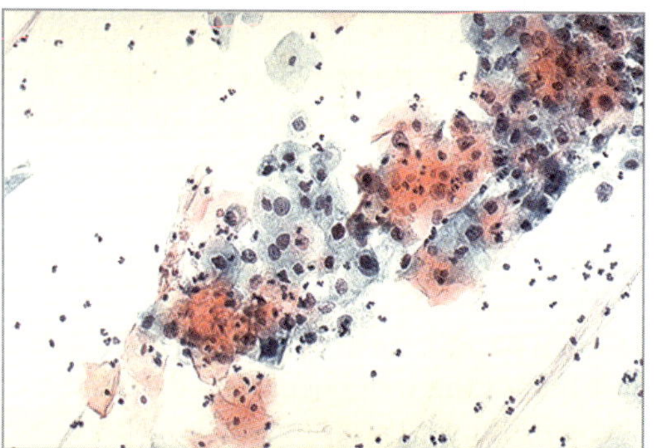

Fig. 12.4B: Exfoliative cytology smear of severe dysplasia of cervix (Papanicolaou stain).

Invasive Cervical Cancer

The incidence of invasive cancer of cervix is coming down both in the developed and developing countries due to the effective cancer screening program and detection of cases at a very early stage of the disease. The peak incidence of cervical cancer is in 4–6 decades of life.

Grossly, it presents like an ulcerative, fungating or infiltrating mass involving the adjacent vaginal wall. The tumor usually arises from the transitional zone and then involves the ectocervix.

Histologically, the most common type of tumor is squamous cell carcinoma. It may be a keratinizing squamous cell carcinoma with the synthesis of keratinizing **(Fig. 12.5)** or non-keratinizing type without keratin. Other histological forms of cervical cancer include adenocarcinoma, small cell carcinoma and adenosquamous carcinoma.

The tumor undergoes a direct spread to the vagina, uterine musculature, urinary bladder and rectum. Involvement of the regional lymph nodes and distant metastasis to lungs, liver and bone marrow are also seen.

Uterus

Normal Structure

It comprises of a lining endometrium and underlying myometrium.

Endometrium

The endometrium is a hormone responsive lining epithelium with the cells showing changes according to the influence of the dominant hormone. The endometrium comprises of glandular epithelium and a supporting stroma **(Fig. 12.6)**.

The glandular epithelium under the influence of estrogen will show proliferative activity in the first half of the menstrual cycle (proliferative phase) and then under the influence of progesterone the glands will show secretory activity during the next half of the menstrual cycle (secretory phase) and it is followed by a menstrual phase characterized

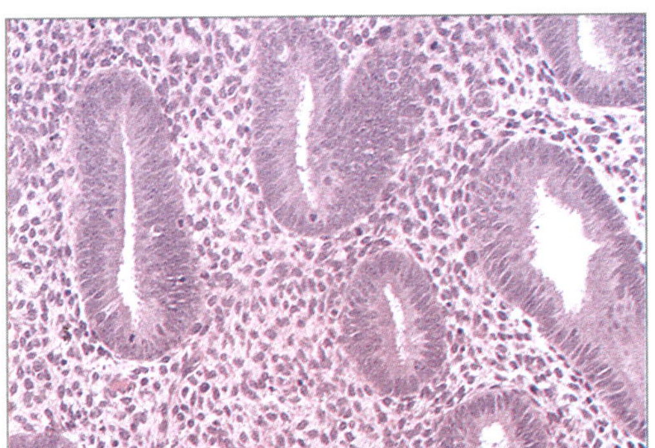

Fig. 12.6: Histomicrograph of normal endometrium with glands and stroma.

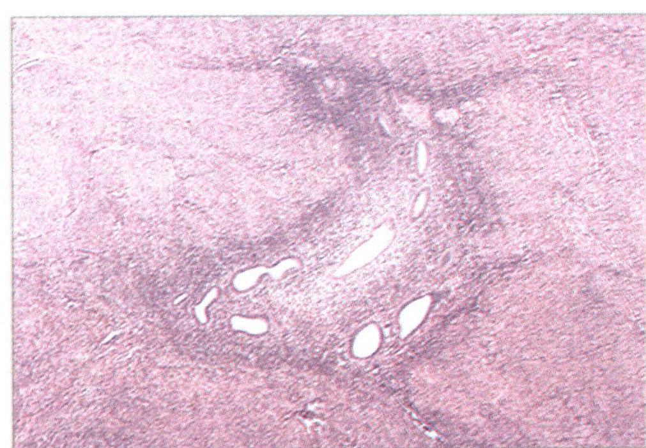

Fig. 12.7: Histomicrograph of adenomyosis of uterus.

by sloughing of the endometrium (menstrual phase). The endometrial stroma is composed of plump spindle to oval cells with round to oval nuclei which appears compact during the proliferative phase and it becomes loose and edematous in the secretory phase of the cycle. During pregnancy, there is an interruption to the menstrual cycle and the endometrial stroma cells become more polygonal with abundant granular cytoplasm and round nuclei, the change referred to as decidual reaction. After menopause, the glands become small and atrophic with a lining by low cuboidal cells and the glands may also show cystic dilatation.

The myometrium is made up of smooth muscle bundles which shows physiological hyperplasia and hypertrophy during pregnancy.

Pathology of Uterus

Common pathological lesions of the uterus include:

- *Inflammatory conditions:* Acute and chronic endometritis
- *Hormone-induced changes:* Dysfunctional uterine bleeding
- Endometrial hyperplasia
- Adenomyosis and endometriosis
- *Tumors:* Endometrial polyp. leiomyoma
- *Malignant lesions:* Endometrial carcinoma, endometrial stromal sarcoma, leiomyosarcoma and others.

Adenomyosis: It is defined as the abnormal presence of the endometrial tissue within the myometrium. It is seen in 20–25% of all the hysterectomy specimens. Grossly, the uterus is enlarged and the cut section shows tiny hemorrhagic spots with prominent trabeculations of the myometrium.

Histologically, it is composed of presence of well-define islands of the endometrial tissue within the myometrium accompanied by hyperplasia of the myometrium **(Fig. 12.7)**. Clinically, it may present with dysfunctional uterine bleeding, polymenorrhea or dysmenorrhea.

Endometriosis: It refers to the presence of the endometrial tissue in extrauterine sites. The most common sites for endometriosis include the ovary, fallopian tubes, uterine ligaments, rectovaginal septum, laparotomy scar (scar endometriosis), umbilicus, vagina, vulva and in the hernial sac.

Pathogenesis: The endometrial tissue may reach these sites through regurgitation from the fallopian tubes or metaplasia of the coelomic epithelium or due to vascular dissemination of the endometrial tissues.

Grossly, the involved tissue shows grayish brown lesions with variable fibrosis. In ovaries they present as a cystic mass greyish brown in color and are referred to as the chocolate cysts of ovary **(Fig. 12.8)**. Histologically, it shows

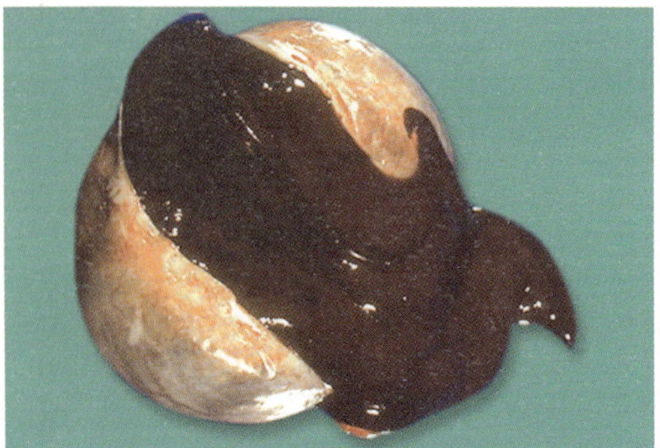

Fig. 12.8: Gross photograph of chocolate cyst of ovary (endometriosis of ovary).

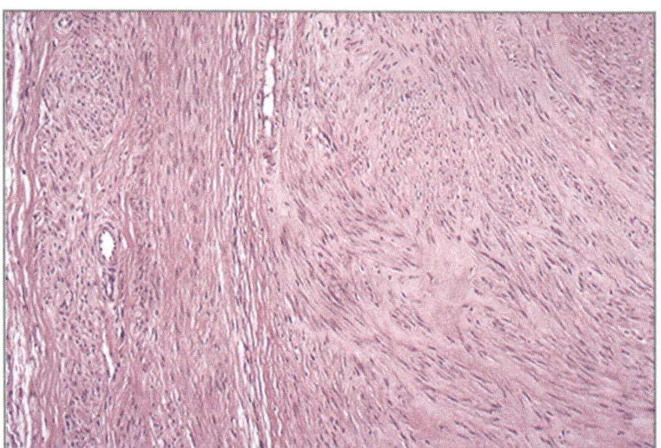

Fig. 12.10: Histomicrograph of leiomyoma, composed of interlacing smooth muscle cells.

functioning endometrial tissue with stroma, areas of hemorrhage and areas of fibrosis.

Leiomyoma: This is the most common benign smooth muscle tumor of the myometrium. It is conventionally referred to as the fibroid tumor. These tumors are located well within the myometrium (intramural leiomyoma), beneath the serosa (subserosal leiomyoma), underneath the mucosa (submucosal leiomyoma). Rarely, the leiomyomas may present as polypoidal masses with a long stalk.

Grossly, it may be single or multiple, well circumscribed, firm nodular masses located within the uterine musculature. The cut section of these tumor shows a whorled appearance **(Fig. 12.9)**.

Histologically, it is made up of interlacing fascicles of spindle-shaped smooth muscle cells with short blunted cigar-shaped nuclei with scanty stromal tissue **(Fig. 12.10)**. The stroma may show varying patterns of degeneration, such as hyaline change, cystic change, calcification, ischemic change and vascular degeneration (red degeneration of leiomyoma). The red degeneration is common during leiomyoma occurring in pregnant uterus.

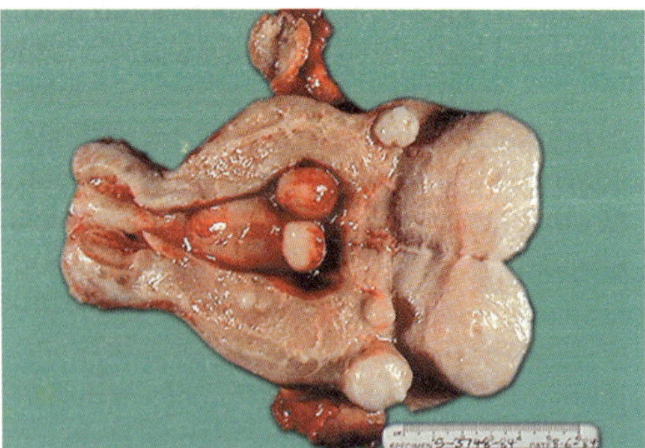

Fig. 12.9: Gross photomicrograph of multiple leiomyomata uterus.

Clinically, this is a silent tumor and rarely present with features of dysfunctional uterine bleeding, dysmenorrhea, polymenorrhea, abdominal pain and it may be a cause for female infertility. Less than 0.5% of these tumors undergo malignant transformation to a leiomyosarcoma.

Endometrial carcinoma: It is one of the common malignancies of the female genital tract next to cervical and ovarian cancers. It is seen in women of 5–7th decade of life. The common risk factors include the following:

- Excessive estrogen secretion
- Obesity
- Hypertension
- Diabetes mellitus
- *Endometrial hyperplasia:* The atypical form of endometrial hyperplasia has a higher prevalence of progressing into an invasive carcinoma.

Grossly, it presents like a soft friable grayish tan polypoidal mass rarely extending into the cervical canal.

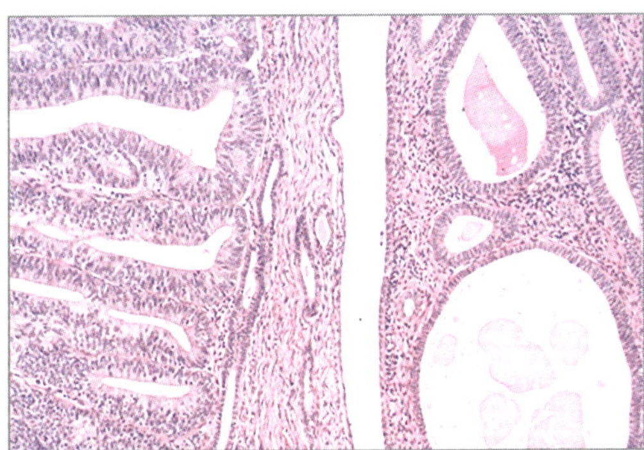

Fig. 12.11: Histomicrograph of endometrial adenocarcinoma.

Histologically, it is an adenocarcinoma composed of closely packed irregular glands lined by irregularly stratified cubo-columnar cells with hyperchromatic nuclei. The tumor infiltrates into the underlying myometrium **(Fig. 12.11)**. The tumor can undergo a local spread to the cervix, vagina, pelvic peritoneum and a lymphohematogenous spread to the regional lymph nodes, lung, liver and bones. Common clinical findings include abnormal uterine bleeding with pain abdomen.

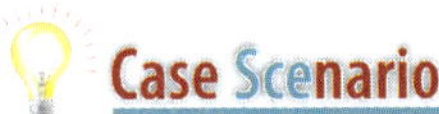

A female patient, a 45-year-old, presents to her gynecologist with complaints of heavy menstrual bleeding and pelvic pain. She reports irregular menstrual cycles and has a history of obesity. Pelvic ultrasound reveals thickening of the endometrium.

Question:

Based on presented symptoms and imaging findings, what condition should be considered as a primary concern?

A. Endometriosis
B. Uterine fibroids
C. Endometrial hyperplasia
D. Ovarian cysts

Answer:

A. Endometrial hyperplasia.

Ovaries

Normal structure: The ovaries are paired organ close to the fallopian tubes. Each ovary measures 3 cm in length and 2 cm in breadth. Histologically, it has a covering by the coelomic epithelium with underlying cortex and medulla. The coelomic epithelium is composed of low cuboidal to columnar cells which is referred to as the surface epithelium. The cortex is made up of numerous follicles. Each follicle contains as central germ cell ovum surrounded by specialized stromal cells called the granulosa cells and the theca cells. These cells secrete estrogen which helps in the development of the follicle and a fully mature follicle is called the Graafian follicle. This Graafian follicle bursts to release the ovum and gets transformed into corpus luteum. The medulla is made up of numerous blood vessels, lymphatics and nerve bundles.

Pathology of ovaries: The common pathological lesions of ovary include the following:

- Non-neoplastic cysts
- Tumors of ovary

Non-neoplastic cysts of ovary: These are one of the most common pathological lesions seen in the ovary. They include:

- Follicular cysts—lined by the granulosa cells. They are usually multiple cysts filled with clear serous fluid seen in the ovarian cortex.
- Luteal cysts—lined by the luteal cells. The wall of these cyst is corrugated and cerebriform and contains yellowish luteal tissue.
- Polycystic ovary disease: It is a characterized by the presence of numerous tiny cysts involving both the ovaries with abundant hyperplastic stroma.

Histologically, the cysts are lined by granulosa cells and represent follicles of varying stages of maturation without formation of corpus luteum **(Fig. 12.12)**. The most common clinical presentation of polycystic ovarian disease is oligomenorrhea, anovulation, infertility, hirsutism and obesity in young women. These patients have a low follicle stimulating hormone levels.

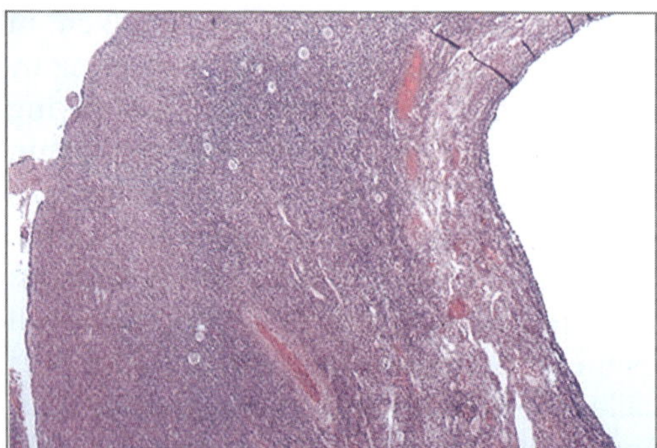

Fig. 12.12: Histomicrograph of polycystic ovarian disease.

Tumors of ovary: The tumors of ovary are one of the common tumors of the female genital tract and they are classified according to the cell of origin of the tumors. The classification is as follows:

- Surface epithelial tumors
- Germ cell tumors
- Sex cord stromal cell tumors
- Others
- Surface epithelial tumors (70–80%):
  - Serous tumors:
    - Serous cystadenoma **(Fig. 12.13)**
    - Borderline serous tumor
    - Serous cystadenocarcinoma
  - Mucinous tumors:
    - Mucinous cystadenoma
    - Borderline mucinous tumors
    - Mucinous cystadenocarcinoma

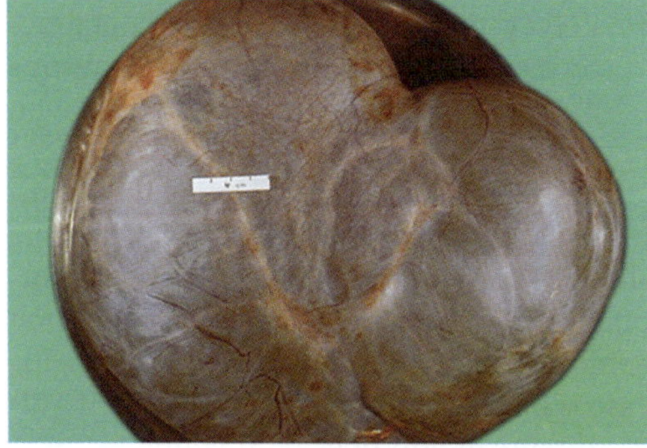

Fig. 12.13: Gross photomicrograph of serous cystic tumor of ovary.

  - Endometrioid tumors
  - Clear cell tumors
  - Brenner and transitional cell tumors
- Germ cell tumors (15–20%):
  - Teratoma: Benign mature, immature, malignant transformation, monodermal specialized teratoma
  - Dysgerminoma
  - Yolk sac tumor
  - Choriocarcinoma
  - Embryonal carcinoma and others
- Sex cord stromal cell tumors (5%):
  - Granulosa cell tumor
  - Fibroma thecoma
  - Sertoli-Leydig cell tumor
- Metastatic tumors (1%)

Clinical features: In general, the benign ovarian tumors are more common. It occurs in age group of 20–40 years. Primary malignant ovarian tumors are common between 4 and 60 years of age. They produce abdominal pain, discomfort, ascites, menstrual irregularities or hormone-induced changes as in certain functional ovarian tumors (granulosa cell tumor secreting estrogen).

Surface epithelial tumors: They constitute the largest number of ovarian tumors (60–70% of benign tumos and 90% of malignant tumors). They have a prominent cystic component and presence of definite solid areas is indicative of malignant change. Benign tumors have a well oriented lining epithelium with papillary projections and no stromal invasion. The borderline tumors have stratification of the lining cells without any stromal invasion **(Fig. 12.14)**. In malignant tumors, there is marked atypia of the lining cells with obvious stromal invasion.

Germ cell tumors : These tumors arise from the germ cells. Around 90% of these tumors are benign. They occur in younger age group. The most common tumor in this category is benign cystic teratoma.

Benign cystic teratoma: It is a tumor which arises from totipotent cells and comprises

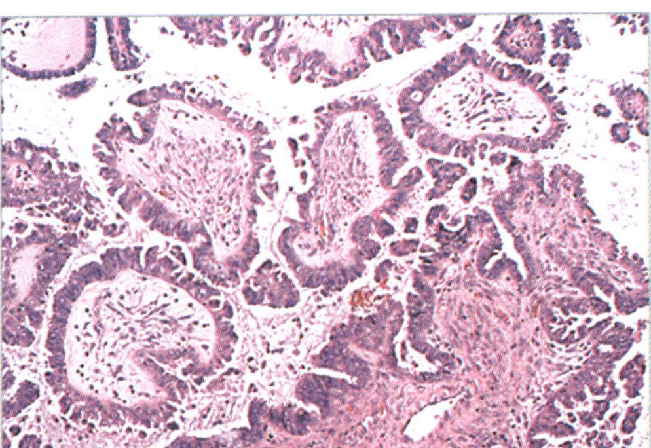

Fig. 12.14: Histomicrograph of serous papillary cystadenocarcinoma ovary.

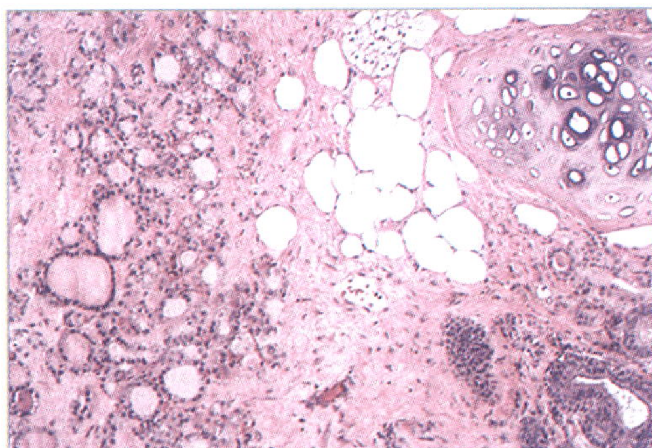

Fig. 12.16: Histomicrograph of benign cystic teratoma.

of elements from more than one germ layer (ectoderm, mesoderm and endoderm). They are conventionally referred to as the dermoid cysts.

Grossly, they present as a cystic mass and the cut section shows paste, such as material, hair tufts, teeth and bony prominences **(Fig. 12.15)**.

Histologically, it is composed of stratified squamous epithelium with adnexal structures and well-defined glandular epithelium, cartilage and bony tissue **(Fig. 12.16)**. The immature teratoma is used to denote a teratoma with immature neurological elements. These tumors are generally solid in contrast to the cystic benign teratoma. Monodermal teratoma is another variant of teratoma which is composed of a single tissue. The most common among this is a teratoma made up of thyroid tissue referred to as struma ovarii.

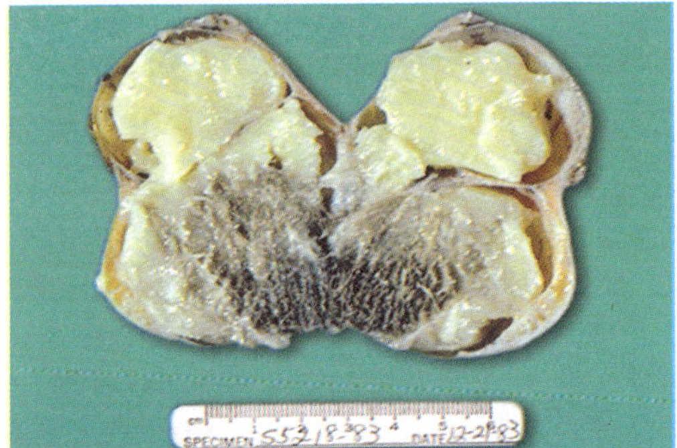

Fig. 12.15: Gross photomicrograph of benign cystic teratoma with hair and pultaceous material.

Dysgerminoma—is the next common germ cell tumor of ovary and it is the female counterpart of seminoma of testis and histologically resembles the tumor.

Sex cord stromal tumors: They constitute around 5% of the ovarian tumors. They arise from specialized stromal cells and most of these tumor will elaborate steroidal hormones and so these tumors are functional in nature. They include the granulosa cell tumor which presents with symptoms of excessive estrogen, such as endometrial hyperplasia, endometrial carcinoma of secretion of androgen, such as substance causes hirsutism, masculinizing effect and others.

Metastatic tumors: Ovaries are involved as a site for metastasis. The tumor cells can reach the ovaries through the lymphohematogenous route of through the transcoelomic spread. The most common primary sites include breast, stomach and hematopoietic malignancies. The metastatic tumors are often bilateral. A distinctive form of metastatic ovarian tumor is Krukenberg tumor which is characterized by the presence of mucin filled signet ring cells. The primary is usually a gastric carcinoma or a breast malignancy.

Trophoblastic diseases: Disease relating to placenta and pregnancy are numerous. Gestational trophoblastic diseases are the one which results from benign or malignant proliferation of the trophoblastic cells. The most common ones are the hydatidiform mole (vesicular mole) and choriocarcinoma.

Hydatidiform mole: It is a condition characterized by the presence of marked hydropic change of the chorionic villi and proliferation of the trophoblastic cells. The incidence of molar pregnancy is common in teen age pregnancies and in elderly primi. Grossly, the uterus is enlarged disproportional to the gestational week with the endometrial cavity showing multiple grapes, such as vesicles **(Fig. 12.17)**.

Histologically, it is made up of large edematous avascular chorionic villi with focal trophoblastic proliferation **(Fig. 12.18)**. Clinically, it presents in 4–5 months of gestation with abnormal uterine bleeding. The serum human chorionic gonadotropin levels are higher than that of the normal pregnancy.

Partial mole: It is a variation of the complete mole in which the uterus is smaller and contains only a few vesicles. Most often a non-viable fetus can be seen in association with this condition.

Choriocarcinoma: It is a highly malignant gestational trophoblastic tumor with widespread rapid metastasis. This may occur following an hydatidiform mole, spontaneous abortion, ectopic pregnancy or rarely after a normal pregnancy. Clinically, it presents with abnormal vaginal bleeding with marked elevation of the serum human chorionic gonadotropin levels. It undergoes rapid metastatic spread through the hematogenous route to the lungs and brain. Other sites include kidneys, vagina, and liver.

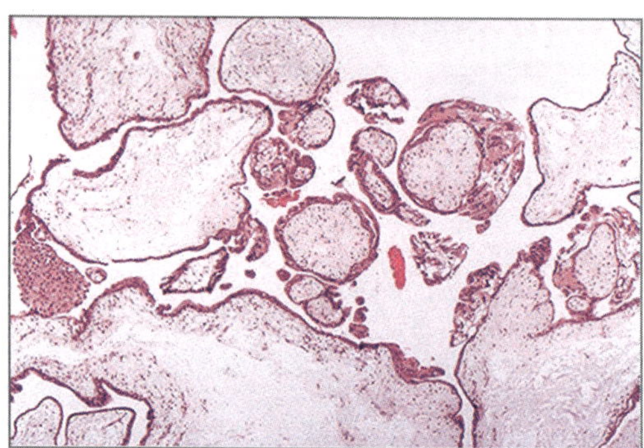

Fig. 12.18: Histomicrograph of hydropic degeneration of chorionic villi.

Grossly the tumor is a hemorrhagic soft fleshy friable mass with wide spread hemorrhagic areas. Histologically, it is made up of clumps of anaplastic cells with no demonstrable chorionic villi. There are wide areas of hemorrhage and necrosis. A proportion of choriocarcinoma can occur without any relation to the gestation (non-gestational choriocarcinoma) **(Fig. 12.19)**. They are seen in the testis, ovaries, mediastinum and other sites.

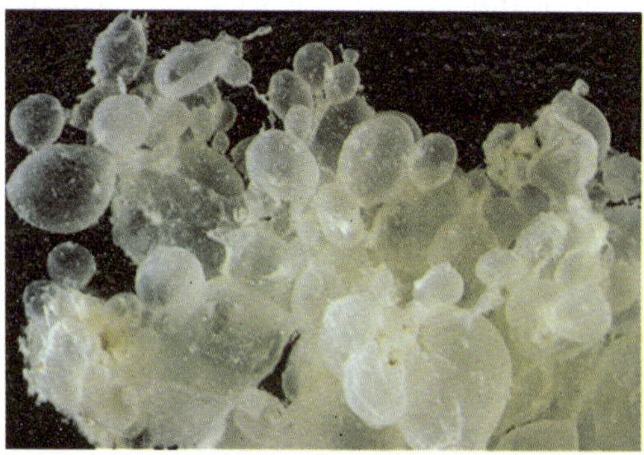

Fig. 12.17: Vesicular mole with multiple grapes, such as vesicles.

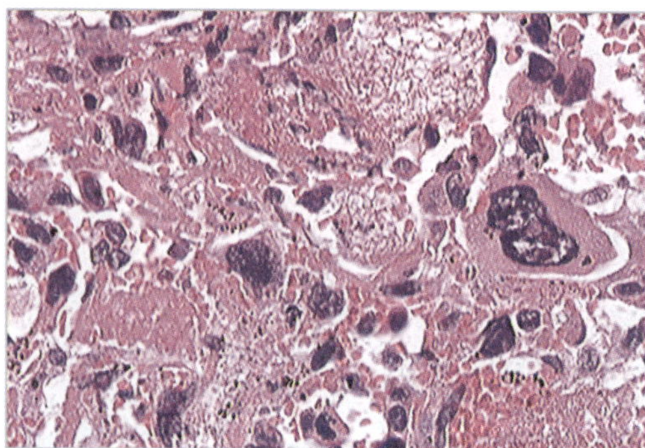

Fig. 12.19: Histomicrograph of choriocarcinoma with highly pleomorphic tumor cells.

Points to Ponder

- The normal anatomical structures of the female genital tract includes the vulva, vagina, uterine cervix, uterus, ovaries and fallopian tubes with supporting tissues.
- The common pathological lesions of cervix include acute and chronic cervicitis, cervical intraepithelial neoplasia and invasive carcinoma of cervix.
- Human papilloma virus is one of the well documented example of virus-induced carcinogenesis. There are various subtypes of the virus involved in cervical cancer. HPV types 6 and 11 are called the low-risk types and serotypes 16, 18, 31, 33 and 35 are termed as high-risk types.
- Exfoliative cytologic studies (Pap screening) are extremely useful in tracking the cases of CIN.
- Adenomyosis defined as the abnormal presence of the endometrial tissue within the myometrium. Endometriosis refers to the presence of the endometrial tissue in extrauterine sites.The most common sites for endometriosis includes the ovary, fallopian tubes.
- Leiomyoma is the most common benign smooth muscle tumor of the myometrium. It is conventionally referred to as the fibroid tumor
- Endometrial carcinoma is one of the common malignancies of the female genital tract next to cervical and ovarian cancers. It is seen in women of 5–7th decade of life.
- The common pathological lesions of ovary include the following non-neoplastic cysts and tumors of ovary.
- The tumors of ovary are one of the common tumors of the female genital tract and they are classified according to the cell of origin of the tumors.
- Disease relating to placenta and pregnancy are numerous. Gestational trophoblastic diseases are the one which results from benign or malignant proliferation of the trophoblastic cells. The most common ones are the hydatidiform mole (vesicular mole) and choriocarcinoma.

ASSESSMENT QUESTIONS

Essay Type Questions

1. **A 60-year-old post-menopausal women was seen in the OPD with foul smelling discharge per vaginum. She was anemic and cachectic. On examination, she had a friable ulcerated growth involving the uterine cervix.**
   a. What is your provisional diagnosis ?
   b. Describe in detail the etiopathogenesis and pathology of this condition.
   c. How will you arrive at a diagnosis in this case?
2. **Classify tumors of ovary. Discuss in detail the pathology of the germ cell tumors of ovary.**

Self Assessment Questions

1. **What are the common risk factors associated with carcinoma uterine cervix?**
2. **Define endometriosis. Enlist the common sites for endometriosis.**
3. **Name the screening methods available for the early detection of carcinoma cervix.**
4. **Define adenomyosis.**
5. **Enlist the common predisposing factors for carcinoma endometrium.**
6. **Name the two hormones produced by syncytiotrophoblast.**
7. **Name the common metastatic sites for choriocarcinoma.**

MULTIPLE CHOICE QUESTIONS

1. **Most common site for endometriosis is:**
   A. Ovary
   B. Fallopian tube
   C. Broad ligament
   D. Pouch of Douglas
2. **Chocolate cyst of ovary is a type of:**
   A. Follicle cyst
   B. Luteal cyst
   C. Mucinous cyst
   D. Endometriotic cyst
3. **The most common benign tumor of uterus is:**
   A. Rhabdomyoma
   B. Stromal nodule
   C. Leiomyoma
   D. Fibroma
4. **Psammoma bodies are commonly seen in:**
   A. Mucinous carcinoma
   B. Clear cell carcinoma
   C. Brenner tumor
   D. Serous papillary carcinoma
5. **Most common histological type of teratoma is:**
   A. Benign
   B. Immature
   C. Struma ovarii
   D. Teratoma with malignant transformation
6. **Most common site for ectopic gestation is:**
   A. Fallopian tube
   B. Ovary
   C. Intra-abdominal
   D. Cornua
7. **The most common genetic anomaly is complete vesicular mole is:**
   A. Diandrogenesis
   B. Aneuploidy
   C. Non-disjunction
   D. Tetraploidy
8. **Most common site for metastasis of choriocarcinoma is:**
   A. Liver
   B. Lungs
   C. Bone
   D. Brain
9. **The histological indicator for ovulation in an endometrial biopsy is:**
   A. Prominent spiral arteriole
   B. Subnuclear vacuolations
   C. Stromal edema
   D. Stromal neutrophils
10. **Prominent spiral arterioles are seen in—phase of menstrual cycle:**
    A. Early secretory
    B. Mid secretory
    C. Late secretory
    D. Early proliferative
11. **Dermoid cyst is a type of:**
    A. Mucinous cyst
    B. Functional cyst
    C. Mature teratoma
    D. Monodermal teratoma
12. **The most common causes for hematosalpinx is:**
    A. Endometriosis
    B. Torsion
    C. Ectopic gestation
    D. Pelvic inflammatory disease

Answer Key for MCQs

1	2	3	4	5	6	7	8	9	10	11	12
A	D	C	D	A	A	A	B	B	C	C	C

CHAPTER

Breast

Learning Objectives

At the end of reading this chapter, the student shall be able to:
- Classify and describe epidemiology, pathogenesis, morphology, pathology, prognostic features and spread of carcinoma breast.

CARCINOMA OF BREAST

It is one of the most common cancers seen in women next to cancer of uterine cervix. The incidence and mortality are on a rise both in the developed and developing nations. This is more common in the perimenopausal age group.

Etiopathogenesis

The exact etiological factor leading to carcinogenesis is unclear. But a large number of risk factors have been identified. They include:

- *Genetic factors:* Family history—cancer breast is more common in women with the first degree relative, such as mother and sister having cancer breast.
  Mutations in *BRCA 1* gene located in chromosome 12, *BRCA 2* gene in chromosome 13 and p53 antioncogene.
- *Hormonal factors:* Unopposed excessive estrogen levels are commonly associated with breast cancers. This occurs in conditions, such as:
  - Early menarche
  - Late menopause
  - Elderly primi (women with first childbirth at a late age more than 30)
  - Estrogen replacement therapy
  - Estrogen producing tumors of ovary
- *Dietary factors:* They have less common association. The factors include intake of large amounts of animal fat and high calorie food, smoking and alcoholism.
- *Underlying breast lesions:* Patients presenting with fibrocystic lesion with atypical duct epithelial hyperplasia are at the risk of developing carcinoma breast and the incidence is directly proportional to the degree of atypia.

Classification

Carcinoma of breast is more common in left breast than the right. It more commonly involves the upper outer quadrant of the breast. The cancer may be rarely bilateral (less than 4%).

Most of the carcinoma arises from the ductal epithelium (ductal carcinoma) and a smaller portion arise from the lobular units (lobular carcinoma).

Based on the pattern of infiltration the tumors are again grouped into non-invasive (intraductal) and invasive carcinoma.

Some of the common tumors are listed below:

- *Non-invasive cancer:*
  - Ductal carcinoma in situ
  - Lobular carcinoma in situ

- *Invasive cancers:*
  - Invasive ductal carcinoma (not otherwise specified)
  - Invasive lobular carcinoma
  - Medullary carcinoma
  - Colloid/mucinous carcinoma
  - Papillary carcinoma
  - Tubular carcinoma
  - Inflammatory carcinoma
  - Secretory carcinoma
  - Other rarer types

Pathological Features

Grossly, the tumor present as an irregular grayish white friable mass of varying sizes with irregular infiltrative margins. The consistency is firm to hard. In cases of medullary and mucinous carcinomas, the mass is well circumscribed with soft fleshy cut surface. The tumor mass may infiltrate the underlying chest wall and overlying skin. This produces puckering of the skin with retraction of the nipple. In some cases, the mass may ulcerate and present grossly as an irregular fungating mass.

Histologically, the tumor is made up of ductal cells with variable degree of cellular and nuclear pleomorphism with cells forming solid nests, cords, trabeculae, and well-defined glandular structures (**Fig. 13.1**). The cells if invasive lobular carcinoma presents with Indian file pattern in which the tumor cells are arranged in a row of targetoid pattern in which the cells are arranged around a ductule. The stroma is usually desmoplastic (**Fig. 13.2**). In certain types of breast cancer like that of the medullary, the cells are large and polygonal with the stroma showing dense lymphoplasmacytic infiltration. In mucinous carcinoma, there are pools of extracellular mucin.

The tumor cells may show invasion of the lymphatic spaces and perineural spaces.

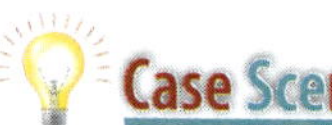

Case Scenario

A 40-year-old woman presents to her primary care physician with a lump in her left breast that she discovered during a self-breast examination. She reports no family history of breast cancer but has noticed changes in the size and shape of the lump over the past few weeks. On physical examination, a firm, immobile mass is palpable in the upper outer quadrant of her left breast.

Question:

Based on woman presentation, what is the most appropriate initial diagnostic imaging modality to assess the breast lump?

A. Magnetic resonance imaging (MRI)
B. Mammography
C. Ultrasound
D. Computed tomography (CT) scan

Answer:

B. Mammography.

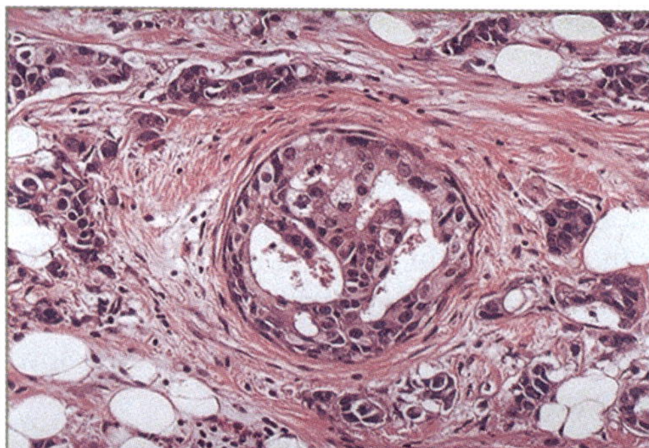

Fig. 13.1: Histomicrograph of invasive ductal carcinoma breast.

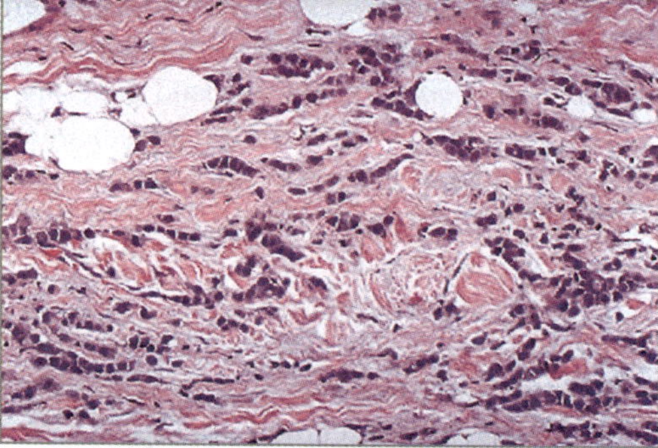

Fig. 13.2: Histomicrograph of invasive lobular carcinoma.

Spread of Breast Cancer

The breast cancer usually spreads through the lymphatic channels to produce enlargement of the regional lymph nodes mostly the axillary nodes followed by internal mammary nodes and others (**Fig. 13.3**). The tumor may also undergo a hematogenous dissemination to opposite breast, lungs, liver, bone, ovaries and brain.

Clinical Profile and Diagnosis

Clinically carcinoma breast presents with a painless, solitary, palpable mass firm to hard in consistency in one of the quadrants of breast. In the initial stages, the mass is mobile and in advanced disease the mass in fixed to the underlying chest wall or the overlying skin with ulceration and fungation. The nipple and areola may be normal or appear retracted due to tumor infiltration. Examination of both sided axillary region for palpable lymph nodes and opposite breast is very much essential.

Diagnosis

The diagnosis of carcinoma breast can be made by the following modalities:

- Clinical examination
- Mammography
- Fine needle aspiration cytology (**Figs. 13.4 and 13.5**)

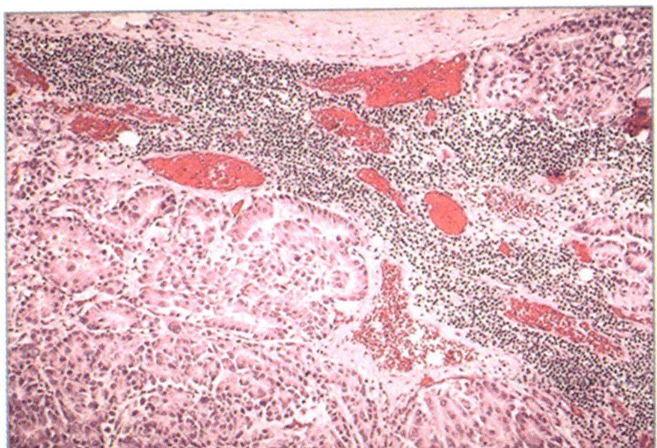

Fig. 13.3: Histomicrograph showing metastatic tumor deposits in axillary lymph node.

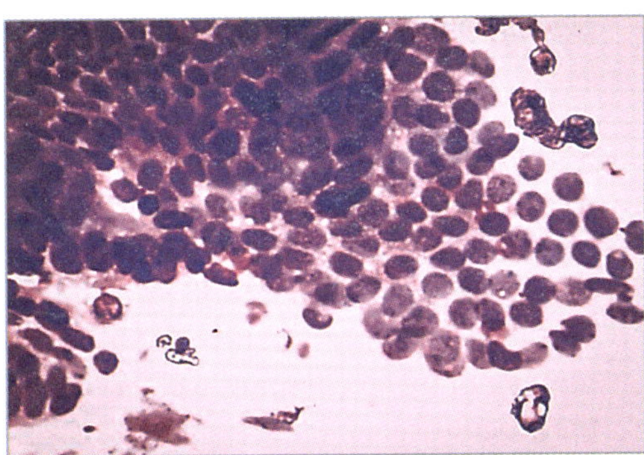

Fig. 13.4: Fine needle aspiration cytology of fibroadenoma (uniform cells).

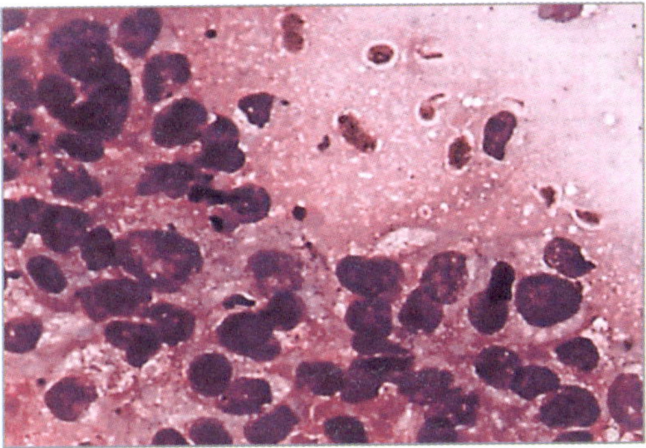

Fig. 13.5: Fine needle aspiration cytology of ductal carcinoma (pleomorphic cells).

- Intraoperative imprint cytology
- Stereotactic biopsy
- Frozen section
- Excision biopsy

Prognostic Factors

There are various prognostic factors which could predict the behavior of the tumor. They include:

- *Histological type of the tumor:* Generally intraductal and lobular carcinoma, medullary carcinoma, papillary carcinoma, tubular carcinoma has a better prognosis when compared with the others.
- *Histological grade of the tumor:* The breast cancers can be histologically grade into three grades I, II, and III based on the formation of tubules, cellular

pleomorphism and mitotic count. This is called the Scarf Modification of the Bloom and Richardson's Grading system. Grade I tumors have a better prognosis.

- *Axillary node status:* This is a single most common factor influencing the prognosis. The survival rate depends on the number and level of nodes involved. More the number of involved nodes worser will be the prognosis.
- *Other factors:* Tumor size, clinical stage of the disease, etc.
- *Estrogen and progesterone receptors in breast cancer:* Evaluating the presence of estrogen and progesterone receptors is of therapeutic importance in breast cancers.

  Tumors which are positive for estrogen receptors are sensitive for subsequent therapy when compared with estrogen negative tumors (**Fig. 13.6**).

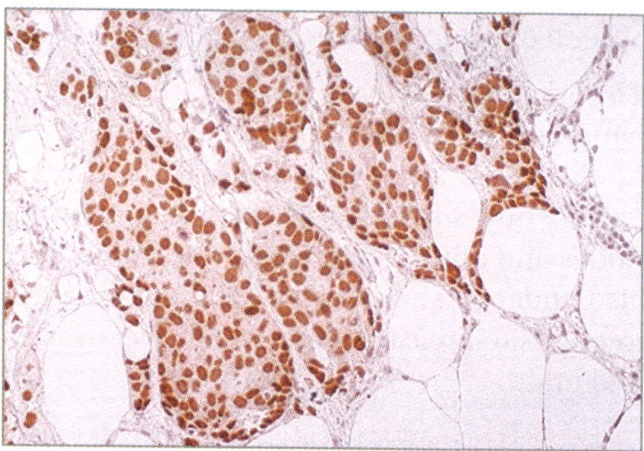

Fig. 13.6: Ductal carcinoma positive for estrogen receptors.

- Assessment of the biological indicators such as mitotic index, AgNORs, DNA ploidy, tumor angiogenesis, Her 2 neu levels, cathepsin D levels also contribute to the evaluation of prognosis.

Points to Ponder

- Carcinoma breast is one of the most common cancers seen in women next to cancer of uterine cervix. A large number of risk factors have been identified including genetic and hormonal causes.
- Most of the carcinoma arises from the ductal epithelium and a smaller portion arise from the lobular units.
- Based on the pattern of infiltration, the tumors are again grouped into non-invasive intraductal carcinoma and invasive carcinoma.
- The breast cancer usually spreads through the lymphatic channels to produce enlargement of the regional lymph nodes mostly the axillary nodes followed by internal mammary nodes and others.
- The diagnosis of carcinoma breast can be made by clinical examination with other laboratory investigations, such as mammography, fine needle aspiration cytology.
- Stereotactic Tru cut biopsy and excision biopsy.
- There are various prognostic factors which could predict the behavior of the tumor which include the histological type, grade, stage of the disease and hormone receptor status.

ASSESSMENT QUESTIONS

1. **Enumerate the common predisposing factors for carcinoma breast.**
2. **How do you broadly classify carcinoma breast?**
3. **Name the common prognostic indicators for a case of carcinoma breast.**
4. **Enlist the common immunohistochemical markers used in the evaluation of carcinoma breast.**
5. **Name the most common oncogenes involved in carcinoma breast.**

MULTIPLE CHOICE QUESTIONS

1. **The most common histological type of breast carcinoma is:**
   A. Invasive ductal NOS type
   B. Medullary
   C. Tubular
   D. Cribriform
2. **Presence of tumor cells in an Indian file pattern is typical of:**
   A. Invasive lobular carcinoma
   B. Medullary carcinoma
   C. Papillary carcinoma
   D. Cribriform carcinoma
3. **One of the following breast tumor is frequently bilateral:**
   A. Invasive lobular carcinoma
   B. Medullary carcinoma
   C. Papillary carcinoma
   D. Cribriform carcinoma
4. **All of the following are referred to as triple markers for breast cancer, *except*:**
   A. Estrogen receptor
   B. Her 2 neu
   C. Progesterone receptor
   D. E-cadherin
5. **The single most important prognostic marker for breast carcinoma is:**
   A. Age of the patient
   B. Tumor size
   C. Axillary node status
   D. Involvement of margins

Answer Key for MCQs

1	2	3	4	5
A	A	A	D	C

CHAPTER 14 Skeletal System

Learning Objectives

At the end of reading this chapter, the student shall be able to:

- Classify and describe the etiology, pathogenesis, clinical features of osteoporosis.
- Describe the etiology, pathogenesis, clinical features and complications of osteomyelitis.
- Classify tumors of bone and discuss in detail the etiology, pathology and radiological findings of common bone tumors.
- Describe the etiology, pathogenesis , clinical features and complications of osteoarthritis, rheumatoid arthritis and gout.

GENERAL FEATURES

The normal skeletal system includes bone and cartilage. The cartilaginous tissue is responsible for the growth and development of bone and formation of the articular surfaces of the joints. Bone is a specialized connective tissue which imparts mechanical support to the body and also plays a vital role in the calcium metabolism. The histomorphology of lamellar bone with marrow elements is depicted in **Figure 14.1**.

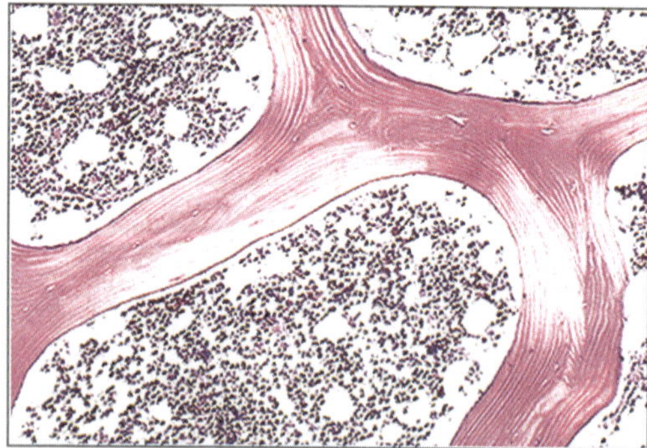

Fig. 14.1: Normal histomorphology of lamellar bone with marrow elements.

The bone is divided into two main components—(1) the compact bone which is responsible for the structural rigidity and (2) trabecular bone which plays a major role in calcium homeostasis. The anatomical structure of bone is shown in **Figure 14.2**.

PATHOLOGY OF BONE

The common disorders of the bone include:

- *Developmental disorders*: Achondroplasia, osteopetrosis, osteogenesis imperfecta
- *Infections*: Osteomyelitis (OM)
- *Metabolic bone disease*: Osteomalacia, rickets, hyperparathyroidism, Paget's disease of bone
- *Tumor like lesions*: Fibrous dysplasia, bone cyst
- *Tumors of bone*: Benign and malignant tumors.

Osteomyelitis

It is defined as an inflammatory pathology of the bone. There are two main forms of OM— (1) acute pyogenic OM, and (2) chronic tuberculous OM.

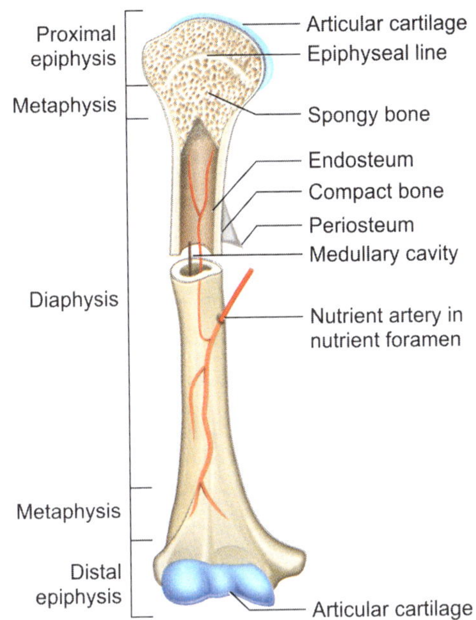

Fig. 14.2: Anatomical structure of bone. Partially sectioned humerus (arm bone).

Pyogenic OM

It is generally caused by spectrum of bacterial organisms, such as *Staphylococcus aureus*, streptococci, *Klebsiella*, *Pseudomonas* and Salmonella. It is common in the long bones of young children between the age of 5 and 15 years. The most common route of infection is direct extension of infection, as a complication of fractures and hematogenous spread from an infective foci. The common predisposing factors include malnutrition, sepsis, immunocompromised states, diabetes mellitus and general debilitation. Tuberculous OM generally involves the thoracic spine (Pott's disease) and long bones of the extremities. In few cases, the caseous necrotic material may track down to the sheath of the psoas muscle producing cold abscess.

Pathology

The infection usually begins at the metaphyseal end of the long bones with infiltration by acute inflammatory cells and this leads to devitalization of the involved bone producing necrosis of the bone called as sequestrum. Later in pathogenesis, new bone formation occurs beneath the periosteum which covers the dead bone and this new bone is called involucrum.

Clinical Profile

Acute OM produces sever pain and swelling of the affected bone associated with fever, malaise and elevated leukocyte count. The bony lesion may form discharging sinuses which my let out necrosed bony particles.

Complications of OM

The common complications include septicemia, extension of infection into the joint spaces—infective arthritis, pathological fractures and secondary amyloidosis.

Osteoporosis

It is a term used to denote a quantitative reduction in the bony tissue mass. This leads to fragile bones prone for easy fractures and deformities. It is mostly seen in elderly individuals. Generally women have a higher incidence of osteoporosis.

The osteoporosis can be of two types—primary and secondary. The primary disease occurs without any known cause. The various causes which may lead to osteoporosis includes gender, genetic factors, reduced physical activity, lack of estrogen and calcitonin, deficiency of vitamin D, hyperparathyroidism, hypogonadism, chronic anemia, long-term use of corticosteroids, anticonvulsant drugs and others. In all these causes, the fine balance between formation of bone and resorption of bone is disturbed with excessive bone resorption.

The most common clinical presentation of osteoporosis is **fracture of the neck of femur, vertebral crush fractures, fracture of wrist and arm and others**. Radiologic evidence becomes prominent only when there is a reduction of more than 30% of the bony mass. Bone densitometry studies are more helpful

TABLE 14.1: Classification of common tumors of bone.

Histological type	*Benign tumors*	*Malignant tumors*
Bone forming	♦ Osteoma ♦ Osteoid osteoma ♦ Osteoblastoma	Osteosarcoma
Cartilage forming	♦ Osteochondroma ♦ Enchondroma	Chondrosarcoma
Hemopoietic	—	♦ Plasmacytoma ♦ Lymphoma
Vascular	Hemangioma	Angiosarcoma
Fibrogenic	Non-ossifying fibroma	Fibrosarcoma
Notochordal		Chordoma
Unknown	Giant cell tumor	♦ Giant cell tumor ♦ Ewing's sarcoma

in making an early diagnosis of osteoporosis and thereby early treatment.

Tumors of Bone

Tumors of bone are generally infrequent tumors as compared to other visceral tumors. They are pathologically grouped under various heading based on the most common tissue pattern seen in the tumor. Diagnosis of bone tumors depends on three major factors—(1) clinical picture, (2) radiological appearance, and (3) pathological features supplemented by other investigations.

The bone tumors are generally grouped as depicted in **Table 14.1**.

We shall now discuss some of the common bone tumors.

Osteogenic Sarcoma

It is the most common malignant tumor of bone. This occurs in young individuals between the age of 10 and 20 years. The most common sites of occurrence include lower end of femur, upper end of tibia, upper humerus, pelvis and rarely jaw bones.

Etiopathogenesis: There are various etiological factors attributed to the occurrence of osteosarcoma. They include mutations in chromosome 13, radiation or preexisting bone diseases, such as fibrous dysplasia, Paget's disease, chronic OM and bone infarcts.

Gross pathology: These are highly aggressive tumors with irregular growth pattern. They initially involve the metaphysis with destruction of the bony structure and extends into the adjacent soft tissue by lifting the periosteum. This pattern of growth gives this tumor "leg of mutton" appearance (**Fig. 14.3**).

Histologically, the tumor is composed of highly pleomorphic stromal cells with

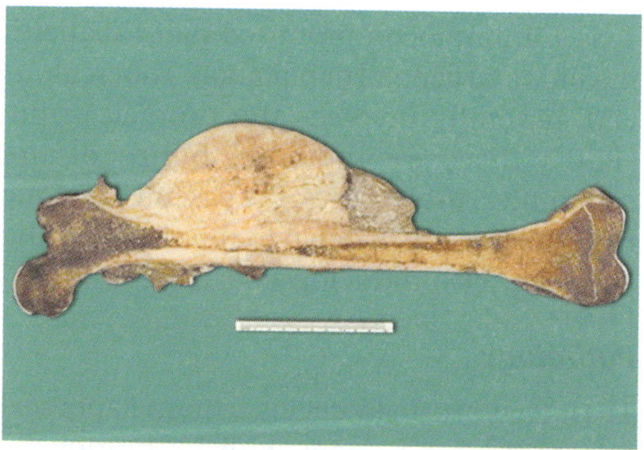

Fig. 14.3: Gross photograph of osteogenic sarcoma with fleshy mass destroying the bone.

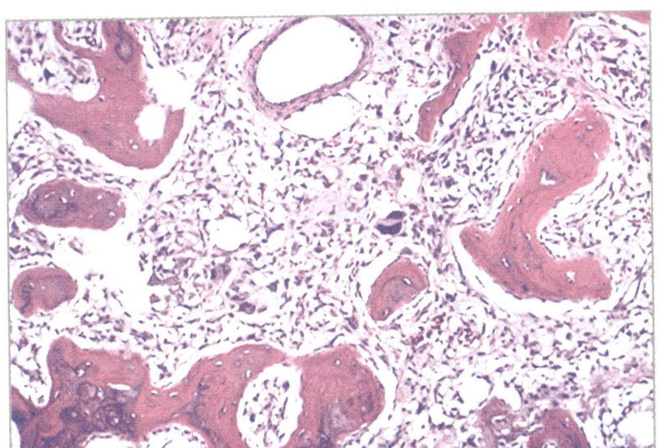

Fig. 14.4: Histomicrograph of osteogenic sarcoma with pleomorphic tumor cells and tumor osteoid.

formation of lace such as tumor osteoid (**Fig. 14.4**).

X-ray of the affected bone shows a sunburst appearance and formation of a Codman's triangle due to lifting of the periosteum.

Clinical features: The patient presents with an irregular swelling with associated severe pain and tenderness. This tumor spreads very rapidly to the lungs and brain.

Osteochondroma

Also referred to as exostosis. It is one of the commonest benign cartilage forming tumor. They mostly arise from the metaphysis of long bones, such as femur and tibia.

The tumors protrude exophytically as a mushroom shaped lesion with cartilaginous cap and underlying lamellar bone (**Fig. 14.5**).

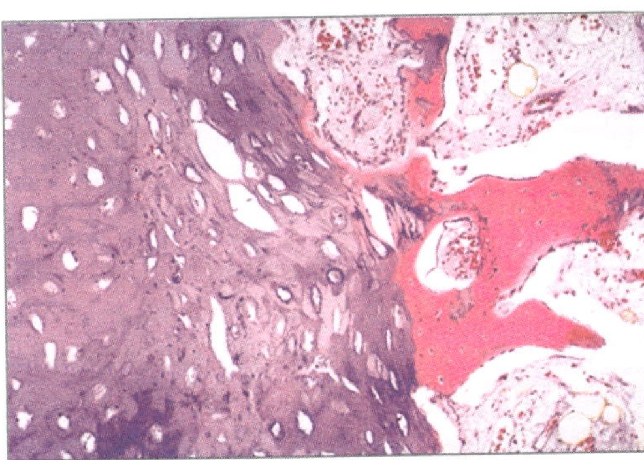

Fig. 14.5: Histomicrograph of osteochondroma with cartilaginous cap.

Giant Cell Tumor (Osteoclastoma)

This tumor arised from the epiphysis of long bones, such as lower end of femur, upper end of tibia and fibula. This tumor is common in age between 20 and 40.

Grossly, it presents as a well circumscribed grayish tan eccentric mass. Cut section of the mass gives a honey comb appearance (**Fig. 14.6**). Radiologically, it is referred to as "soap bubble" appearance.

Microscopically, it is composed of many multinucleated osteoclastic type giant cells with plump spindle shaped stromal cells (**Fig. 14.7**).

Ewing's Sarcoma

It is a highly malignant small round cell tumor involving the diaphysis of long bones in young adults. Most of the individuals present

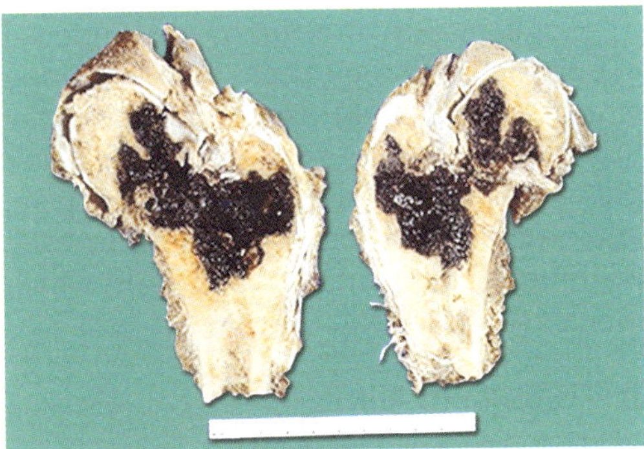

Fig. 14.6: Gross photograph of giant cell tumor of bone.

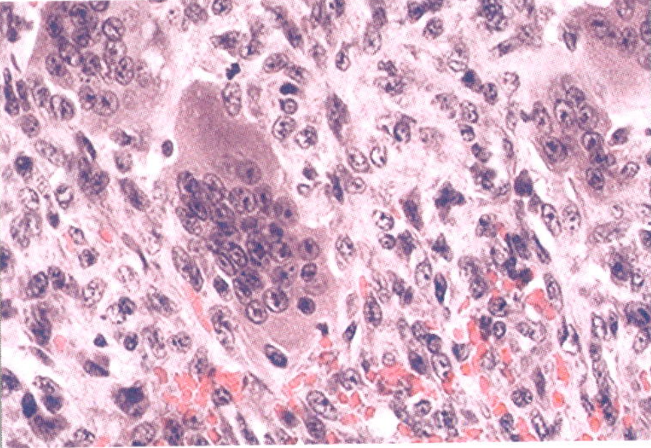

Fig. 14.7: Histomicrograph of giant cell tumor bone.

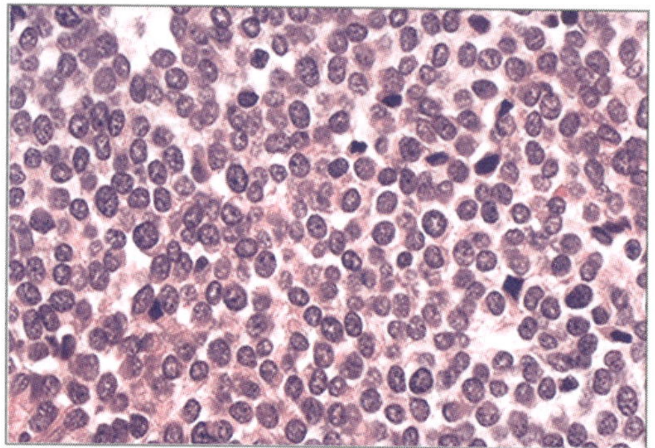

Fig. 14.8: Histomicrograph of Ewings sarcoma composed of small uniform round cells.

with a translocation of chromosome t (11:12) (q24: q12).

Grossly, it presents as a mass in the diaphysis producing expansion of the bone. Radiologically, it is referred to as onion skin appearance.

Histologically, the tumor is composed of uniform small round cells with formation of rosettes (**Fig. 14.8**). The cytoplasm of the tumor cells contains glycogen. Clinically, it presents as a bony mass associated with pain, tenderness, fever, leukocytosis and raised erythrocyte sedimentation rate (ESR) which mimics that of an OM.

PATHOLOGY OF JOINTS

Each joint comprises articular surfaces of the bones and a space lined by synovial membrane. This membrane contains lining synoviocytes and loose fibrovascular connective tissue. This space contains synovial fluid which lubricates the joint space. This fluid is rich in hyaluronic acid.

There are many diseases that affect the joints which are collectively referred to as arthritis. We shall now discuss the features of some of the common forms of arthritis.

Osteoarthritis

This is a degenerative joint disease characterized by gradual degradation of the joint structures of the weight bearing joints. It is more common in the elderly women. It commonly involves hip joint, knee joint, vertebrae and smaller interphalangeal joints. There is progressive gradual loss of the cartilaginous matrix proteins, leading to degradation of the articular cartilage. The underlying bone is also denuded with formation of microcystic spaces. The articular end of the bones shows spiky projections called the osteophytes.

Clinically, it presents with joint stiffness, restricted mobility, discomfort, pain. The degenerative changes in the interphalangeal joints leads to the formation of nodules called the Heberden's nodule in the base of fingers. The osteophytes formed in the vertebrae may compress upon the nerves producing root pain.

Rheumatoid Arthritis

It is an inflammatory polyarthritis involving the peripheral smaller joints in a symmetric pattern. It may be associated with other systemic manifestations involving the blood vessels, lungs and neurological system. It is more common in women between 3–4 decade of life.

Pathogenesis

In more than 80% of the individual's patients have circulating rheumatoid factor (RA factor) indicating an immune mediated inflammatory damage to the synovial membrane. The damage is induced by the release of proinflammatory cytokines elaborated by activated T and B lymphocytes.

Pathology

It initially involves the smaller joints of the hand and feet. Later it involves wrist, ankle, elbow and knee joint. The proximal interphalangeal and metacarpophalangeal joints are severely affected.

Histologically, it is characterized by diffuse synovitis with vascularization of

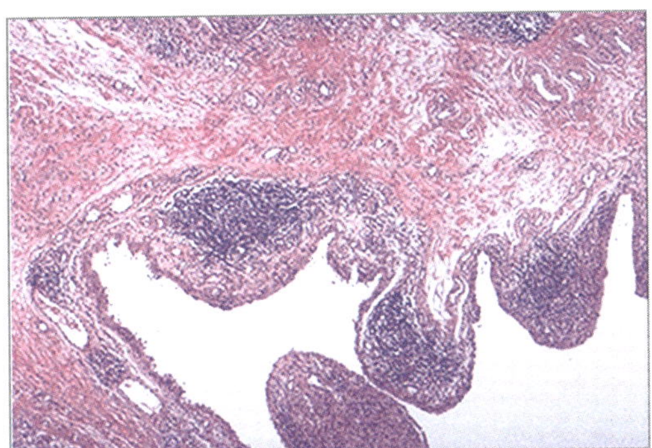

Fig. 14.9: Histomicrograph of synovium in rheumatoid arthritis.

the articular cartilage (Pannus) (normally the articular cartilage is avascular in nature). There is marked thickening of the synovium with villous projections and dense lymphoplasmacytic infiltration with variable areas of fibrinoid necrosis (**Fig. 14.9**). The extra-articular lesions involve blood vessels, lungs, pleura, pericardium, lymph nodes, skin and eyes.

Clinically, it presents with gradual fatigue, malaise, weakness and stiffness of joints. This is followed by pain and joint swellings of the hand and feet. Deformities of the hand in case of rheumatoid arthritis is shown in **Figure 14.10**. Patients will have a mild anemia, raised ESR, leukocytosis and hypergammaglobulinemia.

Case Scenario

Ms Parul, a 35-year-old woman, presents to her rheumatologist with complaints of joint pain, swelling, and morning stiffness in her wrists and hands. She reports experiencing these symptoms for the past several weeks. On examination, the rheumatologist observes synovitis in multiple joints, with a predilection for the small joints of the hands. Laboratory investigations show elevated levels of rheumatoid factor and anti-cyclic citrullinated peptide (anti-CCP) antibodies.

Question:

Based on Ms Parul clinical presentation and laboratory findings, what is the most likely diagnosis?

A. Osteoarthritis
B. Rheumatoid arthritis (RA)
C. Systemic lupus erythematosus (SLE)
D. Gout

Answer:

B. Rheumatoid arthritis (RA).

Gouty Arthritis

This is rarer form of arthritis due to excessive abnormal accumulation of uric acid leading to precipitation of urate crystals within the joint space and subsequent inflammation. Patients may also have other manifestation of hyperuricemia, such as renal disease and uric

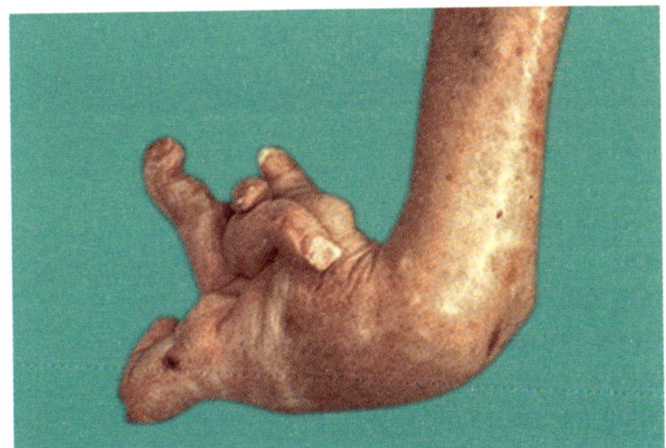

Fig. 14.10: Deformities of the hand in a case of rheumatoid arthritis.

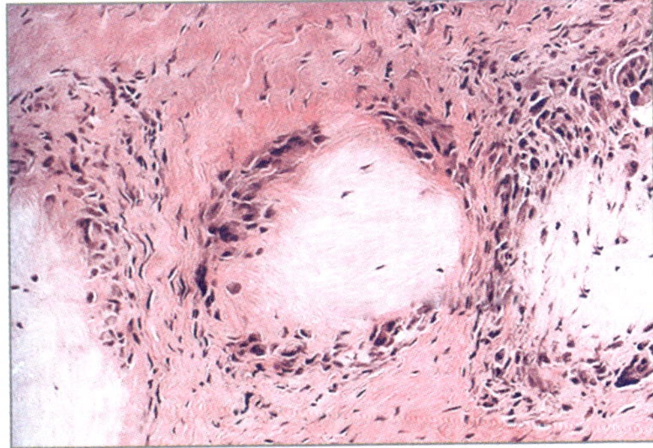

Fig. 14.11: Histomicrograph of a gouty tophi.

acid calculi in the kidneys. A serum uric acid level more than 7 mg/dL indicates increase risk of gout. It is usually a monoarticular arthritis involving the lower limbs mostly the great toe.

There will be acute synovitis with precipitation of needle shaped urate crystals with associated inflammation. This lesion is called *tophi.* The tophi can be seen within the joint space or in the adjacent soft tissue. The histomicrograph of gouty tophi is depicted in **Figure 14.11**.

Points to Ponder

- The common disorders of the bone includes developmental disorders—achondroplasia, osteopetrosis, osteogenesis imperfect, infections—osteomyelitis. Metabolic bone disease—osteomalacia, rickets, hyperparathyroidism, paget's disease of bone. Tumor like lesions—Fibrous dysplasia, bone cyst and tumors of bone—benign and malignant tumors.
- Osteoporosis is a term used to denote a quantitative reduction in the bony tissue mass. This leads to fragile bones prone for easy fractures and deformities. It is mostly seen in elderly individuals. Generally, women have a higher incidence of osteoporosis.
- Osteomyelitis is an inflammatory pathology of the bone. There are two main forms of osteomyelitis acute pyogenic and chronic tuberculous
- Osteogenic sarcoma is the most common malignant tumor of bone. This occurs in young individuals between the age of 10–20 years. The most common sites of occurrence includes lower end of femur, upper end of tibia, upper humerus, pelvis and rarely jaw bones. Other tumors include giant cell tumor, Ewings's sarcoma and osteochondroma.
- Osteoarthritis is a degenerative joint disease characterized by gradual degradation of the joint structures of the weight bearing joints. It is more common in the elderly women. It commonly involves hip joint, knee joint, vertebrae and smaller interphalangeal joints.
- Rheumatoid arthritis is an inflammatory polyarthritis involving the peripheral smaller joints in a symmetric pattern. It may be associated with other systemic manifestations involving the blood vessels, lungs and neurological system. It is more common in women between 3 and 4 decade of life.
- Gouty arthritis is rare form of arthritis due to excessive abnormal accumulation of uric acid leading to precipitation of urate crystals within the joint space and subsequent inflammation.

ASSESSMENT QUESTIONS

1. **What is a sequestrum?**
2. **Define Brodie's abscess.**
3. **Enlist the common causes for secondary osteoporosis.**
4. **Enlist most common malignant bone tumors.**
5. **Enumerate the radiological findings in osteogenic sarcoma.**
6. **Enumerate the radiological findings in giant cell tumor.**
7. **Write in detail about the pathological findings in giant cell tumor.**
8. **Which portion of the bone is involved in Ewing's tumor?**
9. **What are the predominant synovial changes in rheumatoid arthritis?**
10. **What is a tophus?**

MULTIPLE CHOICE QUESTIONS

1. **The type of collagen seen in bone is:**
   - A. I
   - B. II
   - C. III
   - D. IV
2. **The most common malignancy seen in Paget's disease is:**
   - A. Osteosarcoma
   - B. Chondrosarcoma
   - C. Giant cell tumor
   - D. Ewing's sarcoma
3. **Osteomyelitis seen in patients with sickle cell disease is due to infection with:**
   - A. Staphylococci
   - B. Streptococci
   - C. *Salmonella*
   - D. *Pseudomonas*
4. **The most common primary bone malignancy is:**
   - A. Osteosarcoma
   - B. Chondrosarcoma
   - C. Giant cell tumor
   - D. Ewing's sarcoma
5. **Sunburst appearance in X-ray is typical of:**
   - A. Osteosarcoma
   - B. Chondrosarcoma
   - C. Giant cell tumor
   - D. Ewing's sarcoma
6. **The tumor cell in a giant cell tumor is:**
   - A. Osteoblast
   - B. Osteoclast
   - C. Stromal cell
   - D. Reticulum cell

Answer Key for MCQs

1	2	3	4	5	6
A	A	C	A	A	C

CHAPTER

Central Nervous System

Learning Objectives

At the end of reading this chapter, the student shall be able to:

- Define hydrocephalus and enlist the causes.
- Describe the etiology, pathogenesis and cerebrospinal fluid findings in various types of meningitis.
- Enumerate the causes for cerebrovascular accidents and describe them.
- Classify tumors of the brain and describe the pathology of the common tumors.

GENERAL FEATURES

The central nervous system (CNS) comprises the delicate brain and spinal cord encased in a bony skull and vertebral cage. There are four main anatomic regions of the brain: (1) cerebrum, (2) cerebellum, (3) pons, and (4) medulla. Histologically, there are two main components the neurons and neuroglia. The neurons are specialized cells which are involved in conduction of impulses. The neuroglia are cells which support the neurons they include astrocytes, oligodendrocytes and ependymal cells. The astrocytes having multiple complex cytoplasmic processes. The ependymal cells are the one which line the ventricular spaces. In addition to the above cells, there are other cells called the microglia, which constitute the mononuclear macrophage system of the brain. The brain is covered by tough fibrous sheath called the dura mater and leptomeninges which includes pia mater and arachnoid mater.

PATHOLOGY OF CENTRAL NERVOUS SYSTEM

The common disorders of CNS include the following:

- *Developmental anomalies*: Spina bifida, meningocele, meningomyelocele
- *Infections and inflammations*: Meningitis, encephalitis, abscess
- *Cerebrovascular disease*: Thrombosis, hemorrhage, hematoma
- *Demyelinating disorders*: Multiple sclerosis
- *Tumors*: Meningioma, astrocytoma, medulloblastoma

Hydrocephalus

Definition

It is defined as an increased volume of cerebrospinal fluid (CSF) within the brain. It is divided into internal and external hydrocephalus. In the internal type, there is irregular dilatation of the ventricular spaces with increased intracranial pressure and in the external type there is localized collection of CSF in the subarachnoid space. CSF is normally produced by the choroidal plexus of the lateral, third and fourth ventricles. The total volume is 120–150 mL.

Causes

Hydrocephalus occurs due to the following reasons:

- *Obstruction to the CSF flow*: Stenosis of aqueduct, Arnold-Chiari malformation tumors adjacent to ventricles
- *Overproduction of CSF*: Due to tumors like choroid plexus papilloma
- *Deficient reabsorption of CSF*: As in meningitis.

Pathological Changes

There are irregular dilatation of ventricles with thinning and stretching of brain.

Infections

The brain and spinal cord are prone for a wide range of infections. The infections reach the brain through blood stream (hematogenous), local spread from adjacent infective foci and along nerve roots (viral infections).

The general pattern of inflammations include meningitis (inflammation of meninges), encephalitis (inflammation of the brain parenchyma) and meningoencephalitis (both).

Meningitis

Inflammatory condition involving the meninges.

Causative organisms: Based on the etiologic agents the meningitis is grouped in **Table 15.1**.

Clinical profile: The general clinical features include fever, severe headache, vomiting, drowsiness, stiffness of the neck, convulsions, stupor and coma. The diagnosis is made based on the examination of CSF.

Cerebrospinal fluid findings in various forms of meningitis (**Table 15.2**).

TABLE 15.1: Common types of meningitis with the causative organisms.

Type of meningitis	*Causative organisms*
Acute pyogenic	*E. coli, H. influenzae, Neisseria meningitidis*, pneumococci
Acute aseptic	*Enterovirus*, echovirus, *Coxsackievirus*, Epstein-Barr virus
Chronic meningitis	Tuberculous, cryptococcus

Encephalitis

Inflammation of the brain parenchyma due to bacterial, viral and fungal infections. The most common clinical entities are brain abscess, which are localized suppurative inflammatory conditions of the brain, tuberculoma a manifestation of tuberculosis of brain, neurosyphilis which is seen in the tertiary form of syphilis. Viral infections CNS usually causes encephalitis. The most common viral agents include HIV, herpes zoster virus, cytomegalovirus, poliovirus.

The common fungal organisms include cryptococci, aspergillus, histoplasma and other fungi.

TABLE 15.2: Comparison of the CSF findings in common type of meningitis.

CSF findings	*Pyogenic meningitis*	*Aseptic meningitis*	*Chronic meningitis*
Naked appearance	Cloudy/purulent	Clear	Clear with formation of cob web
Pressure	Elevated	Elevated	Elevated
Predominant cells	Neutrophils	Lymphocyte	Lymphocyte
Protein level	Increased	Normal	Increased
Sugar content	Decreased	Normal	Reduced
Bacteriological study	Organisms demonstrable	Sterile	Acid-fast bacillus staining

Cerebrovascular Diseases

There are two main forms of cerebrovascular diseases they include:

1. Diseases due to ischemic brain damage
2. Diseases due to intracranial hemorrhage.

The cardinal clinical feature of the cerebrovascular disease is stroke syndrome, which is a sudden onset of neurological deficit manifesting as hemiplegia or coma.

Ischemic Brain Damage

Brain is very sensitive for hypoxic injury and it results in irreversible cell death. Hypoxia can be induced by the following reasons:

- *Arterial occlusion:* Due to occlusive thrombi of the cerebral vessels or occlusion by emboli originating from heart or other sites. Inflammatory conditions, such as arteritis form rarer cause of occlusion.
- Other causes include that of venous occlusion and compression of the vessels by tumors.

Hypoxic injury to brain results in infarct of the brain.

The infarct may be anemic or hemorrhagic. The affected area is soft and swollen and after 3 days undergoes cystic degeneration. Histologically, it presents with neuronal damage, laminar necrosis and ischemic encephalopathy (**Fig. 15.1**).

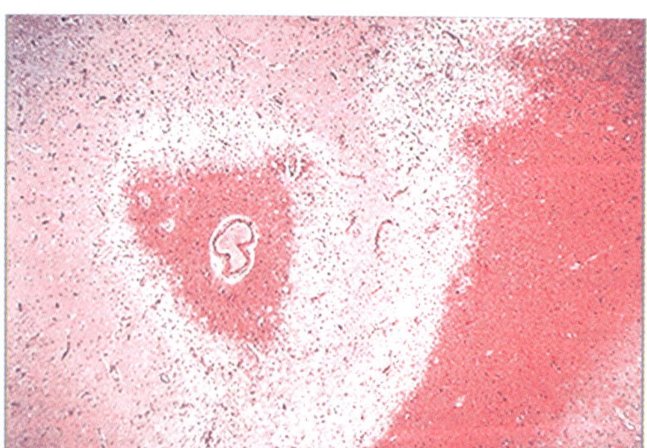

Fig. 15.1: Histomicrograph of infracted brain tissue.

Intracranial Hemorrhage

The gross image of intracerebral hemorrhage is shown in **Figure 15.2**. There are two types of intracranial hemorrhage—intracerebral and subarachnoid. The most common causes for intracranial hemorrhages include:

- *Hypertension*: Due to the rupture of microaneurysms, the hemorrhage is seen in the basal ganglia, pons and cerebral cortex (**Fig. 15.3**).
- *Rupture of aneurysms*: Most common type is rupture of berry aneurysm of the circle of Willis.
- Arteriovenous malformations
- *Traumatic*: Trauma generally leads to epidural and subdural hematoma.

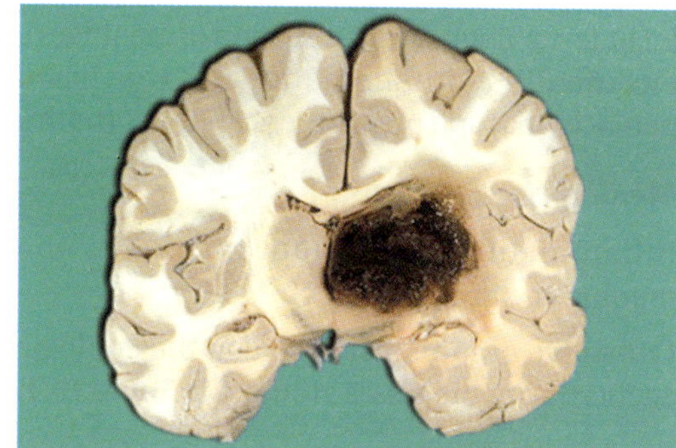

Fig. 15.2: Gross photograph of intracerebral hemorrhage.

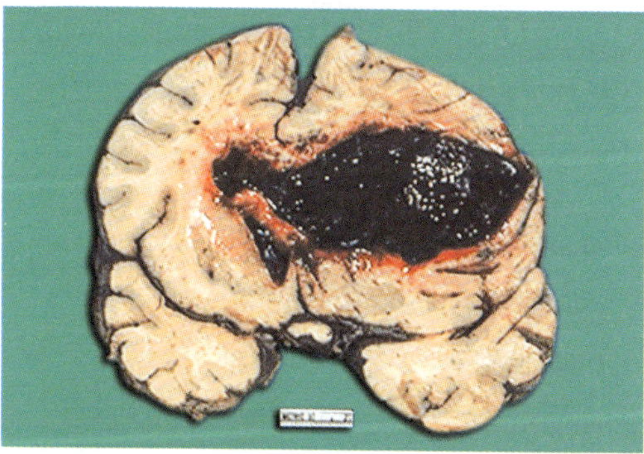

Fig. 15.3: Gross photograph of intracerebral hemorrhage in hypertension.

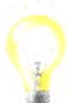

Case Scenario

Mr Aman, a 65-year-old man, is brought to the emergency department with a sudden onset of severe headache, vomiting, and altered consciousness. His family reports that he had been complaining of dizziness and confusion earlier in the day. On examination, he has a Glasgow Coma Scale (GCS) score of 8, unequal pupils, and signs of right-sided hemiparesis. Non-contrast CT scan of the head reveals a hyperdense area consistent with a hemorrhage in the left basal ganglia.

Question:

What is the most likely type of intracranial hemorrhage in Mr Aman, based on the location described in the CT scan?

A. Epidural hematoma
B. Subdural hematoma
C. Subarachnoid hemorrhage
D. Intracerebral hemorrhage

Answer:

D. Intracerebral hemorrhage.

Tumors of Brain

Tumors of the CNS may originate from the brain and spinal cord. The tumors can arise from the primary parenchymal cells of the brain or the supporting tissues. Some of the common tumors are listed below:

- *Tumors of neuroglia*: Astrocytoma, oligodendroglioma, ependymoma
- *Tumors of neurons*: Neuroblastoma, ganglioneuroma
- *Embryonal tumors*: Medulloblastoma
- Tumors of meninges: Meningioma
- *Nerve sheath tumors*: Schwannoma, neurofibroma
- Metastatic tumors
- Others: CNS lymphomas, vascular tumors

Astrocytomas

Most common glial tumor of brain. They are usually seen in adults in 5–6 decade. It occurs in the cerebral hemispheres.

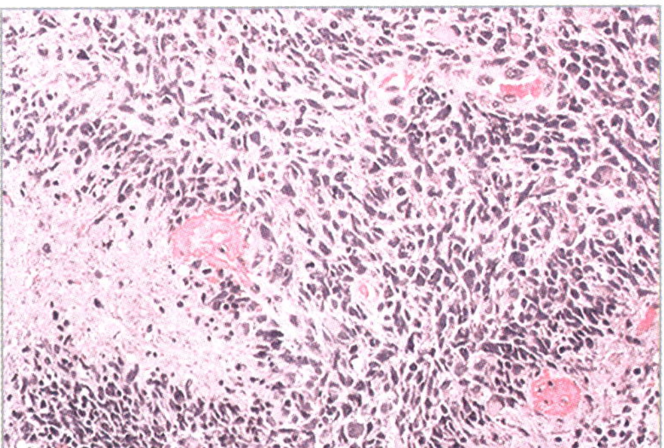

Fig. 15.4: Histomicrograph of highly malignant glioblastoma multiforme.

There are various histological forms of astrocytoma namely pilocytic, protoplasmic, gemistocytic, fibrillary and anaplastic. A highly anaplastic type of astrocytoma is termed as glioblastoma multiforme (**Fig. 15.4**). Other glial tumors are generally uncommon.

Medulloblastoma

It is the most common type of primitive neuroectodermal tumor of brain. Seen in children. The most common location is the cerebellum.

It is a highly malignant tumor composed of clusters of small round cells with formation of rosettes (**Fig. 15.5**). It generally invades locally and through the CSF.

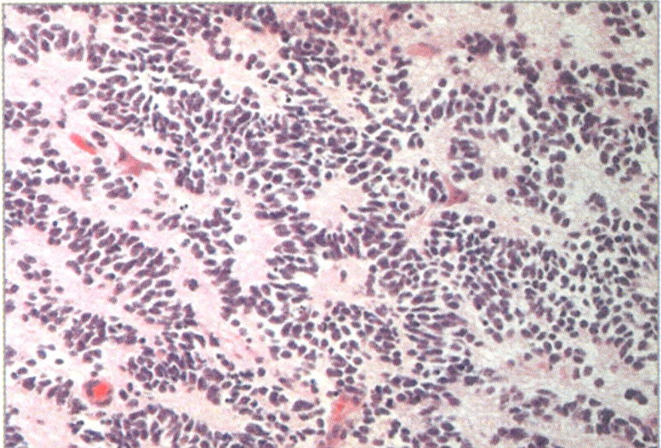

Fig. 15.5: Histomicrograph of medulloblastoma, small round cell tumor with rosettes.

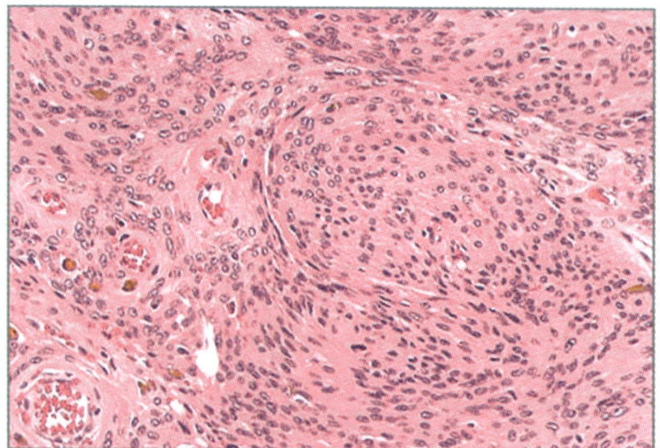

Fig. 15.6: Histomicrograph of meningothelial meningioma.

Meningioma

They constitute around 20% of the intracranial neoplasms. They arise from the arachnoid cap cells. Most common sites include the cerebral convexities, olfactory groove, foramen magnum, cerebellopontine angle and spinal cord. Most of the tumors benign and occur in women between the age of 20 and 60 years.

Grossly, they are well circumscribed grayish white solid mass firmly attached to the dura.

Microscopically, the tumor is made up of fascicles of plump spindle to oval cells with an oval nuclei and finely granular cytoplasm (**Fig. 15.6**). Most of the meningiomas are characterized by the presence of Psammoma bodies, which are laminated calcified spherules. There are various histological types of meningioma: fibroblastic, meningotheliomatous, transitional, angioblastic, xanthomatous, psammomatous and anaplastic type.

Points to Ponder

- Hydrocephalus is defined as an increased volume of cerebrospinal fluid (CSF) within the brain. It is divided into internal and external hydrocephalus.
- The general pattern of inflammations include meningitis (inflammation of meninges), encephalitis (inflammation of the brain parenchyma) and meningoencephalitis (both).
- Meningitis: Inflammatory condition involving the meninges.
- The clinical features include fever, severe headache, vomiting, drowsiness, stiffness of the neck, convulsions, stupor and coma. The diagnosis is made based on the examination of CSF.
- Cerebrovascular diseases include. Diseases due to ischemic brain damage and diseases due to intracranial hemorrhage.
- The cardinal clinical feature of the cerebrovascular disease is stroke syndrome, which is a sudden onset of neurological deficit manifesting as hemiplegia or coma.
- Tumors of the CNS may originate from the brain and spinal cord. The tumors can arise from the primary parenchymal cells of the brain or the supporting tissues.

ASSESSMENT QUESTIONS

1. **Enlist the major functions of astrocytes.**
2. **What are the common causes for hydrocephalus?**
3. **Enumerate the common microorganisms associated with meningitis.**
4. **Enumerate the CSF findings in acute pyogenic, tuberculous and viral meningitis.**
5. **What are the common causes for intracranial hemorrhage?**
6. **Name the common malignant tumors of brain.**
7. **Discuss the pathology of meningioma.**

MULTIPLE CHOICE QUESTIONS

1. **The mononuclear phagocyte cell of CNS is:**
   A. Oligodendroglia
   B. Ependymal cell
   C. Microglia
   D. Red neuron
2. **Most common causes for intracerebral hemorrhage is:**
   A. Hypertension
   B. Vascular tumors
   C. Malignancy
   D. Bleeding disorders
3. **Exudation in pneumococcal meningitis is seen in:**
   A. Basal portion
   B. Parasagittal
   C. Ventricles
   D. Cerebral
4. **Tuberculoma in children is seen usually in:**
   A. Frontal lobe
   B. Posterior fossa
   C. Parietal lobe
   D. Meninges
5. **The most common type of adult CNS tumor is:**
   A. Medulloblastoma
   B. Glioblastoma
   C. Pilocytic astrocytoma
   D. Fibrillary astrocytoma
6. **Cobweb appearance of CSF is typically seen in:**
   A. Viral meningitis
   B. Pyogenic meningitis
   C. Tuberculous meningitis
   D. None of the above
7. **What is the most common cause of spontaneous intracerebral hemorrhage?**
   A. Trauma
   B. Hypertension
   C. Ischemic stroke
   D. Cerebral aneurysm rupture
8. **What is the recommended approach to blood pressure management in the acute phase of intracerebral hemorrhage?**
   A. Allow blood pressure to remain elevated
   B. Aggressively lower blood pressure with antihypertensive medications
   C. Administer intravenous fluids to increase blood pressure
   D. Perform urgent carotid endarterectomy
9. **Which diagnostic test is commonly used to identify the underlying cause of intracerebral hemorrhage?**
   A. Lumbar puncture
   B. Carotid ultrasound
   C. Transcranial Doppler ultrasound
   D. Digital subtraction angiography (DSA)
10. **In managing elevated intracranial pressure in intracerebral hemorrhage, which intervention is contraindicated?**
    A. Hyperventilation to decrease $PaCO_2$
    B. Osmotic therapy with mannitol
    C. Elevating the head of the bed
    D. Administering anticoagulant medications

Answer Key for MCQs

1	2	3	4	5	6	7	8	9	10
A	A	D	B	D	C	B	B	D	D

UNIT 3

Clinical Pathology—Hematology

Section Outline

CHAPTER 16

Introduction to Practical Hematology and Collection of Blood and Preservation

Learning Objectives

At the end of reading this chapter, the student shall be able to:

- Describe the composition and functions of blood.
- Enlist the methods of collection of blood and the anticoagulants used.

BLOOD

Blood is a specialized connective tissue which circulates in a closed system of blood vessels. It contains cells like the erythrocytes, leukocytes and platelets suspended in a fluid called plasma. The total volume of blood comprises 8% of the total body weight. The main functions of blood are:

- Transport of oxygen from the lungs to the tissues and that of carbon dioxide from the tissue to the lung
- Transport of metabolic wastes
- Transport of amino acids, fatty acids, hormones, ions and metabolites
- Regulation of acid-base balance and temperature
- Defense against infections
- Coagulation of blood

HEMATOLOGY

Hematology comprises the study of blood components and coagulation system. It includes:

- Analysis of the concentration, structure and functions of the component cells and plasma in the peripheral blood
- Analysis of the hemopoiesis and precursor cells in the bone marrow
- Study of the proteins involved in the coagulation system
- Identifying blood groups and immunohematology.

COLLECTION OF BLOOD

Collection of Capillary Blood by Skin Puncture

Site: In adults, it is done in fingertip. And in infants, the site is preferably great toe or heel.

Method: The selected site is cleaned with 70% alcohol or spirit and a quick stab is made by a sharp needle or a lancet. The first drop of the blood is wiped off and the subsequent drop of blood is used for analysis. The site should not be squeezed for collection.

Tests done: The capillary blood obtained can be used to determine the following:

- Hemoglobin concentration,
- Counts of erythrocytes, leukocytes and platelets
- Bleeding time
- Blood grouping and typing
- Reticulocyte count

- Peripheral smear study
- Thick and thin smear studies for hemoparasites

Collection of Blood by Venipuncture

Sites: Usually, the median cubital vein in arm is preferred. Other veins of the dorsum of hand, femoral vein and cephalic vein can also be used. The area selected must be free of any scars and healed hematomas.

Method: The patient must be made comfortable and explained about the procedure. A tournicquet is applied without exerting much pressure, the vein is identified and after strict asepsis, blood is drawn in a clean dry sterile syringe without exerting much pressure. The blood collected is immediately transferred to the specific containers for subsequent tests.

Tests done: The venous blood thus obtained is generally used for:

- Complete hemogram
- Erythrocyte sedimentation rate
- Hematocrit
- Clotting time
- Tests for coagulation
- Estimation of biochemical components of plasma and serum
- Special hematological tests, such as osmotic fragility test, LE preparation, Coomb's test and others.

ANTICOAGULANTS

Anticoagulants are substances that prevent clotting of blood when mixed in appropriate amounts with the blood sample. They mostly act on calcium and converts it to a unionized form. So, blood clotting is prevented. Heparin is an anticoagulant which prevents formation of thrombin, which in turn prevents blood clotting. Some of the properties of commonly used anticoagulants are summarized below.

Anticoagulant	*Mechanism*	*Tests performed*
EDTA	Powerful calcium chelator	All routine hematological tests
Trisodium citrate	Calcium chelator	Determination of ESR, coagulation tests, blood storage in blood bank
Double oxalate (Ammonium oxalate and Potassium oxalate)	Calcium chelator	Determine hematocrit, ESR and routine hematological tests
Heparin	Antithrombin action	For urgent estimation of blood sugar, electrolytes

Points to Ponder

- Blood is a specialized connective tissue which circulates in a closed system of blood vessels. It contains cells like the erythrocytes, leukocytes and platelets suspended in a fluid called plasma.
- The common samples of blood are capillary sample and venous blood sample. Arterial blood is rarely sample and is done for doing a blood gas analysis.
- Anticoagulants are substances that prevent clotting of blood when mixed in appropriate amounts with the blood sample. They mostly act on calcium and converts it to an unionized form. So, clotting is prevented.

ASSESSMENT QUESTIONS

1. **What are the common functions of blood?**
2. **Enumerate the differences between plasma and serum.**
3. **What are the common preferred sites for venipuncture?**
4. **Enlist the common anticoagulants used in a hematology laboratory.**

MULTIPLE CHOICE QUESTIONS

1. **The anticoagulant of choice in coagulation experiments is:**
   A. Heparin
   B. Double oxalate
   C. Trisodium citrate
   D. EDTA
2. **Which of the following is a direct oral anticoagulant (DOAC)?**
   A. Warfarin
   B. Heparin
   C. Rivaroxaban
   D. Aspirin
3. **What is the primary mechanism of action of warfarin?**
   A. Inhibiting vitamin K epoxide reductase
   B. Enhancing antithrombin activity
   C. Inhibiting factor Xa
   D. Activating protein C
4. **Which laboratory test is routinely monitored in patients taking warfarin?**
   A. Activated partial thromboplastin time (aPTT)
   B. Prothrombin time (PT)
   C. Anti-Xa assay
   D. Platelet count
5. **In the event of an acute bleed, which anticoagulant has a readily available specific reversal agent?**
   A. Rivaroxaban
   B. Apixaban
   C. Warfarin
   D. Dabigatran
6. **What is the primary advantage of direct oral anticoagulants (DOACs) over warfarin?**
   A. No need for routine monitoring
   B. Lower cost
   C. Longer half-life
   D. No risk of bleeding

Answer Key for MCQs

1	2	3	4	5	6
C	C	A	B	C	A

CHAPTER 17

Determination of Hemoglobin

Learning Objectives

At the end of reading this chapter, the student shall be able to:
- Describe the structure and function of hemoglobin.
- Enlist the common methods of estimating hemoglobin.

INTRODUCTION

Hemoglobin (Hb) is a conjugated protein synthesized within the bone marrow by the erythroid precursor cells. It consists of two components—heme and globin. Heme is composed of iron and protoporphyrin and globin is composed of amino acids. Each molecule of hemoglobin has one globin unit and four heme units. The molecular weight is 68,000 Daltons. The globin unit is composed of four polypeptide chains and there are different types of hemoglobin based on the nature of the amino acid chains.

Hemoglobin A : Alpha and Beta chains
Hemoglobin A2 : Alpha and Delta chains
Hemoglobin F : Alpha and Gamma chains

At birth, the hemoglobin content is 18 g/dL and the gradually declines and reaches the adult value of 14–16 g/dL. Men generally have a slightly higher value than women.

ESTIMATION OF HEMOGLOBIN

The estimation of hemoglobin is one of the basic laboratory tests in hematology and a significant decrease in its concentration is indicative of anemia. There are various tests available for the estimation of Hb. They are categorized based on the principle involved in estimation. They are:

- *Colorimetry*: Visual and photocolorimetry
- Specific gravity method
- Oxygen binding capacity
- Iron binding capacity

The most commonly used methods belong the colorimetry group. Here the color product of the test sample is compared with that of the standard and value of hemoglobin is derived. Some of the commonly used colorimetric tests are:

- *Tallquist method:* Here the sample of blood is allowed to dry in a strip of filter paper and the color is compared with a comparator scale and the value is read directly. This is a highly error prone method for estimating Hb.
- *Sahli's acid hematin method:* This is one of the most widely used methods for estimating Hb. The blood is added to 0.1N hydrochloric acid. The Hb is converted into acid hematin and the resulting color is compared with that of the standard color and the value is obtained. Since, this test is based on visual color comparison, it is not a sensitive test.
- *Cyanmethemoglobin method:* This a photo calorimetric method of estimating Hb and is considered to be a very sensitive test for estimation. The Hb in the given sample of blood is converted to cyanmethemoglobin by the addition of Drabkin's reagent.

This reagent contains potassium ferricyanide, potassium cyanide and potassium dihydrogen phosphate.

The intensity of the color is proportional to the concentration of hemoglobin.

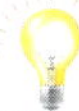

Case Scenario

A 12-year-old school going female child not attentive in classes with complaints of tiredness, eating chalk. Frequent pain abdomen. O/E pallor ++, angular cheilosis, flat nails, no hepatosplenomegaly.

Question:

What is your provisional diagnosis?

Answer:

Iron deficiency anemia

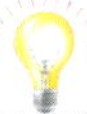

Case Scenario

A 55-year-old female with complaints of pain abdomen, tiredness, feel of pins and needle in legs, loss of appetite and loss of weight. O/E pallor +, mild icterus + liver, spleen normal pedal edema +

Question:

What is your provisional diagnosis?

Answer:

Macrocytic anemia (B_{12}/folic acid deficiency)

OTHER METHODS FOR ESTIMATING HEMOGLOBIN

Specific gravity method: This is used as a screening test for detecting a cutoff value of hemoglobin in blood donation camps. In this copper sulfate solutions of varying specific gravity are used. Normally, a solution with specific gravity of 1.055 is prepared for men and 1.053 for women. A drop of blood is suspended in the solution and if the drop sinks to the bottom, then the hemoglobin value is normal. If the drop of blood floats it indicates a low hemoglobin concentration.

Iron binding capacity and oxygen binding capacity methods (Gasometry): These are used as methods of standardization for calibrating instruments for estimation of Hb.

Normal values of hemoglobin is summarized in the table below:

Age group/Gender	*Normal value (g/dL)*
Men	14–18
Women	11.5–15.5
Infants	13.5–19.5
Children (up to 1 yr)	11–14
Children (10–14 yrs)	11.5–13.5

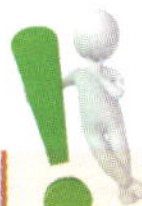

Points to Ponder

Estimation of hemoglobin is one of the basic laboratory tests in hematology and a significant decrease in its concentration is indicative of anemia. There are various tests available for the estimation of hemoglobin.

ASSESSMENT QUESTION

1. **Enumerate the common causes for anemia.**

Blood Cell Counts

CHAPTER 18

Learning Objectives

At the end of reading this chapter, the student shall be able to:

- Describe the basic mechanism of counting of the blood cells and the calculations used in them.
- Describe the basic mechanism of the functioning of the automated blood cell counters.
- Enumerate the various conditions with increase and decrease in blood cell counts.

INTRODUCTION

The cellular compartment of blood contains erythrocytes, leucocytes and the platelets. We shall briefly see the morphology of these cellular elements.

ERYTHROCYTES (ERYTHROS-RED, CYTOS-CELL)

The red blood corpuscles are biconcave anucleate cell of **size 7.5 micron with a thickness of 2 micron**. It contains hemoglobin and is the heaviest of all the cellular elements of blood. The normal red cells have got a finite lifespan of **120 days +/- 20 days**

The normal red cell count is **4.5–5.5 million cells/cumm**.

LEUKOCYTES

White blood cells are nucleated cells and the number varies between **4000 to 11,000 cells/cumm**.

Type of cell	*Components*	*Numbers*
Granulocytes	Neutrophils	50–70%
	Eosinophils	1–4%
	Basophils	0–1%
Agranulocytes	Lymphocytes	25–45%
	Monocytes	2–8%

This classification is based on the morphological properties of the cell. The morphology and functions of the various leucocytes are depicted below:

Cell	*Morphology*	*Functions*
Neutrophils (10–12 microns)	Multilobed nuclei with fine purplish cytoplasmic granules	Cell of acute inflammation phagocytosis
Eosinophils (10–12 microns)	Bilobed nuclei with coarse azurophilic granules	Immune hyper-sensitivity reactions, parasitic killing (major basic proteins)
Basophils (8–10 microns)	Round to oval nuclei with coarse basophilic granules	Secrete histamine, serotonin (vasodilators)

Contd...

Contd...

Cell	Morphology	Functions
Lymphocyte–small (8–10 micron) and large (12–15 micron)	Round to oval nuclei filling the entire cell	Cells of immunity, secrete immuno-globulins
Monocyte (16–22 micron)	Indented nuclei with vacuolated cytoplasm, fine pinkish violet granules	Cell of chronic inflammation, phagocytic cells

PLATELETS

Platelets are tiny anucleate cells of size **2–4 microns**. The normal number of platelets varies from **2,00,000 cells to 4,00,000 cells/cumm**. The lifespan of the cells is between **7–14 days**. Of the total number of platelets two thirds are seen in active circulation and the rest one third is stored in the spleen (splenic reserve). The major function of platelet is to maintain hemostasis, they play a pivotal role in the primary hemostasis.

LABORATORY DETERMINATION OF CELL COUNTS

The technique of counting of the blood cells is known as *Hemocytometry*. This method involves manual counting of the cells after diluting it with the suitable diluting fluid and the counts are made in specialized counting chambers with rulings.

COUNTING CHAMBER

The most widely used counting chamber is the Thoma's chamber with improved Neubauer ruling, preferably called as the **Neubauer's chamber**.

It has a counting **area of 9 sqmm and a depth of 0.1 mm**. The **9 sqmm** area is further divided into **9 squares**. Each square measures an area of **1 sqmm**. The four corner squares are further divided into **16 smaller squares** and the central square is divided into **25 smaller squares**. Each square measure **1/400 sqmm** in area.

Other counting chambers that can be used are the Fuchs-Rosenthal chamber and Speirs-Levy counting chambers. The depth and counting area of these chambers are more, so they are used to count fluids with a smaller number of cells as in cerebrospinal fluid. The special type of chamber is used for counting the spermatozoa is called the Makler chamber.

RED CELL COUNT

Sample

EDTA or Double oxalated blood or capillary sample.

Instruments

Neubauer counting chamber, RBC pipette and RBC diluting fluid.

RBC Pipette

It has a larger bulb with a red glass bead. The stem has got three markings 0.5.1.0 and 101. The function of the red bead is to ensure proper mixing of the sample with the diluting fluid, to ensure that the bulb is dry and to identify the pipette.

RBC diluting fluid **(Hayem's fluid)**—It contains sodium citrate, formalin, mercuric chloride and distilled water.

Procedure

The blood sample is drawn upto **0.5 mark** and the diluting fluid upto **101 mark**. This makes a **dilution of 1 in 200**. The sample is mixed well and the sample from the stem of the pipette is discarded. The chamber is cleaned and the sample is introduced under the coverslip and allowed to settle for 2–3 minutes. The red cells seen in the four corners and the center of central square of the chamber is counted.

Calculation of Red Cell

Number of cells counted: N
Dilution factor : 1 in 200
Area of counting : 80 small squares each with an area of 1/400 sqmm

Total area is 80/400 = 1/5 sqmm

Depth of the chamber: 1/10 mm

Volume of the counting area: $1/5 \times 1/10 = 1/50$ cumm

Total number of blood cells/cu m =

$$\frac{\text{Number of cell counted} \times \text{Dilution factor}}{\text{Volume of the chamber}}$$

$$\frac{N \times 200}{1/50}$$

Total number of blood cells/cumm is

$$N \times 200 \times 50 = N \times 10000$$

Normal Values

Male : 4.5–6.0 million cells/cumm
Female : 4.0–5.0 million cell/cumm

Decreased RBC count	*Increased RBC counts*
Anemia	Polycythemia
Pregnancy	Cyanotic heart diseases
Other causes	Hemoconcentration

WHITE CELL COUNT

Sample

EDTA or double oxalated blood or capillary sample.

Instruments

Neubauer counting chamber, WBC pipette and WBC diluting fluid.

WBC Pipette

It has a bulb with a white glass bead. The stem has got three markings 0.5.1.0 and 11. The function of the bead is to ensure proper mixing of the sample with the diluting fluid, to ensure that the bulb is dry and to identify the pipette.

WBC Diluting Fluid (Turk's Fluid)

It contains gentian violet (to stain the nuclei of the white cells) and glacial acetic acid (to lyse the red cells).

PROCEDURE

- The blood sample is drawn upto 0.5 mark and the diluting fluid upto 11 mark.
- This makes a dilution of 1 in 20.
- The sample is mixed well and the sample from the stem of the pipette is discarded.
- The chamber is cleaned and the sample is introduced under the coverslip and allowed to settle for 2–3 minutes.
- The white cells seen in the four large peripheral squares are counted.

Calculation of White Cell Count

Number of cells counted: N

Dilution factor : 1 in 20

Area of counting : 4 squares each with an area of 1 sqmm

Depth of the chamber: 1/10 mm

Volume of the counting area: $4 \times 1/10 = 4/10$ cumm

Total number of blood cells/cu m =

$$\frac{\text{Number of cell counted} \times \text{Dilution factor}}{\text{Volume of the chamber}}$$

$$\frac{N \times 20}{0.4}$$

Total number of blood cells/cumm is $= N \times 50$

Normal Values

Adults : 4000–11,000 cells/cumm
Children : 6000–18,000 cells/cumm

Decreased WBC count (leukopenia)	Increased WBC counts (leukocytosis)
Aplastic anemia	Physiological—muscular exercise, pregnancy, children
Drug-induced suppression	Acute infections
Megaloblastic anemia	Chronic infections
Typhoid infection	Leukemoid reaction
Certain viral infections	Leukemia

PLATELET COUNT

Sample

EDTA or deouble oxalated blood (preferred) or capillary sample.

Instruments

Neubauer counting chamber, RBC pipette and platelet diluting fluid.

Platelet Diluting Fluid

It contains procaine hydrochloride, sodium chloride and distilled water.

Procedure

- The blood sample is drawn upto 0.5 mark and the diluting fluid upto 101 mark.
- This makes a dilution of 1 in 200.
- The sample is mixed well and the sample from the stem of the pipette is discarded.
- The chamber is cleaned and the sample is introduced under the coverslip, the chamber is placed in a Petri dish with moist filter paper and left for 15 minutes.
- The platelets are counted in all the 25 small central squares.

Calculation

Number of cells counted: N
Dilution factor : 1 in 200
Area of counting : 1 sqmm
Depth of the chamber: 1/10 mm
Volume of the counting area: 1 × 1/10
= 1/10 cumm

Total number of platelets/cumm =

$$\frac{\text{Number of cell counted} \times \text{dilution factor}}{\text{Volume of the chamber}}$$

$$\frac{N \times 200}{0.1}$$

Total number of blood cells/cumm = $N \times 2000$

Normal Values

2,00,000–4,00,000 cells/cumm.

Decreased count (thrombocytopenia)	Increased counts (thrombocytosis)
Immune mediated destruction	Essential thrombocythemia
Aplastic anemia	Muscular exercise
Megaloblastic anemia	Post-splenectomy
Acute leukemia	Cases of chronic myeloid leukemia
Hypersplenism	

Points to Ponder

- The technique of counting of the blood cells is known as hemocytometry. This method involves manual counting of the cells after diluting it with the suitable diluting fluid and the counts are made in specialized counting chambers with rulings.
- Chemotaxis is the process by which white blood cells move toward the site of infection or injury.

ASSESSMENT QUESTIONS

1. **Enumerate the various types of counting chambers used to count blood cells.**
2. **Name the various diluting fluids used in counting red blood cells.**
3. **Name the various diluting fluids used in counting white blood cells.**
4. **Name the various diluting fluids used in counting platelets.**
5. **What is the normal red blood cell count? How will you call increase in count and decrease in count respectively?**
6. **Enlist the advantages of using an automated blood cell counter.**

MULTIPLE CHOICE QUESTIONS

1. **One of the following is a diluting fluid used in counting platelets:**
   A. Hayem's fluid B. Turk's fluid
   C. Rees Ecker fluid D. Heparin
2. **What is another name for platelets?**
   A. Erythrocytes B. Thrombocytes
   C. Leukocytes D. Lymphocytes
3. **Where are platelets produced in the body?**
   A. Liver B. Spleen
   C. Bone marrow D. Kidneys
4. **Which type of white blood cell is associated with the release of histamine during allergic reactions?**
   A. Neutrophil B. Basophil
   C. Monocyte D. Lymphocyte
5. **Which WBC is the most numerous and is known for its role in phagocytosis?**
   A. Lymphocyte B. Monocyte
   C. Neutrophil D. Eosinophil

Answer Key for MCQs

1	2	3	4	5
C	B	C	B	C

Study of Blood Smear and Differential Leukocyte Count

Learning Objectives

At the end of reading this chapter, the student shall be able to:

- Describe in detail the method of preparing a peripheral blood smear, the procedure of staining and methods of interpretation.
- Describe the various alterations in the morphology of the blood cells in a peripheral smear.

STUDY OF BLOOD SMEAR

The peripheral blood smear is preferable to use a capillary blood sample for making a peripheral smear rather than a venous sample. The smear should be immediately stained for proper evaluation of the cell morphology.

PROCEDURE

A thin smear is made by keeping a small drop of blood near the edge of the slide and with the spreader placed at an angle of 30 on the blood drop and a gentle push if given to make a smooth thin smear without ragged edges. The film is allowed to dry and taken for staining immediately.

STAINING PROCEDURE

The blood film is usually stained by dyes of the Romanowsky family. All the members of this family will have an acid dye and a basic dye dissolved in a solvent. The common stains of this family are Leishman's stain, Giemsa stain, Wright's Jenner stain and May Grunwald stain. They can used as single stains or as a combination of two stains, e.g., May Grunwald-Giemsa, Wright Giemsa and others. Combination of two Romanowsky stains gives the advantage of improved staining with a spectrum of colors. They are referred to as panoptic staining.

Steps in Staining

- The smear is placed flat on a staining rack.
- The film is covered well with the stain and allow it to stand for 1 minute.
- Double the quantity of buffer solution (Sorensen's Buffer pH 6.8) or distilled water is added to the stain and both the solutions are mixed thoroughly by gentle blowing. It is allowed to stand for 10 minutes.
- After 10 minutes, the smear is washed well in running tap water without taking the slide from the rack.
- The slide is allowed to dry.

EXAMINATION OF BLOOD FILMS

Introduction

The examination of a well made and well stained peripheral blood smear is probably the single most important laboratory test as it helps to:

- Estimate approximately the numbers of each of the three cellular elements

- Study the morphology of these cells
- Look for blood parasites and abnormal cells
- Study the response of the body to various disease processes.

It is therefore important to observe all the cellular elements when you study the blood smear.

Uniform Grading of Blood Picture

It is very important to remember that the smear must be well made, properly stained and examined systematically. Operator's skill influences the quality of a blood film. A poorly made blood smear will have ruptured and distorted cells as well as uneven distribution of cells. Coverslip preparation and the new spin methods give much better distribution of cells. Poor staining can also make it very difficult to identify cells and accurately interpret the smear.

Blood picture study involves examination of the smear under:

- Low power objective
- High dry objective
- Oil immersion objective

Low Power Examination

This is a very important aspect of blood smear examination because this gives an overall picture. It is something like an aerial view of a landscape by which you get to know the total picture of the landscape though finer details cannot be made out. The whole smear has to be scanned under low power to assess the following:

- The quality of the film and staining
- Look for the approximate number of RBCs as to whether they are normal, decreased (anemia) or increased (polycythemia)
- Degree of rouleaux formation
- Presence of autoagglutination
- Look for the approximate number of WBCs as to whether they are normal, decreased (leukopenia) or increased (leukocytosis)
- Presence of atypical cells, such as immature blast cells
- Distribution of platelets
- Presence of parasites, such as microfilaria, trypanosomes and malaria
- Proper field selection for oil immersion study.

Examination Under High Dry Objective

This is to assess approximately the total white cell count. Observe at least 6 fields in the thick portion of the smear where the red cells overlap and estimate the number of WBCs per high power field.

No. of WBCs/hpf	*Approx. total count per cumm*
2–4/hpf	4,000–7,000/cumm
4–6/hpf	7,000–10,000/cumm
6–10/hpf	10,000–13,000/cumm
10–20/hpf	13,000–18,000/cumm

Examination Under Oil Immersion Objective

Proper field selection: In selecting the field, one should choose an area where the red bloods cells are just beginning to overlap. There should be approximately 200 cells per 1000 × magnification.

Study of RBC

Various aspects of the RBC, such as size, shape, degree of hemoglobinization and color are studied and graded in addition to the study of red cell inclusions and nucleated RBCs.

Grading system: Many different types of grading systems are used to indicate abnormalities in a blood picture. It is not enough to just indicate the abnormality but the degree of abnormality should also be mentioned. Grading may be as mild, moderate or marked or by using the "plus" system. In either method the technician must have a definite criterion for describing the morphology. When hematological abnormalities are graded, the total picture must be presented so that the physician can see the peripheral blood smear in his mind as he reads the report. The grading system utilizing a scale of 1 plus to 4 plus is described below, however it is not mandatory to follow the "plus" system of grading the peripheral smear.

Variation in the size of RBC

Anisocytosis: The normal size of RBC is 7.2 microns and a normal RBC is referred to as a normocyte. Anisocytosis is a term which refers to an abnormal variation in the size of erythrocytes. This may include normocytes **(Fig. 19.1)**, macrocytes, and microcytes. Two factors must be considered when using a grading system of 1 to 4. The amount of anisocytosis depends upon the degree of variation and the number of cells that vary in size.

1 + Anisocytosis	Most red cells in the average oil immersion field appear uniform in size but 5–10 cells per field (2–5%) are easily distinguished from the predominant cell line
2 + Anisocytosis	Most red cells in the average oil immersion field appear uniform in size but 10–15 cells / field (5–7%) are easily distinguished from the predominant cell line
3 + Anisocytosis	Most red cells in the average oil immersion field appear uniform in size but 15–25 cells / field (7–12%) are easily distinguished from the predominant cell line
4 + Anisocytosis	Most red cells in the average oil immersion field are uniform in size but at least 26–50 cells/field (12–25%) are easily distinguished from the predominantly cell line

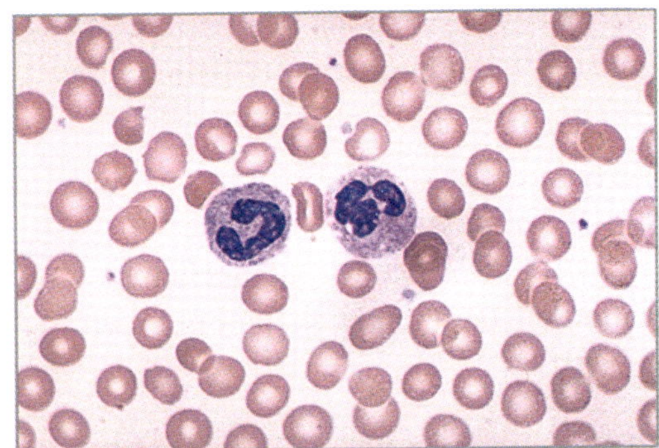

Fig. 19.1: Normocytic red cells with neutrophils.

Microcytosis: Red cells less than 6 microns in diameter are termed microcytes. When microcytes are present it is usually accompanied by a low MCV

1 + Microcytosis	5–20% of the red cells per oil immersion field are microcytes
2 + Microcytosis	21–50% of the red cells per oil immersion field are microcytes
3 + Microcytosis	51–75% of the red cells per oil immersion field are microcytes
4 + Microcytosis	76–100% of the red cells per oil immersion field are microcytes

Microcytes are seen in iron deficiency anemia, thalassemia and sideroblastic anemia.

Macrocytosis: Erythrocytes greater than 8 microns in diameter are termed macrocytes. When macrocytes are present there is usually an increase in MCV

1 + Macrocytosis	2–10% of the red cells per oil immersion field appear larger than normal
2 + Macrocytosis	11–25% of the red cells per oil immersion field appear larger than normal
3 + Macrocytosis	26–50% of the red cells per oil immersion field appear larger than normal
4 + Macrocytosis	More than 50% of the red cells per oil immersion field appear larger than normal

Macrocytes are seen in megaloblastic anemia, hemolytic anemia with excessive erythropoiesis, chronic liver disease, etc.

Variation in shape of RBC: Normal shape of RBC is described as biconcave disc.

Poikilocytosis: Erythrocytes which slow abnormal variation in shape from a normal biconcave disc are termed poikilocytes. RBCs that can be classified as poikilocytes are spherocytes, oval macrocytes, target cells, acanthocytes, schistocytes, sickle cells, burr cells, teardrop cells, pencil cells and ovalocytes **(Table 19.1)**. If more than 5% (10 poikilocytes per field) of one type is present then report the percentage of that type.

TABLE 19.1: Different types of poikilocytes.

Terminology	*Description*	*Associated disease states*
Echinocytes (Crenated cells)	Crenation is the term applied to the shrinkage of a red cell through loss of water in a hypertonic medium. This appears to make the cell membrane wrinkled	As an artifact due to slow drying of smear or smears made several hours after collection and uremia
Burr cells	Burr cells are very small irregular shrunken cells with rounded and pointed projections of varying sizes. They derive their name from their resemblance to the small thorny 'burrs' which come from certain grasses	Uremia, chronic liver disease, pyruvate kinase deficiency
Acanthocyte (spike)	Irregularly speculated hyperchromic RBC with variable irregular projections	Abetalipoproteinemia, alcoholic liver disease, post-splenectomy, malabsorptive states, pyruvate kinase deficiency, chronic liver disease
Stomatocyte	Central area of pallor appears like a slit	Hereditary stomatocytosis. Alcoholism, cirrhosis, obstructive liver disease
Spherocyte	Spherocytes are spherical red cells which have rounded up so that they no longer have the biconcave shape **(Fig. 19.2)**. In smear it appears, smaller than normal with no central pallor. The normal red blood cells morphology is seen in **Figure 19.1**	Hereditary spherocytosis, auto immune hemolytic anemia, post-transfusion state
Schistocyte (helmet cell or fragmented cell) **(Fig. 19.3)**	These are fragmented RBCs	Microangiopathic hemolytic anemia (DIC, vasculitis, glomerulonephritis, prosthetic or pathologic valves), severe burns
Elliptocyte (Ovalocyte)	Oval to elongated cell blunt ends	Hereditary elliptocytosis, thalassemia, iron deficiency, myelophthisic anemia and megaloblastic anemia
Drepanocyte (Sickle cell) **(Fig. 19.4)**	Cells containing Polymerized hemoglobin S. They are sickle shaped or elliptical with pointed ends	Sickle cell disorders (SS, S-trait, SC, SD S-thalassemia, etc.)

Contd...

Contd...

Terminology	*Description*	*Associated disease states*
Codocyte (bell, target cell)	These are cells which tend to be somewhat enlarged but which characteristically have a central round area of staining surrounded by a ring of pallor and then an outer border which is stained again. They are thinner than normal cells and look as if the size of the membrane is too much for the amount of hemoglobin. They look like a target	Obstructive liver disease, hemoglobinopathies (S, C), thalassemia, iron deficiency, post-splenectomy
Dacrocyte (teardrop cell)	Cells with a single elongated or pointed extremity shaped like tear or a pear	Myelofibrosis with myeloid metaplasia, myelophthisic anemia, thalassemia
Leptocyte (thin)	Thin, flat cell with hemoglobin at periphery with a large area of central pallor	Thalassemia, obstructive live disease

1 + Poikilocytosis	2–6 cells per oil immersion field vary from the normal shape
2 + Poikilocytosis	7–10 cells per oil immersion field vary from the normal shape
3 + Poikilocytosis	11–20 cells per oil immersion field vary from the normal shape
4 + Poikilocytosis	21 or more cells per oil immersion field vary from the normal shape

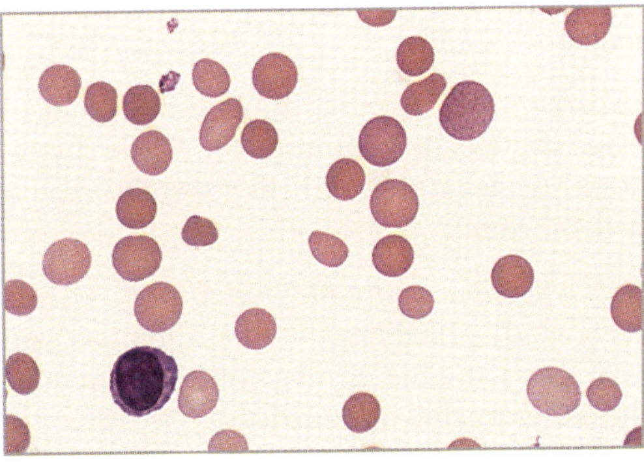

Fig. 19.2: Spherocytes in peripheral blood smear.

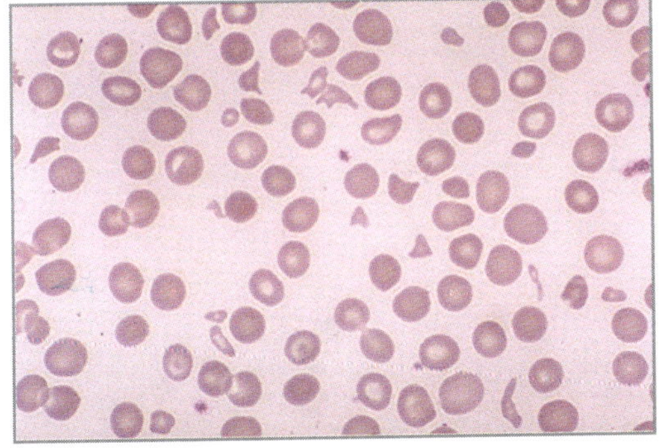

Fig. 19.3: Schistocytes (fragmented red cells).

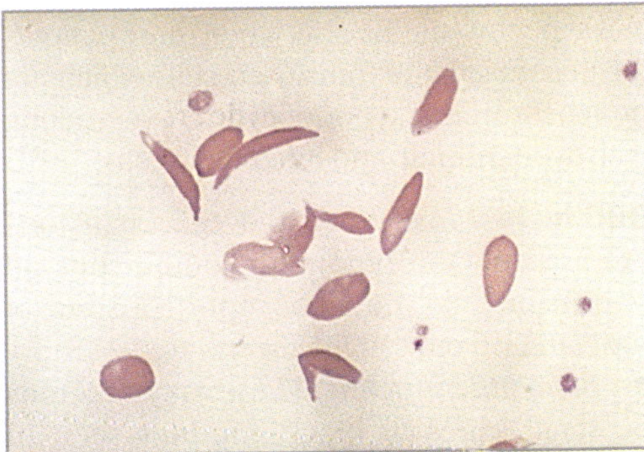

Fig. 19.4: Sickle cells.

Color of RBC: Normal RBC is referred to as normochromic. Normal RBC has a small area of central pallor.

Hypochromia: This is an abnormal decrease in the hemoglobin content of the red cell. This is often difficult to grade and depends much on the quality of the smear. MCHC is usually decreased when hypochromia is present and can be used in assessing the degree of hypochromia along with the blood smear.

Polychromatophilia: Polychromatophilic RBCs are immature, non-nucleated RBCs with the presence of some residual RNA in them. They are seen as larger than the normal RBC, with various shades of blue combined with tinges of pink.

Increased number of polychromatophilic red cells are associated with elevated reticulocyte count.

Hyperchromia: Hyperchromia is a term used when there is no central pallor. Spherocytes, acanthocytes and sickle cells generally appear hyperchromic.

Anisochromia or double population: This is seen when deficiency anemias (such as iron deficiency anemia or megaloblastic anemia) are either treated or transfused. Two different populations of RBCs are seen. When iron deficiency anemia is treated, newly formed cells are fully hemoglobinized and of normal size but the already existing cells are microcytic and hypochromic. So also, when these patients are transfused, the transfused cells which are normochromic and normocytic are seen along with hypochromic and microcytic cells.

RBC inclusions: When red cell inclusions are present, the type and number per oil immersion field should be reported. Some of the common red cell inclusions are:

- *Basophilic stippling:* These are numerous small blues of black granules seen in red cells on Romanowsky staining. They are more often seen in cells which are polychromatophilic. This is found in patients with heavy metal poisoning, especially associated with lead and sometimes with mercury and bismuth. They may also be seen in megaloblastic anemia and in some hemolytic anemias like thalassemia.
- *Howell-Jolly bodies:* These inclusions appear as small, round, densely staining, dark blue particles, 0.5–1 micron in diameter **(Fig. 19.5)**. They are often located towards the periphery of the cell. They are composed of deoxyribonucleic acid (DNA) and are actually remnants of the nucleus of the precursor normoblast. They are seen in certain hemolytic anemias, megaloblastic anemia, hyposplenic states and also are characteristically found after splenectomy.
- *Cabot rings:* These are seen as pale rings or as 'figure of eight; within the red cell cytoplasm, they appear to be remnants of the spindle. They are seen in hemolytic anemias, megaloblastic anemia, and sometimes after splenectomy.
- *Siderosomes and pappenheimer bodies:* In pathological state, the iron granulations are larger and more numerous. Siderosomes are found in the periphery of the cell whereas basophilic stippling tends to be distributed uniformly throughout the cell. Pappenheimer bodies are siderosomes that stain with Wright's stain.
- *Malaria parasites:* These are intra-erythrocytic parasites. Different stages of malarial parasites such as trophozoites,

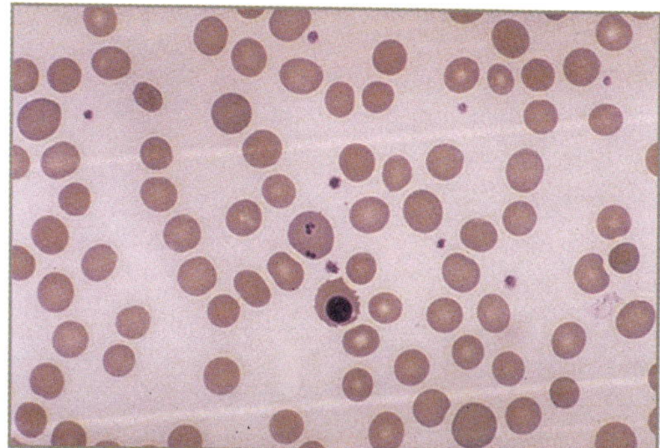

Fig. 19.5: Howell-Jolly bodies and a nucleated red cell.

schizonts and gametocytes of the different species of *Plasmodium* can be seen depending on the type of infection in our country. *Plasmodium vivax* and *Plasmodium falciparum* is commonly seen.

Nucleated RBC (Normoblast): If only an occasional nucleated RBC (nRBC) is seen when scanning the white blood cells under low power then this is reported as occasional. If nucleated RBCs are seen during the differential count, they are reported as a given number per 100 WBCs. If more than 3 nucleated RBCs are seen during the differential count of 100 WBCs then the WBC count must be corrected. Presence of nRBC indicates increased erythroid activity in the bone marrow.

Study of leukocytes: Under oil immersion, the differential count, morphological variations and abnormalities of WBC are studied.

Differential count: The differential WBC count is a method whereby the number of different types of white blood cells present in the blood sample of a given patient are counted by examining a well stained peripheral smear. The WBCs of different types are then expressed as a percentage of the total number of cells counted. Usually, 100 WBCs are counted. When the count is very high as in cases of leukemia, ideally 500 WBCs are counted to get a better idea of the pattern of distribution of various types of WBCs.

Technique: The differential count is done in the area of the smear where the RBC morphology is well made out (RBCs are separated without overlapping). The WBCs is this area shows good morphological details. There is uneven distribution of WBCs in the peripheral smear, i.e., the larger cells monocytes and granulocytes occupy the edges and the tail of the smear while relatively smaller lymphocytes occupy the center.

Follow one of the following three methods:

1. Going back and forth side on the smear including both the edges and the center.
2. Going back and forth lengthwise on a smear including both body and tail.
3. Battlement method

One starts at the edge of the smear and moves towards the center for 4–5 oil fields lengthwise, then return to the edge counting the cells as you go. Then moving on along the edge, you again move towards the center and then along the back to the edge.

Normal counts:

Normal total WBC count	
Adults	4000–11000/cu mm
Newborn	10000–26000/cu mm
Infants (up to 1 year)	6000–18000/cu mm
Children (4–7 years)	5000–15000/cu mm
Children (8–12 years)	4500–131500/cu mm
Normal differential count	
Adults	
Neutrophil **(Fig. 19.6)**	4000–11000/cu mm
Lymphocytes **(Fig. 19.7)**	20–45%
Monocytes **(Fig. 19.8)**	2–10%
Eosinophils **(Fig. 19.7)**	1–6%
Basophil **(Fig. 19.8)**	0–1%
Newborn (approximately)	
Neutrophil	61%
Lymphocytes	31%
Monocytes	6%
Eosinophils	2%
Basophil	<1%
Children	
Neutrophil	40–75%
Lymphocyte	30–60%
Monocytes	2–10%
Eosinophil	1–6%
Basophil	<1%

Variations in the leukocyte counts: Increase in the total WBC count of more than 11,000/cumm is known as 'leukocytosis,' while counts less than 4,000/cumm is called 'leukopenia.'

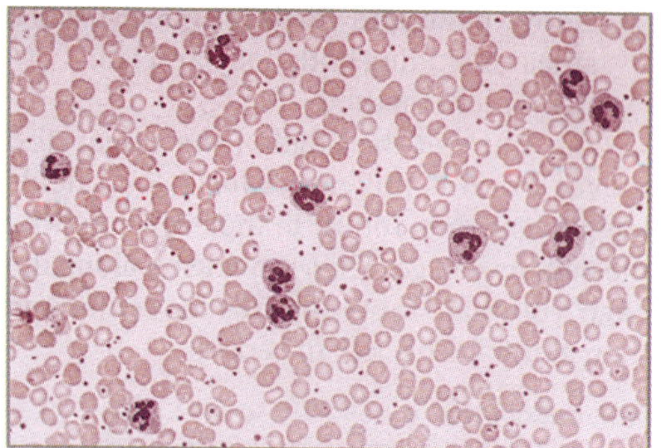

Fig. 19.6: Neutrophils and platelets.

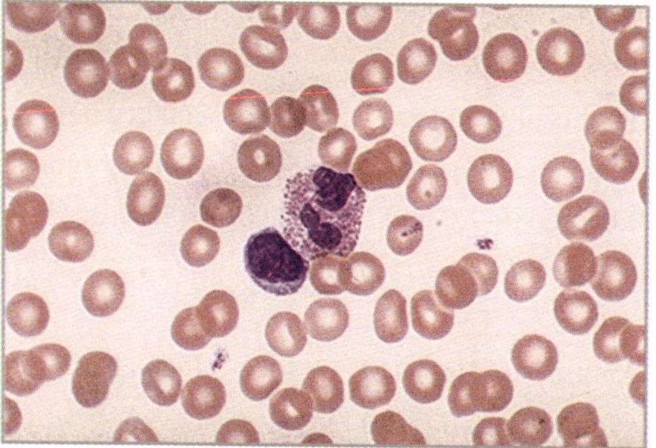

Fig. 19.7: Eosinophil and lymphocyte.

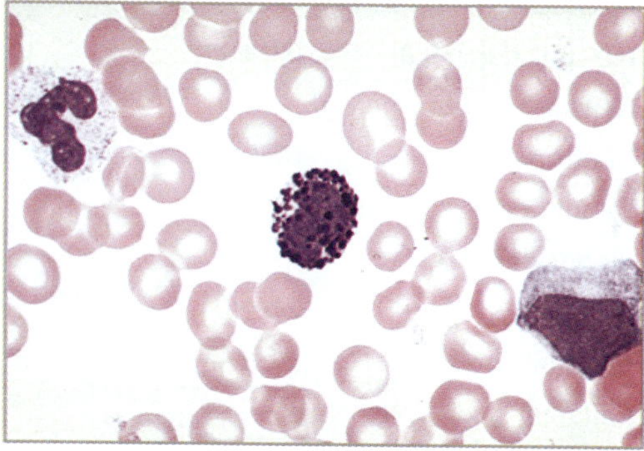

Fig. 19.8: Basophil and monocyte.

Variations in neutrophils:

- *Neutrophilia:* Indicates a condition in which there is increase in the percentage of neutrophils in the differential WBC count. All the physiological causes that give rise to leukocytosis also give rise to neutrophilia. Pyogenic bacterial infection is the most common cause of neutrophilia. The severity of the infection and the degree of response of the body are indicated by the degree of neutrophilia.
- *Neutropenia:* The infections which cause leukopenia (e.g., typhoid, viral infections, such as measles, influenza and dengue) also cause a neutropenia. It can also occur in iron deficiency anemia, megaloblastic anemia, aplastic anemia and bone marrow suppression from drugs or irradiation. A very severe form of neutropenia is referred to as agranulocytosis.

Variations in lymphocytes:

- *Lymphocytosis:* Indicates increase in the lymphocytes in the peripheral blood. It may be relative or absolute.

  The main causes are:
  - Age—in children, the lymphocyte counts are higher.
  - Bacterial infections—whooping cough, typhoid, tuberculosis and syphilis.
  - Viral infections—mumps, measles and influenza.
  - Infectious mononucleosis—there may not only be lymphocytosis but also morphological changes in the lymphocytes.
  - Chronic lymphocytic leukemia.
- *Lymphopenia:* Seen in the acute stages of infections irradiation and AIDS.

Variation in other white blood cells:

- *Monocytosis:* Seen in kala-azar, typhoid, tuberculosis, malaria and in subacute bacterial endocarditis.
- *Eosinophilia:* Seen in parasitic infection, such as filariasis, trichinosis and hook-worm.

  Allergic diseases, such as hay fever and asthma. Skin conditions, such as eczema and psoriasis. Hypereosinophilic syndrome, such as Loeffler's syndrome and eosinophilic leukemia.

- *Basophilia:* Seen in myeloproliferative disorders—chronic myeloid leukemia, myelofibrosis and polycythemia vera.

Abnormal cells: In various leukemias, we see blasts and immature cells. Sometimes we see plasma cells in the peripheral blood in multiple myeloma. These cells can be picked up on low power scanning and details studied under oil immersion objective. All immature forms of white blood cells and lymphocytes should be reported.

Quantitative and qualitative changes in leukocytes: Quantitative changes are leukocytosis and shift to left (appearance of immature forms of neutrophils). Quantitative changes in leukocyte morphology include toxic granulations, Dohle bodies and cytoplasmic vacuolations. These changes are seen during infections.

- *Toxic granulation:* The neutrophil granules often become larger and stain darkly and appear more basophilic. These are called "toxic granules". These granules or they may be scattered in between the more normal small pinkish granules or they may be in sufficient number to nearly replace the normal granules. Good staining is required to see the toxic granules.
- *Dohle bodies:* The cytoplasm may show focal areas of bluish staining bodies in the otherwise pink cytoplasm. These are called "Dohle bodies".
- *Cytoplasmic vacuolation:* Presence of cytoplasmic vacuoles indicate a reactive state of a neutrophil.
- *Hypersegmented neutrophils:* Normally neutrophils has 2–4 nuclear lobes. Neutrophils with 5 or more than 5 lobes are called hypersegmented neutrophils. This can be seen in megaloblastic anemia. A normal individual usually has approximately 76% two or three lobed neutrophils, 17% four lobe neutrophils and 2% five lobe neutrophils and the remaining 5% will be non-segmented neutrophils.

Study of platelets

Estimation of number of platelets: It is very important to give an accurate estimation of the number of platelets as well as the description of the morphology. Platelet estimate can usually be made on a peripheral smear, as each platelet in an average oil immersion field represent 15,000 platelets per cu mm. It is important to remember that these estimates are only reliable when the blood has been mixed well with EDTA and the slides are prepared within an hour. This estimate should be used when the smear has been made from capillary blood using finger prick method.

The normal platelet count is 150,000 to 400,000 cells/cumm of blood.

When the platelet count is reduced it is called Thrombocytopenia. It can be seen in acute leukemias, idiopathic thrombocytopenic purpura, aplastic anemia, megaloblastic anemia, hypersplenism, etc. Platelet counts more than 4.5 lakhs/cumm is referred to as thrombocytosis. It is seen in infections, immediately after hemorrhage, trauma or surgery, in chronic myeloid leukemia and in essential thrombocythemia.

Morphology of platelets: Platelet anisocytosis, presence of giant platelets (up to 7 to 9 micron) and the abnormal forms must be reported. Giant platelets are seen in Bernard-Soulier syndrome. Absence of platelet aggregation on a finger prick smear is seen in Glanzmann's thrombasthenia.

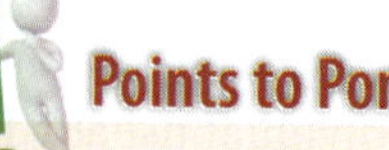

Points to Ponder

- The examination of a well made and well stained peripheral blood smear is probably the single most important laboratory test as it helps to.
- Estimate approximately the numbers of each of the three cellular elements.
- Study the morphology of these cells.
- Look for blood parasites and abnormal cells.
- Study the response of the body to various disease processes.
- The normal size of RBC is 7.2 microns and a normal RBC is referred to as a normocyte. Anisocytosis is a term which refers to an abnormal variation in the size of erythrocytes. This may include normocytes, macrocytes, and microcytes.
- Erythrocytes which slow abnormal variation in shape from a normal biconcave disc are termed poikilocytes.
- Increase in the total WBC count of more than 11,000/cumm is known as 'leukocytosis', while counts less than 4,000/cumm is called 'leukopenia'.

ASSESSMENT QUESTIONS

1. **Define leukocytosis.**
2. **What do you mean by leukopenia?**
3. **Define thrombocytopenia. Mention two common causes for it.**
4. **What is the function of a platelet?**
5. **Name the common stains used for staining a peripheral smear.**
6. **Give examples for hemoparasites.**
7. **Name the stains used to demonstrate malarial parasites in a blood film.**
8. **Enlist the conditions in which you see target cells in a blood film.**
9. **What are toxic granules ? In which condition do you see them?**
10. **Name the two types of granules seen in platelets.**
11. **Enlist the common causes for neutrophilia.**
12. **Enlist the common causes for neutropenia**
13. **Enlist the common causes for eosinophilia.**
14. **Enlist the common causes for lymphocytosis.**
15. **What is a reticulocyte ?**
16. **Define Buffy coat. Mention its composition.**
17. **What is agranulocytosis ?**
18. **Mention the common diseases transmitted through blood.**
19. **What do you mean by leukemia?**

MULTIPLE CHOICE QUESTIONS

1. **Half-life of neutrophil is:**
   A. 6-7 hours
   B. 2-3 days
   C. 100 hours
   D. 120 days
2. **The most common cause of neutropenia is:**
   A. Typhoid
   B. Drugs
   C. Viral infection
   D. Protozoal infection

3. The most common stain used to stain peripheral smear is:

A. Leishman
B. Jenner
C. Wrights
D. Giemsa

4. Eosinophil cell count is increased in one of the following infections:

A. Bacterial
B. Viral
C. Fungal
D. Parasitic

5. Thrombocytopenia refers to decrease in the number of:

A. Platelets
B. Lymphocytes
C. Neutrophils
D. Red blood cells

Answer Key for MCQs

1	2	3	4	5
A	B	A	D	A

CHAPTER 20

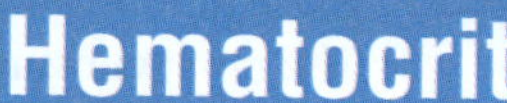

Hematocrit

Learning Objectives

At the end of reading this chapter, the student shall be able to:

- Describe the basic methodology of doing a packed cell volume (PCV) in a given sample and its interpretation.

DEFINITION

The hematocrit [Packed cell volume (PCV)] of a sample of blood is the ratio of the volume of erythrocytes to that of the whole blood.

It is expressed as a percentage or as a decimal fraction.

METHODS

The two methods of direct measurement of PCV are:

1. Macro method using Wintrobe's tube
2. Micro method using capillary tubes

Macro Method or Wintrobe's Method

- *Instrument:* Wintrobe's hematocrit tube is a special thick walled glass tube 11 cm long, with an internal diameter of 2.5 mm and a flat inner base. It is calibrated at 1 mm intervals to 105–110 mm and holds about 1 mL blood.
- *Blood sample:* Venous blood anticoagulated with EDTA, Wintrobe's mixture, or heparin can be used.
- *Procedure:* Thoroughly mix the blood in the bottle by repeated inversion or by a mechanical rotator. Draw the blood into a long Pasteur pipette. Fill the Wintrobe's tube up to the 100 mm mark, starting from the bottom and gradually withdrawing the pipette as blood is expressed. This is to avoid air bubbles, which can get trapped in the column of blood. Centrifuge the tube at 2000–2300 rpm for 30 minutes.
- *Reading and interpretation:* The height of the red cells column is taken as the PCV, i.e., the volume occupied by the red cells expressed as a fraction of the total volume of blood. Other fractions noted are—above the pack of red cells a thin grayish-red layer of leukocytes and a creamy layer of platelets above that and just below the plasma. These two together constitute the "buffy coat". The column of plasma is seen uppermost.
- Other information that can be gained apart from PCV:
  - Buffy coat: The buffy coat layer is an approximate indication of the number of white cells and platelets. Normally, 0.1 mm of this layer corresponds to about 1000 WBC/cu mm. The white cells from the buffy coat could be smeared to detect the

presence of immature cells when the cell count is very low and this can be used in LE (lupus erythematosus) cell preparation. Occasionally, an increase in buffy coat could be due to marked increase in platelets.

- Plasma color
  Yellow color of plasma indicates jaundice.
  Opaque plasma is due to lipemia.
  Pink color denotes hemoglobinemia.

❖ *Normal values*

Men	40–54%
Women	36–47%
At birth	44–62%

❖ *Clinical significance:* A value below an individual's normal or below the reference range for the age and sex indicates anemia and a higher value indicate polycythemia. Hematocrit reflects the ratio of red cells to plasma and not the total red cell mass.

Microhematocrit Method Using Capillary Tubes

❖ *Instruments:*
- Capillary hematocrit tube about 7 cm, long with uniform bore size of about 1 mm is used.
- Heparinized capillary tubes are used for capillary blood collection.
- Special centrifuge or centrifuge head to accommodate the capillary tube.

❖ *Procedure:* Two-thirds of the tube is filled with blood. The empty end is closed by plasticine or modeling clay. Blood fills by capillary action. The filled tubes are placed in the radial grooves of the micro hematocrit centrifuge head with the sealed end away from the center. Centrifuge at the speed of 10,000 to 12,000 G for five minutes.

❖ *Reading:* As the tubes are not graduated, they are measured using millimeter rule. The total length of blood including plasma and the length of red cell column are measured separately and the ratio calculated. A better and convenient way of taking the reading is by using the special chart provided by the manufacturer.

❖ *Advantages:*
- Only small amount of blood is needed for the test.
- Even capillary blood can be sampled.
- Less time is needed for the test.
- Easier procedure.
- Amount of trapped plasma is much less.

MEASUREMENT OF PCV IN AUTOMATED INSTRUMENTS

This is the method employed in some electronic cell counters. It is calculated by multiplying MCV by red cell count. The values are slightly less than that of the macro and micro methods.

Points to Ponder

- The hematocrit **(packed cell volume)** of a sample of blood is the ratio of the volume of erythrocytes to that of the whole blood.
- It is expressed as a percentage or as a decimal fraction.

ASSESSMENT QUESTION

1. What do you mean by hematocrit? Give indications for doing this test.

MULTIPLE CHOICE QUESTIONS

1. **Normal MCV is:**
   A. 70–90 µm³ C. 90–96 µm³
   B. 82–92 µm³ D. 75–95 µm³
2. **What role do red blood cells play in hematocrit measurement?**
   A. They carry oxygen C. They make up the plasma
   B. They clot the blood D. They contribute to the volume of blood
3. **Which of the following medical conditions may result in an elevated hematocrit?**
   A. Anemia C. Polycythemia
   B. Hemorrhage D. Leukemia
4. **Which condition is characterized by a low hematocrit value?**
   A. Polycythemia C. Thrombocytosis
   B. Leukocytosis D. Anemia
5. **What does the term "hematocrit" refer to in a blood test?**
   A. Red blood cell count C. Platelet count
   B. White blood cell count D Plasma volume

Answer Key for MCQs

1	2	3	4	5
B	D	C	D	A

21

CHAPTER

Erythrocyte Indices

Learning Objectives

At the end of reading this chapter, the student shall be able to:

- Define the common erythrocyte indices.
- Describe the formula used to calculate these indices.
- Enlist the clinical significance of this indices.

INTRODUCTION

Based on the results of tests which measure hemoglobin, packed cell volume and total red cell count, several calculations have been described which give quantitative information about the red cells. It was Wintrobe who introduced these calculations; hence, they are also known as Wintrobe's constant. The purpose of calculating these values is mainly for the classification of anemia.

The red cell indices are

- Mean corpuscular volume or MCV
- Mean corpuscular hemoglobin or MCH
- Mean corpuscular hemoglobin concentration or MCHC

Since these values are calculated from Hb, PCV and red cell count, meticulous care should be taken while doing these tests to get correct indices.

MEAN CORPUSCULAR VOLUME

It is the mean value of the red cell volume.

It is calculated using the formula:

$$MCV = \frac{\text{PCV/liter of blood}}{\text{Red cell count/liter of blood}}$$

PCV is expressed as percentage or per 100 mL and the red cell count as per cubic mm.

Mean corpuscular volume (MCV) is expressed in femtoliters **(fl) [1 L = 10^{-15} fl]**.

In practice, the **PCV (0.45) is divided by the red cell count in million (5) and multiplied by 1000**. The answer is expressed in femtoliters.

MEAN CORPUSCULAR HEMOGLOBIN

The mean corpuscular hemoglobin (MCH) is defined as the amount of hemoglobin in the average red blood cell or the average amount of Hb in all the red cells.

The basic formula is:

$$MCH = \frac{\text{Hb/liter of blood}}{\text{Red cell count/liter of blood}}$$

For convenience the value expressed in picograms [1 g = 1000 × 1000 × 1000 pg].

So, for practical purposes the formula for **MCH is Hb in g dL (15) divided by RBC count in millions (5), multiplied by 10,** expressed in picograms.

MEAN CORPUSCULAR HEMOGLOBIN CONCENTRATION

The mean corpuscular hemoglobin concentration (MCHC) is defined as the concentration of hemoglobin in the average red blood cell or that portion of the average red cell composed of hemoglobin. This is expressed as a percentage. The formula is:

$$\text{MCHC} = \frac{\text{Hemoglobin} \times 100}{\text{PCV}}$$

NORMAL VALUES

Mean Corpuscular Volume

Adults	-	85 ± 9 fl
Full term/cold blood	-	106 fl (mean)
Children 1 year	-	78 ± 8 fl
Children 10-12 years	-	85 ± 7 fl

Mean Corpuscular Hemoglobin

Adults—29.5 ± 2.5 pg.

Mean Corpuscular Hemoglobin Concentration

Adults and children—33 ± 2%.

CLINICAL SIGNIFICANCE

The values are altered in anemia. The indices are used to classify anemias morphologically.

Macrocytic Anemia

- MCV is increased up to 150 fl.
- MCH is slightly increased.
- MCHC is normal or diminished.

Microcytic Hypochromic Anemia

- MCV is diminished up to 50 fl. Or lower.
- MCH is diminished to 15 pg or lower.
- MCHC is diminished to 25% or less.
- Red cell distribution width (RDW) is increased.

Spherocytosis

- MCV is diminished
- MCHC is elevated—Spherocytosis is the only condition where MCHC is elevated.

OTHER INDICES

Color Index

The color index is an old method of estimating the average amount of hemoglobin in red cells in comparison to normal.

Color index = Hb % of normal/RBC % of normal.

100% Hb is taken as 14.5 g/dL and RBC count as 5 millions/cumm.

Normal range—0.85 to 1.15.

Mean Cell Diameter (MCD)

Previously measured by Haden Hauser Halo meter.

It can also be measured by calibrated micrometer discs on a blood film. About 200-500 cells are measured and their average calculated.

Normal range—7.2-7.5 m

Red Cell Distribution Width (RDW)

This is an estimate of variation in size of erythrocytes. It is measured in automatic cell counters by measuring the size of each red cell as it passes the counting aperture. This index is useful in differentiating iron deficiency anemia and thalassemia.

Normal range—11.6-14.6%

Points to Ponder

The red cell indices are
- Mean corpuscular volume of MCV.
- Mean corpuscular hemoglobin or MCH.
- Mean corpuscular hemoglobin concentration or MCHC.
- Since these values are calculated from Hb, PCV and red cell count, meticulous care should be taken while doing these tests to get correct indices.

ASSESSMENT QUESTION

1. **Enumerate the common erythrocyte indices used in laboratory.**

MULTIPLE CHOICE QUESTIONS

1. **One of the following indices gives an idea on the size of the red blood cells:**
   A. Mean corpuscular volume
   B. Mean corpuscular hemoglobin
   C. Color index
   D. Mean corpuscular hemoglobin concentration
2. **What are erythrocyte indices used for in a blood test?**
   A. Measuring red blood cell count
   B. Assessing white blood cell function
   C. Evaluating platelet activity
   D. Analyzing plasma composition
3. **MCHC is an abbreviation for:**
   A. Mean corpuscular hemoglobin content
   B. Mean corpuscular hemoglobin concentration
   C. Mean corpuscular hematocrit
   D. Mean corpuscular cell
4. **What is the normal range for MCHC?**
   A. 25 to 35 g/dL
   B. 30 to 40 g/dL
   C. 32 to 36 g/dL
   D. 36 to 42 g/dL
5. **What does a low MCV value typically indicate?**
   A. Microcytic anemia
   B. Macrocytic anemia
   C. Normocytic anemia
   D. Polycythemia

Answer Key for MCQs

1	2	3	4	5
A	A	B	C	A

22 CHAPTER Erythrocyte Sedimentation Rate

Learning Objectives

At the end of reading this chapter, the student shall be able to:

- Describe the basic methodology of doing a erythrocyte sedimentation rate (ESR) in a given sample and its interpretation.

DEFINITION

When the mixed venous blood is placed in a vertical tube, the red cell sediment or fall to the bottom. The length of fall to the top of the column of RBCs in a given interval of time is called erythrocyte sedimentation rate (ESR).

STAGES IN ERYTHROCYTE SEDIMENTATION RATE

Three stages are observed:

1. *Rouleaux formation or aggregation:* In the first ten minutes, the RBCs come together in rouleaux formation, i.e., like piles of coins, one on top of another. The more the rouleaux, the faster will be the next stage.
2. *Settling or sedimentation:* For the next 40 minutes, the RBCs settle at a constant rate.
3. *Packing:* In the final 10 minutes, sedimentation slows and the cells pack at the bottom of the tube.

METHODS

- Westergren method (modified)
- Wintrobe's method
- Micro ESR method—useful in infants and small children.

Modified Westergren Method

This Westergren tube is a straight pipette, 30 cm long, with an internal diameter of 2.5 mm, calibrated in millimeters from 0–200. It holds 2 mL of blood. A Westergren rack holds the pipettes vertical. It has a rubber band on which the pipette's tip is placed. A spring clip holds the upper end of the pipette so that no blood escapes.

Procedure

The preferred anticoagulant is 3.8% sodium citrate.

- 3.8% sodium citrate
  1.6 mL of blood is collected in 0.4 mL of anticoagulant to maintain a ratio of 1:4 (Westergren)
- EDTA (1.5 mg/mL) to collect 2 mL of blood.

Method

- Draw the anticoagulated blood into the Westergren tube upto the 0 mark, the outside wiped clean and the tube is set up in the rack perfectly vertical. Ensure that there are no air bubbles in the blood column.
- Start a stop watch or clock and take reading at 1 hour. The reading corresponding to the upper layer of the RBC column in the pipette is taken.

Wintrobe Method

The Wintrobe tube is filled with anticoagulated blood (EDTA) using a special long capillary pipette up to the 0.0 mark, near the top of the tube, making sure that there are no air bubbles in the column. The tube is then placed vertically in a stand and at the end of one hour, the reading of the top of the red cell column is taken in millimeters, marked on the tube.

Micro ESR Method

A plastic ESR tube, 230 mm long with one millimeter internal bore is filled with 0.2 mL of blood.

The tube is placed vertically and reading taken of the top of the red cell column at the end of one hour. This method is useful in infants and small children, since the volume of blood needed for the test is small.

Normal values (Westergren Method)

Age	*Men*	*Women*
Below 50 yrs	15 mm/hr	20 mm/hr
Above 50 yrs	20 mm/hr	30 mm/hr
Above 85 yrs	30 mm/hr	40 mm/hr

FACTORS AFFECTING ESR

Physiological Factors

- *Plasma factors:* An increase in plasma fibrinogen, globulins and cholesterol increase the ESR by decreasing the negative charge on RBCs. This negative charge prevents the RBCs from coming together to form rouleaux. Increase in albumin levels, decrease the ESR.
- *Red cells factors:* Decrease in the number of RBCs as in Anemia, increases the ESR, while in polycythemia, it is decreased. Smaller or microcytic RBCs and RBCs having less hemoglobin in them as in hypochromic anemia led to decreased ESR. Red cells with abnormal shapes as in sickle cell anemia do not form rouleaux and the ESR is decreased.
- *Age:* In infants, the ESR is low and it gradually increases to adult levels by puberty. In old age, the ESR is higher.
- *Sex:* Women have a slightly higher than men, perhaps because their PCV is lower.
- *Pregnancy:* The ESR begins to increase about the third month and returns to normal by four weeks after delivery.

Laboratory Factors

Errors in the test are commonly due to one of these factors.

1. *Temperature:* The test should be done at 20°C to 25°C. If the blood has been refrigerated, it should be brought to room temperature before the test is set up, since a low temperature can alter the result. Care should be taken to see that the tubes are not exposed to direct sunlight or to a source of heat.
2. *Time:* The test should be done within 2 hours of drawing of blood. If it has to be kept longer, the anticoagulant should be EDTA and the sample kept at 4°C.
3. *Anticoagulant:* Sodium citrate or EDTA or balanced oxalate solution may be used but in the proper concentration of anticoagulant to blood. Heparin alters the cell membrane potential and should not be used.
4. *Tube factors:* Length and diameter of ESR tube: The ESR is greater with longer tubes. The longer Westergren tubes is therefore preferred. The inner diameter should be 2.5 mm or more to overcome capillary attraction.
5. *Tilting of tube and movement:* If the tube is not perfectly vertical. The ESR increases as the RBCs slide down along the lower side. Similarly, if the tube is not perfectly still, the ESR will change. Hence the tube rack should not be on a surface which is disturbed easily or where any vibratory equipment like centrifuge is kept.

INTERPRETATION

This is a non-specific test but has its uses. An increase in ESR is usually an indication of disease. Usually, the diseases are chronic inflammatory conditions, such as tuberculosis, rheumatoid arthritis or malignancy. The test can also be useful in following disease activity or response to treatment once a diagnosis is made.

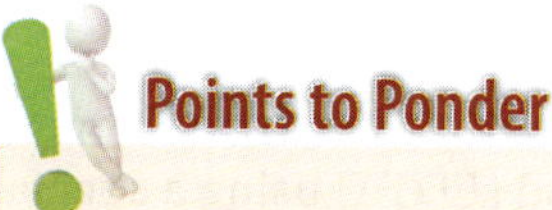

Points to Ponder

The length of fall to the top of the column of RBCs in a given interval of time is called erythrocyte sedimentation rate (ESR).

ASSESSMENT QUESTIONS

1. **What is erythrocyte sedimentation rate? Enlist the stages of ESR.**
2. **Name two conditions in which ESR is increased.**

MULTIPLE CHOICE QUESTIONS

1. **The most common anticoagulant used in the determination of ESR is:**
   - A. EDTA
   - B. Heparin
   - C. Trisodium citrate
   - D. Ammonium oxalate
2. **What does the Modified Westergren Method primarily measure?**
   - A. White blood cell count
   - B. Platelet count
   - C. Erythrocyte sedimentation rate (ESR)
   - D. Hematocrit
3. **What is the age-dependent reference range for ESR in the elderly?**
   - A. Higher than in younger adults
   - B. Lower than in younger adults
   - C. No significant difference
   - D. Varies widely
4. **What method is commonly used to measure ESR in a laboratory setting?**
   - A. Hemoglobin electrophoresis
   - B. Enzyme-linked immunosorbent assay (ELISA)
   - C. Westergren method
   - D. Polymerase chain reaction (PCR
5. **Which blood component plays a significant role in the rate of ESR?**
   - A. Platelets
   - B. White blood cells
   - C. Red blood cells
   - D. Plasma proteins

Answer Key for MCQs

1	2	3	4	5
C	C	A	C	C

CHAPTER 23

Bone Marrow Examination

Learning Objectives

At the end of reading this chapter, the student shall be able to:

- Enlist the indications for doing a bone marrow study.

INTRODUCTION

Hematopoiesis is the proliferation of progenitor cells and their differentiation into mature cells in the periphery. Under normal conditions, all the cellular components originate and complete the development within the bone marrow.

In the fetus, hematopoiesis starts in the yolk sac and then migrates to the fetal liver, spleen and finally the bone marrow. Bone marrow becomes the active site for hematopoiesis from the 5th month of gestation and remains to be the major site for blood cell production throughout the life.

At birth, all the bone marrow cavities contain hematopoietic elements as the age advances marrow is replaced from the peripheral long bones to the axial skeleton, such as vertebrae, sternum, iliac bones and proximal end of long bones.

Gross examination of the marrow shows two elements: The red marrow which contains active hematopoietic elements and the yellow marrow which is made up of fat cells. At birth, the marrow is predominantly red in nature as the age advances the yellow marrow gradually infiltrates the red marrow and by the age of 18 about 50% of the marrow is replaced by the fat.

Aspiration and biopsy are the two techniques through which the bone marrow can be examined. A thorough evaluation of bone marrow should include both of them.

INDICATIONS FOR BONE MARROW STUDY

- *Evaluation of increased or decreased number of cells in the peripheral blood:* As in cases of anemia, leukopenia and thrombocytopenia.
- *Diagnosis of acute and chronic leukemia:* Study of bone marrow is diagnostic for most of the acute and chronic leukemia.
- *Evaluation of the iron content of the marrow:* This is useful in the diagnosis of iron deficiency anemia, sideroblastic anemia and to estimate the iron stores.
- *Diagnosis of tumor involvement:* Examination of the bone marrow is useful in staging lymphomas, involvement of marrow in small cell carcinoma and other tumor infiltration of the marrow.
- *Confirmation of infection:* In cases of disseminated tuberculosis, marrow can be examined for presence of caseating granulomas or detection of the presence of intracellular organisms, such as *Leishmania donovani* as in cases of Kala-azar.
- Diagnosis of storage disorders, such as Gaucher's disease, Neimann-Pick disease.
- *Investigation of immunological disorders:* Bone marrow examination is diagnostic in

cases of monoclonal gammopathies, such as multiple myeloma.

INDICATIONS FOR BONE MARROW BIOPSY

Study of the bone marrow biopsy is indicated in the following conditions:

- *Failure to obtain cells in the bone marrow aspiration:* This may be due to technical defects or a dry marrow.
- *Evaluation of pancytopenia:* A bone marrow biopsy along with bone marrow aspiration is very useful in evaluation of pancytopenia and in cases showing leukoerythroblastic picture in the peripheral smear.
- *Evaluation of hematological neoplasms:* As in multiple myeloma and hairy cell leukemia.
- *Evaluation of tumor staging:* As in staging of lymphoma.

COMMON SITES FOR BONE MARROW ASPIRATION

The bone marrow aspiration is done in the following sites: Sternum, posterior superior iliac crest and proximal end of tibia. Other rarer sites include vertebra.

INSTRUMENTS

Bone marrow aspiration can be done by special type of needles which has two parts, the outer needle and inner stillet. The outer needle has got a guard to prevent extensive penetration into the bone.

The common needles used are:

- Salah's bone marrow aspiration needle
- Jamshidi needle
- University of Illinois needle

Bone marrow biopsy is done with a special Tru-Cut needle—Jamshidi bone marrow biopsy needle.

METHOD

The bone marrow aspiration should be done in a hospital with due precautions. The patient must be explained and reassured about the procedure before doing. The site of the aspiration is decided according the indication of the study. Normally, the common sites are the posterior superior iliac crest and sternum. The patient is made to lie down comfortably. The aspiration site is cleaned and the procedure is done under strict asepsis. Local anesthesia is given to the site. After securing anesthesia the needle with the stillet is introduced and once the cortex is reached a firm pressure is applied, securing the needle in the position, the stillet is removed and a 10 cc syringe is fitted to the needle and a firm aspiration is done. The patient will experience an acute pain called the suction pain. The needle is gradually removed and complete hemostasis must be ensured. The aspirated material is blown to glass slides and smears are made in quick succession. The smears should be made without any delay and the smears are air dried and stained with Romanowsky stain for interpretation.

INTERPRETATION

The stained marrow is evaluated for the extent of cellularity. Then evaluation of erythroid, myeloid, megakaryocytes are done in a systematic manner. The marrow is analyzed for the number of cells, morphology of cells and the pattern of maturation **(Fig. 23.1)**. For quantification of the number of cells at least 500 to 1000 cells are counted and a differential is made. Study of the morphology and pattern of maturation is very useful in deriving a

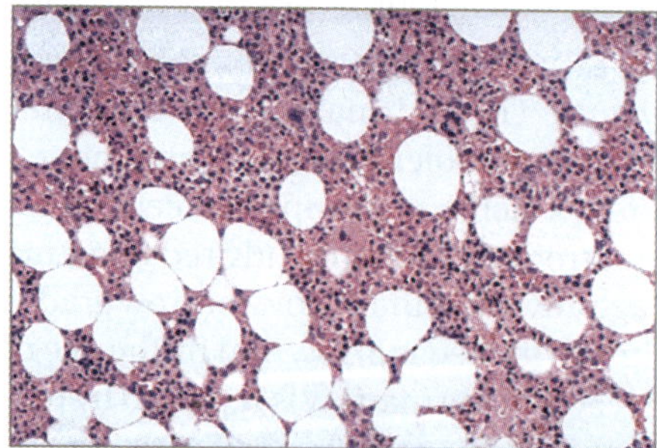

Fig. 23.1: Normal marrow cellular elements.

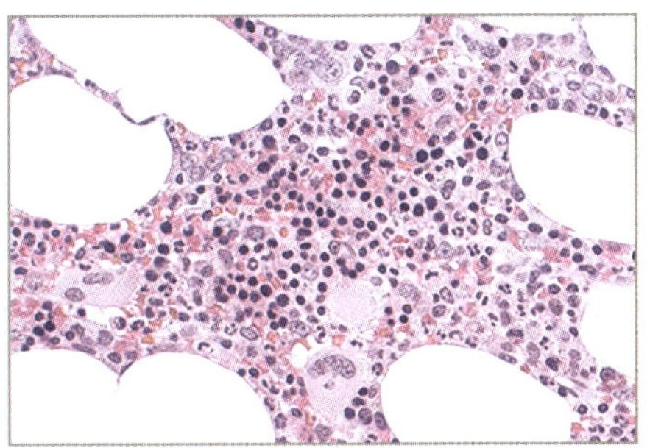

Fig. 23.2: Hemopoietic cells in bone marrow.

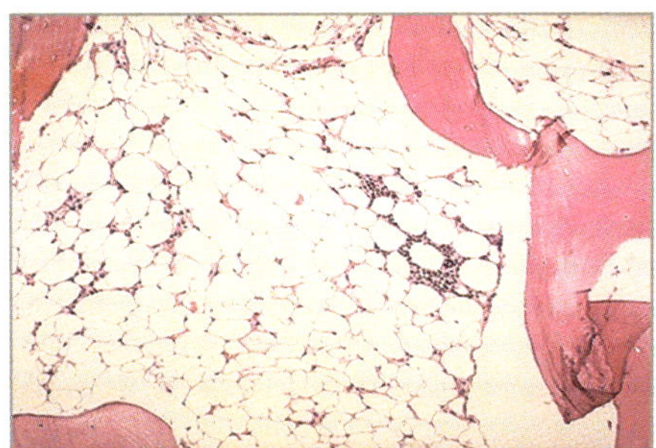

Fig. 23.3: Aplasia of the bone marrow.

diagnosis from the material obtained from the bone marrow. A ratio of the myeloid to the erythroid cells is made which gives an idea about the erythropoiesis and myelopoiesis **(Fig. 23.2)**. Any abnormal cell or presence of a non-hemopoietic cell must be noted carefully. **Figure 23.3** shows bone marrow in case of aplastic anemia.

ASSESSMENT QUESTIONS

1. **Name the various needles used for bone marrow aspiration study.**
2. **Enlist four common indications for doing a bone marrow aspiration study.**

MULTIPLE CHOICE QUESTIONS

1. **Morphology of cells in the marrow is best studied by:**
   A. Bone marrow biopsy
   B. Bone marrow aspiration and smear
   C. Prussian blue staining of marrow
   D. None of the above
2. **The normal myeloid erythroid ratio is:**
   A. 3:1
   B. 1:3
   C. 4:1
   D. 6:1
3. **What is the primary purpose of a bone marrow examination?**
   A. To measure blood clotting factors
   B. To assess kidney function
   C. To evaluate red blood cell count
   D. To examine the cellular composition of the bone marrow
4. **What is the most common site for bone marrow aspiration in adults?**
   A. Femur
   B. Humerus
   C. Iliac crest (pelvic bone)
   D. Tibia
5. **What is the primary purpose of bone marrow aspiration?**
   A. To assess bone density
   B. To evaluate the rate of red blood cell sedimentation
   C. To obtain a sample of bone marrow for examination
   D. To measure clotting factors

Answer Key for MCQs

1	2	3	4	5
B	B	D	C	C

CHAPTER 24 Tests for Hemostasis

Learning Objectives

At the end of reading this chapter, the student shall be able to:

- Describe in detail the laboratory tests for screening abnormalities in hemostasis.

INTRODUCTION

Hemostasis is a complex mosaic of various interrelated systems which function hand in hand to maintain the blood in a fluid state within the vessels and to form a clot whenever the circulation is interrupted. The components include blood vessels, platelets, coagulation factors, inhibitors of coagulation system and fibrinolytic system.

Disorders can be any one of more of the component systems. The most common defects are seen with the platelet number and function and the functioning of the coagulation factors. The most common presenting symptom of these disorders is bleeding. Laboratory plays a very vital role in detecting the abnormalities in the hemostatic machinery. It includes elucidation of a detailed clinical history, a through clinical examination and well performed battery of laboratory investigations.

The laboratory tests can be categorized into screening test, special tests and confirmatory tests.

Screening tests include the following:

- Complete hemogram with blood cell counts
- Examination of blood film
- Biochemical examination

Special tests for hemostasis include the followings:

- Bleeding time
- Whole blood clotting time
- Clot retraction time
- Clot lysis time
- Activated partial thromboplastin time (aPTT)
- Prothrombin time (PT)
- Differential tests for aPTT and PT

Confirmatory tests include the following:

- Platelet function tests
- Quantitative assay of the clotting factors.

BLEEDING TIME

Principle

It is the time taken for the bleeding to stop after a standardized puncture to the capillary bed in other words, it is the time taken for the formation of a primary hemostatic plug. It is a measure of the platelet and vascular integrity.

Method

There are various methods of performing bleeding time. It includes:

Duke's Method

Here the ear lobe is punctured with a lancet. This is not a preferred method because of the pain and formation of a hematoma.

Ivy and Template Method

This a preferred method for estimating bleeding time. In this, the forearm is the site selected for puncturing. The forearm is cleaned with spirit and a blood pressure cuff is tied to the arm and is inflated. Using a special blade called the template two incisions are made parallelly. When the blood appears in the wound the timer is put on and the time at which bleeding stops is noted for both the cuts and the average is taken.

Normal Values

Normal bleeding time 2–6 minutes.

Prolonged Values

Prolonged bleeding time is seen in the following conditions:

- Quantitative and qualitative platelet defects
- Von Willebrand factor deficiency
- Patients on drugs, such as aspirin, heparin

Patients with prolonged bleeding time must be investigated extensively for platelet disorders by estimating platelet count with phase contrast microscope, ultrastructural study of platelets, bone marrow analysis for thrombopoiesis and battery of tests for the platelet function.

WHOLE BLOOD CLOTTING TIME

Principle

It is the time taken for the freshly drawn blood to clot. It measures the integrity of the intrinsic and extrinsic pathways of clotting. This is not a very sensitive test and is poorly reproducible.

Method

The most common method is a Three test tubes method or the Lee and White method. The venous blood is taken by two syringe method and the timer is started as the blood appears in the second syringe. Three mL of blood is withdrawn and each mL is added to three clean dry test tubes placed in preheated water bath maintained at 37°C. The tubes are tilted at every 20 seconds and the time taken to form a clot in the first tube is calculated as the clotting time. The time taken for the other two tubes are also noted and the average value is taken

Normal Value

10–20 minutes

Prolonged Clotting Time

- Deficiency of clotting factors
- Presence of circulating anticoagulants
- Acquired bleeding disorders, such as Disseminated intravascular coagulation

With the clot that is produced in the two more hemostatic tests can be done. They are clot retraction test and clot lysis test.

Clot Retraction Test

Normal blood clot undergoes retraction to 50% of its original volume by the end of 2 hours, due to the presence of a platelet contractile protein called thrombosthenin. Deficiency of this protein leads to defective clot retraction.

Clot Lysis Time

Normal clot does not dissolve for 48 hours. Accelerated lysis of the clot indicates over activity of the fibrinolytic system.

The other important tests done in evaluation of hemostasis are: activated partial thromboplastin time and prothrombin time.

Activated Partial Thromboplastin Time (aPTT)

This test measures the integrity of the intrinsic pathway factors. It is the time taken for the patient's plasma to clot after addition of partial thromboplastin. This activates the intrinsic pathway allows the sample to clot.

Normal aPTT is 25–40 seconds.

Prolonged value is seen in deficiency of the intrinsic pathway factors like factor XII, XI, IX and VIII or in cases of circulating anticoagulants.

Prothrombin Time (PT)

This test measures the integrity of the extrinsic and common pathway clotting factors. It is the time taken for the patient's plasma to clot after adding complete thromboplastin. This activates the extrinsic pathway and allows the sample to clot if the factors are normal.

Normal PT—12–14 seconds

Prolonged prothrombin time occurs in the deficiency of the clotting factors, such as factor VII, X, II, and I. Most of these factors are vitamin K dependent factors. Other causes include diffuse liver disease, vitamin K deficiency, newborn children and presence of circulating anticoagulants and drugs, such as coumarin anticoagulants.

After doing aPTT and PT, the exact factor deficiency can be detected by doing a set of differential tests by adding reagents, such as the aged serum and adsorbed plasma to the patient's sample.

The results can be confirmed by doing a quantitative assay for the appropriate clotting factors.

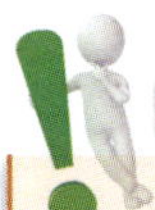

Points to Ponder

Hemostasis is a complex mosaic of various interrelated systems which function hand in hand to maintain the blood in a fluid state within the vessels and to form a clot whenever the circulation is interrupted. Laboratory plays a very vital role in detecting the abnormalities in the hemostatic machinery. It includes collection of a detailed clinical history, a thorough clinical examination and well performed battery of laboratory investigations. The laboratory tests can be categorized into screening test, special tests and confirmatory tests.

ASSESSMENT QUESTIONS

1. **What is bleeding time? Mention the tests done to estimate bleeding time.**
2. **What is whole blood clotting time? Name the tests done to estimate clotting time.**
3. **Give the normal value for activated partial thromboplastin time (aPTT).**
4. **Give the normal value for prothrombin time (PT).**
5. **Enlist the conditions in which prothrombin time is increased.**
6. **Name some common diseases presenting with abnormal bleeding.**

MULTIPLE CHOICE QUESTIONS

1. **Bleeding time is prolonged in all the following, *except*:**
   A. Hemophilia A
   B. Immune thrombocytopenia
   C. von Willebrand disease
   D. Prolonged use of aspirin
2. **What does prothrombin time (PT) measure?**
   A. Red blood cell count
   B. Blood clotting ability
   C. Platelet function
   D. White blood cell count
3. **PT is commonly used to monitor patients on:**
   A. Blood pressure medications
   B. Anticoagulant therapy
   C. Antibiotic treatment
   D. Diabetes medications

4. Which clotting factor is primarily assessed in the PT test?

A. Factor II
B. Factor V
C. Factor VII
D. Factor IX

5. What is the unit of measurement for PT?

A. Seconds
B. Millimeters
C. International normalized ratio (INR)
D. Grams

Answer Key for MCQs

1	2	3	4	5
A	B	B	C	A

CHAPTER 25 Blood Grouping and Typing

Learning Objectives

At the end of reading this chapter, the student shall be able to:
- Describe in detail the method of doing a Blood grouping and Rh typing, methods of Interpretation and compatibility testing.

INTRODUCTION

Transfusion plays an important prominent role in modern medical care. Blood transfusions are essential not only to save the lives of the bleeding patients, but also to the successful outcome of many complex treatments. A proper knowledge about the blood groups is mandatory for a good transfusion.

BLOOD GROUPING SYSTEM

A blood group system consists of a group of red cell antigens produced directly or indirectly by the alleles at a single gene locus. ABO blood group system is the most important blood group system to be considered in transfusion practice and is the only system in which reciprocal antibodies are consistently present in the serum of the individuals.

Biochemical Basis of ABO blood group system

ABO blood group expression depends upon the gene encoded glycosyltransferase enzyme system that links a particular oligosaccharide to the cell wall glycosphingolipid **(Table 25.1)**.

TABLE 25.1: Antigens and antibodies in ABO blood group system.

ABO group	*Red cell antigens*	*Red cell antibodies*
A	A	Anti-B
B	B	Anti-A
AB	A and B	Neither
O	Neither	Anti-A and Anti-B

Group A: The glycosyltransferase enzyme links N-acetylgalactosamine to the precursor oligosaccharide.

Group B: The glycosyltransferase enzyme links Galactose to the precursor oligosaccharide.

Group O: They have neither of these enzymes and so do not express A or B cell antigens.

Group AB: They have both the enzymes and so express both the antigens.

Determination of ABO blood group

In order to determine, the ABO blood group of an individual, it is important to do both the cell grouping (forward) and serum typing (reverse). Both the forward and reverse typing results must match to confirm the true ABO group of the individual.

ABO Blood Grouping Reagents

It consists of antibody reagents, red cell reagents and supplementary reagents.

Antibody Reagents

It consist of monoclonal antibodies directed against the blood group antigens. They are more specific and potent than polyclonal antibodies.

Red Cell Reagents

It consist of pooled A, B and O cells. The red cells are washed in saline to remove the serum and plasma.

Supplementary Reagents

This is generally used in testing the subgroups. It consists of anti-A1 lectin and anti-H lectin.

Procedures

ABO grouping may be performed by:

- Slide or tile method
- Tube method
- Microplate method
- Automatic/semiautomatic method

Slide or Tile Method

This is generally used for emergency blood group determination especially in outdoor. It is not a very sensitive test and another disadvantage is that it dries up quickly.

Method: The slide/tile is labelled to identify the cells. A drop of the reagent antisera is kept on the slide and a drop of red cell suspension is added to it. Both of them are mixed well with a separate applicator stick and the slide is gently rocked and looked for visible agglutination. Normally, the results are read within 2 minutes. The well that shows the agglutination is read as the blood group of the individual. The test results can be summarized as follows:

Group interpretation	*Anti-A antibody*	*Anti-B antibody*
A	++++	Negative
B	Negative	++++
AB	++++	++++
O	Negative	Negative

Tube Method

It has the following advantages over the slide method. It does not allow drying of the sample and it ensures proper incubation of the reagents. There are two different forms of tube testing—immediate spin technique or the saline room temperature technique.

Immediate Spin Technique

Three clean dry test tubes are taken and labelled as A, B and O. Two drops of antisera are added to the prelabelled tubes accordingly. One drop of the red cell suspension is added to all the three tubes. The test tubes are centrifuged for 15–20 seconds. The agglutination is read visually.

Reverse Typing

In this method, the serum sample is used for testing. The serum separated from the patients sample and to this is added known cells. The tubes are incubated at room temperature and then centrifuged to look for agglutination and finally checked under microscope.

The test results can be summarized as follows:

Agglutinations	*Antibody in the test serum*	*Blood group of the sample*
A cell	Anti-A	B
B cells	Anti-B	A
A cell and B cells	Anti-A and B	O
No agglutination	None	AB

Microplate Method

This is an ideal method for testing large number of blood samples. It saves time and cost of the reagents used.

Problems in ABO Grouping

Problems can arise when there is a discrepancy between the forward and reverse blood grouping. The main causes include:

- Improper specimen identification
- Improper technique
- Poor reagents
- Patient factors, such as extremes of age, leukemia, pregnancy, bone marrow transplantation and others
- Excessive rouleaux formation, such as mistaken for agglutination
- Presence of weak antibodies as in immunodeficiency.

Rh TYPING

Introduction

After A and B antigen, the D antigen is an important red cell antigen in transfusion practice. This protein is a part of Rh blood group system, a system complex composed of more than 40 different antigens. Other important Rh antigens include C, E, c and e.

In contrast to the ABO system, the corresponding reciprocal antibody is not present in the serum.

Clinical Significance

The Rh (D) antigen is a potent immunogen. Anti-D antibody is the most common cause for hemolytic disease of newborn, which occurs in Rh-negative woman carrying an Rh-positive fetus.

Rh Grouping Procedures

In most of the laboratories, the Rh grouping is done along with the ABO grouping using the same techniques.

The Rh grouping can be done with slide method or the tube method. The tube method is more sensitive. The antibody used is anti-D antibodies. To a clean dry test tube, a drop of the red cell suspension is taken and to these 2 drops of anti-D antibody is added. The tube is centrifuged for 15 to 20 seconds and looked for agglutination.

COMPATIBILITY TESTING

The term compatibility testing refers to a set of procedures required before the blood is issued by the blood bank as being compatible. The pretransfusion compatibility testing will confirm the ABO compatibility between the donor and the recipient and presence of clinically significant antibodies.

Cross-matching is a part of compatibility testing. It is carried out to ensure that there are no antibodies present in the patients serum that will react with the donor cells when transfused. It is a final check for the ABO compatibility and detection of unknown antibodies missed during screening.

There are two forms of cross-match testing procedures:

1. *Major cross-match:* It consists of mixing the donor red cells with the recipient serum.
2. *Minor cross-match:* It consists of mixing the recipients red cells with the donor serum.

Major Cross-match Technique

The common methods used are:

- Immediate spin technique
- Saline room temperature technique
- Albumin addition technique
- Indirect antiglobulin technique

Immediate Spin Method

It is the more commonly used procedure. In a clean dry test tube two drops of the recipient serum is taken and to this is added two drops of the donor red cells. The contents are mixed well and incubated for 5–10 minutes. The sample is then centrifuged for one minute at a speed of 1000 rpm. The tube is examined for agglutination or hemolysis.

Interpretation of Results

If agglutination is present in the tube, then the cross-match is incompatible.

If agglutination is negative, the cells are washed well with saline and to this added one drop of antihuman globulin (Coombs sera). The tube is incubated and centrifuged and looked for any agglutination. If there is no agglutination then the sample is declared compatible and is fit for transfusion.

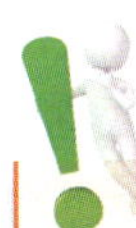

Points to Ponder

- Blood group system consists of a group of red cell antigens produced directly or indirectly by the alleles at a single gene locus. ABO blood group system is the most important blood group system.
- The term compatibility testing refers to a set of procedures required before the blood is issued by the blood bank as being compatible. The pretransfusion compatibility testing will confirm the ABO compatibility between the donor and the recipient and presence of clinically significant antibodies.

ASSESSMENT QUESTIONS

1. **What are blood group antigens? Where do you see them?**
2. **What is Rh typing?**
3. **Mention the common methods of estimating blood group of a given individual.**
4. **What do you mean by cross matching?**
5. **Mention the various methods of cross matching.**
6. **What do you mean by Rh incompatibility?**

MULTIPLE CHOICE QUESTIONS

1. **All of the following are transfusion associated diseases, *except*:**
   A. Hepatitis B infection
   B. Hepatitis C infection
   C. Hepatitis A infection
   D. Hepatitis D infection
2. **Which term is used to describe an individual with Rh-positive blood?**
   A. Rh-positive
   B. Rh-negative
   C. Rh-neutral
   D. Rh-ambiguous
3. **The Rh factor is also known as:**
   A. Antibody
   B. Antigen
   C. Enzyme
   D. Plasma protein
4. **What component of blood is tested for compatibility in a cross-match?**
   A. Red blood cells
   B. White blood cells
   C. Plasma
   D. Platelets
5. **Which blood group combination indicates an individual is Rh-negative?**
   A. A^+
   B. AB^-
   C. O^+
   D. B^-

Answer Key for MCQs

1	2	3	4	5
C	A	B	A	B

UNIT 4

Clinical Pathology—Others

Section Outline

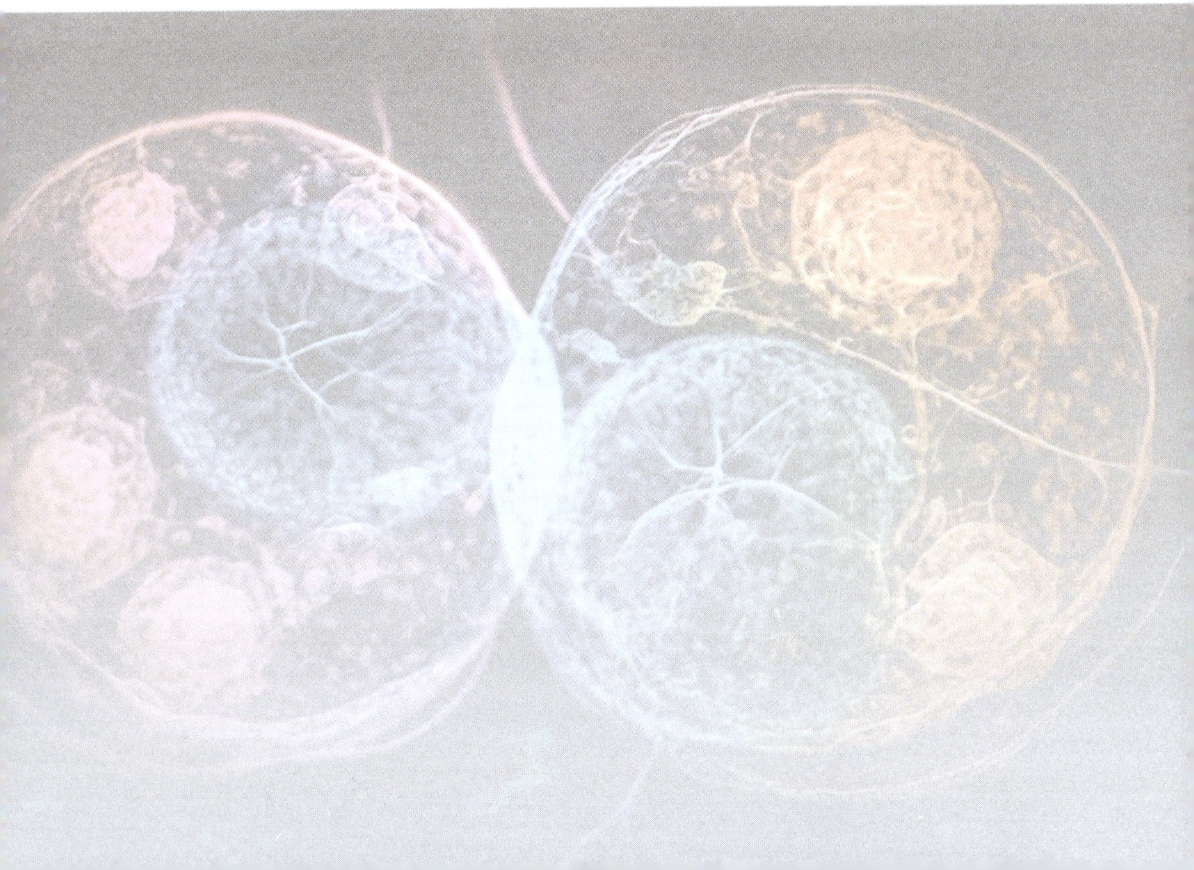

CHAPTER 26 Urine Analysis

Learning Objectives

At the end of reading this chapter, the student shall be able to:

- Describe in detail the mechanism of formation of urine and its composition.
- Describe the methods of collection of urine and the preservatives used in it.
- Enlist the methods of common macroscopic examination of urine sample and interpret abnormalities.
- Perform a systematic chemical analysis of the given urine sample using a battery of laboratory tests and to interpret each of them.
- Prepare a sample for the microscopic examination of urine and enlist the common abnormalities in urine microscopy.

INTRODUCTION

Examination of urine is a basic and an invaluable procedure, and should be carefully performed to obtain the maximum and best test results. Analysis of urine serves two purposes. One is to ascertain the existence of metabolic and endocrine disturbances in the body in which the kidneys function normally and therefore excrete abnormal amounts of metabolic end products specific for a particular disease. The second purpose is to detect intrinsic conditions that affect the kidney and the urinary tract. A diseased kidney cannot function normally in regulating the volume and composition of body fluids and in maintaining homeostasis. Consequently, substances normally retained by the kidney or excreted in small amounts may appear in the urine in large quantities and substances normally excreted may be retained. Structural elements, such as red blood cells, leukocytes, cells from the urinary tract, and casts from the diseased kidneys may appear in the urine.

FORMATION OF URINE

In a normal adult, a large volume of blood, i.e., 25% of the cardiac output (1 liter/min) flows through the kidney. The blood enters the glomerulus of each nephron by passing through the afferent arteriole into the glomerular capillaries. The capillary walls in the glomerulus are highly permeable to water and low molecular weight components of the plasma. They filter through the capillary walls and an ultrafiltrate passes into the tubule where reabsorption of substances, such as simple sugars, fatty acids, amino acids, salt and water (98–99%) take place. In addition to that, secretion of creatinine, potassium, uric acid and hydrogen ions occurs along with concentration of urine. The loop of Henle and the collecting tubules are the principal sites where the urine is concentrated as a mechanism for conserving body water. The filtrate now has a pH of 7.4, an osmolality similar to that of plasma (285 mOsm/kg water) and a specific gravity of 1.007. Its concentration however depends on the state of hydration of the individual.

TABLE 26.1: Average normal composition of urine.

Inorganic constituents	*Gram/liter*
Chloride	9.0
Phosphorus	2.0
Sulfur	1.5
Sodium	4.0
Potassium	2.0
Calcium	0.2
Magnesium	0.2
Iron	.003
Organic constituents	*Gram/liter*
Urea	25
Uric acid	0.6
Creatinine	1.5
Ammonia	0.6
Sugar (not detected by Benedict's test)	Trace
Ketone bodies	Trace
Carbonates, bicarbonates and free carbonic acid	Trace
Mucin and mucin-like substances	Trace
Diastase	Trace

COMPOSITION OF NORMAL URINE

The main constituent of urine is water which accounts for 95% of the urine. The remaining 5% is composed of 2% urea and the balance 3% is divided between organic and inorganic substances **(Table 26.1)**.

The major solutes in the urine are urea and sodium chloride. Excretion of sodium and chloride depends on the dietary intake and are therefore variable.

Variations in diet and exercise can influence and alter the constituents to a considerable degree. The chemical composition of an individual's urine also varies during different parts of the day, in relation to meals, activities and sleep.

COLLECTION OF URINE SPECIMEN

In order for urine analysis to be meaningful, the urine must be properly collected. Improper collection may invalidate the results of the laboratory procedures, no matter how skillfully or carefully the tests are performed.

Containers

Containers used for collecting urine are quite variable in type.

- *Glass bottles:* Wide-mouthed bottles are routinely used but it requires cleaning with soap and water and must be thoroughly dried before the specimens are collected. Care should be taken to label the bottles correctly.
- *Disposable containers (plastic or paper)* are available in many sizes and are provided with lids for covering the specimen to reduce bacterial and other types of contamination. They can also be used for transporting urine samples.
- *Polyethylene bags* are available for collection of urine especially from infants.

Methods of Obtaining Samples

A freshly voided, clean-catch, midstream specimen of urine is sufficient for most urine analysis except for bacteriological examination. The patient should be instructed to void directly into a clean, dry container or into a clean dry bedpan and then transfer he specimen directly into a clean, appropriate container. Specimen from infants and young children can be collected in a disposable collection apparatus, consisting of a plastic bag with an adhesive backing around the opening to fasten it to the child so that he voids directly into the bag. All specimens should be covered immediately and brought without delay to a storage place or laboratory.

Clean-voided Sample

To obtain a sample for bacteriological examination a clean-voided midstream specimen is essential. Bladder catheterization and percutaneous suprapubic aspiration of the bladder may be used, but only in rare and unusual circumstances. To avoid contamination of the voided specimen by organisms in the areas adjacent to the urethral meatus, this area must be thoroughly cleansed before the patient voids. To avoid contamination of the specimen with organisms in the distal urethra, the initial stream of voided urine, which clears these organisms from the urethra, is discarded and the subsequent midstream is collected.

In males, the sample is collected after retracting the foreskin of the penis and cleansing the glans with soap and water, particularly the area surrounding the meatus. With the foreskin still retracted, a small amount of urine is passed into the toilet or bedpan to be discarded. From the subsequent midstream urine a specimen is collected in a sterile container.

In females, the labia is spread and cleansed with soap and water. The washing is accomplished by a front-to-motion. With the labia still held apart, a small amount of urine is passed and discarded, and then a midstream sample is collected in a sterile container which is immediately closed with a sterile cover. For infants and children who are not toilet trained a sterilized disposable collection apparatus can be used to obtain specimens after the perineal region has been suitably cleansed.

Types of Sample

The concentration of urine varies throughout the day depending partly on the person's water intake and partly on his activities. The various types of urine sample include:

- *First morning specimen:* This is the ideal specimen as it is the most concentrated and has an acidic pH which preserves the formed elements and casts. It is best for detection of nitrite, protein and sediment overview.
- *Random specimen:* This type of sample is the most convenient and is good for chemical screening and microscopic examination. However, it alters with fluid intake and traces of dissolved substances such as protein or sugar may be missed if the urine is very dilute.
- *Timed specimen:* The urine is collected in a container for a fixed period usually 12/24 hours.

  24 hours specimen: This is used for true quantitative estimation of protein, sugar, electrolytes, hormones and concentration of acid fast bacilli. The early morning urine is discarded and all the urine during the next 24 hours including the early morning urine the next day is collected.

  12 hours specimen: It is useful for quantitative cell (Addis) count and urobilinogen.

  2 hours specimen: This is good for detection of urobilinogen and glucose.
- *Postprandial specimen:* Collection of urine 2 hours after lunch or dinner is helpful for detection of glycosuria.

Preservation

Ideally, examination of urine should be done immediately or within 1–2 hours on a fresh sample. When urine examination is delayed for periods longer than 1 hour, special precautions must be taken both to avoid deterioration of chemical and cellular elements and to prevent multiplication of bacteria that may be present in the collected urine with resultant alteration in urinary constituents. If allowed to stand for a few hours especially in hot weather, decomposition and bacterial growth occurs. To prevent this, the sample should be refrigerated at 5°C or preservatives should be added. Preservatives are also added to urine when the samples are to be sent to a distant laboratory or when a 24 hours urine sample is required.

Preservatives: Qualitative and quantitative chemical determinations, cells and casts are best preserved at an acidic pH in a refrigerator without preservatives **(Table 26.2)**.

No preservatives should be added for if the urine is to be sent for culture.

Routine Examination of Urine

Physical Examination of Urine

The tests include:
- Volume
- Appearance: Color and turbidity
- Odor
- pH
- Specific gravity

Volume: The amount of urine voided per day varies inversely with the amount of fluid eliminated by the lungs, skin, intestine and physiological factors, such as fluid intake, diet, exercise, environmental temperature and humidity, body weight and age. Infants and children excrete 3–4 times more urine than adults, for their body weight. The average normal urine output an adult is 1.2–2 L/day and the volume of urine during the day is 3–4 times the volume during night. The amount of urine excreted in the night is usually less than 400 mL.

'Polyuria' is an increase in urine output, i.e., >2000 mL/day. The causes include:

Physiological: Cold weather and increases intake of fluids.

Pathological:
- Diabetes mellitus: Excess glucose excreted causes a solute diuresis.
- Chronic renal failure: There is loss of functioning renal tissue and thereby the kidney loses its ability to concentrate urine.
- Drugs: Caffeine, alcohol, diuretics.
- Diabetes insipidus: Reduced antidiuretic hormone (ADH) results excess urine output.

'Oliguria' is decrease in urine output, i.e., <500 mL/day. The causes are:
- Reduced water intake
- Hot weather—due to excess sweating
- Dehydration due to excess vomiting, diarrhea, febrile states
- Acute and chronic glomerulonephritis
- Obstruction to urinary flow, e.g., hydronephrosis enlarged prostate, etc.

'Anuria' is total suppression of urine, the output falling to less 100 mL per day. The causes are:
- Chronic renal disease
- Acute glomerulonephritis

TABLE 26.2: Urine preservatives.

Preservative	*Concentration*	*Uses*	*Limitations*
Boric acid	0.5 g/60 mL	Hormone estimation	Precipitates uric acid
Formaldehyde	2–4 drops/30 mL	Addis count	♦ False positive for Benedict's test ♦ Precipitates protein
Thymol	0.1 g/100 mL or 1 crystal to urine	Sediment cytology	False positive for sugar, ketones and proteins
Toluene	2 mL/100 mL, forming a thin layer on the surface	Chemical constituents (Best preservative)	False positive sulfosalicylic acid test
Chloroform	5 mL/100 mL or 1 drop/30 mL	Sediment cytology	False positive for sugar
Conc. Hcl	10 mL/24 hours specimen	Catecholamine, VMA, calcium, nitrogen	
Sodium fluoride	0.5 g in 3–4 liter container	24 hours glucose estimation	Inhabits strip test for glucose

- Mismatched blood transfusion
- Absence of kidneys

'**Nocturia'** is increased nocturnal excretion of urine by an adult of >500 mL of urine with a specific gravity of <1.018. It may due to:

Physiological: Excess fluid intake.

Pathological:
- Reduced renal osmotic concentration
- High sodium excretion
- Solute diuresis
- Reduced bladder capacity
- Irritable bladder
- Partial bladder obstruction

Appearance:
Color: The color of normal urine is amber yellow and is due to presence of uroerythrin and urochromes. It depends on quantity of urine voided. Abnormal color can be due to either excess of endogenous pigments, such as hemoglobin, myoglobin, bile pigments, porphyrin, etc., or exogenous substances which alter the color of the urine.**Table 26.3** enlists a few condition which present abnormal color of urine.

Turbidity: Normal freshly voided urine is clear. Turbidity in urine may be due to:
- Amorphous phosphates and carbonates
- Crystals, cellular exudates, bacteria and fungus which can be removed by centrifugation.
- Chyle and fat cannot be removed by centrifugation.
- Pus which clears on filtering
- Amorphous urates

Odor: Normal fresh urine has an aromatic odor which is due to volatile acids. On standing, there is decomposition of urea forming ammonia which gives a strong ammoniac smell. If freshly voided urine smells ammoniac, it is important to suspect infection by urea splitting organisms, such as proteus **(Table 26.4)**.

TABLE 26.3: Conditions presenting abnormal color of urine.

Color	*Conditions*
Colorless	Very dilute urine: Polyuria, diabetes mellitus
Yellow orange (high colored)	Concentrated urine: Excess urobilin bile pigments, intake of carrots
Red/smoky	Hemoglobin/RBC myoglobin, porphyrins beetroot/ aniline dyes menstrual contamination
Cloudy	Phosphates and carbonates, urates and uric acid, pus cells, bacteria yeast, spermatozoa
Milky	Pyuria, fat (chyluria) lipiduria
Brown black	Methemoglobin, homogentisic acid (alkaptonuria), melanin
Orange	Bile pigments, drugs: Rifampicin

TABLE 26.4 : Conditions presenting abnormal odor in urine.

Abnormal odor	*Conditions*
Fruity	Ketoacidosis
Mousy	Phenylketonuria
Rotting fish	Trimethylaminuria
Rancid	Tyrosinemia

pH: Reflects the ability of the kidney to maintain normal hydrogen ion concentration in plasma and extracellular fluid. Normal kidneys are capable of producing urine the pH of which varies from 4.5 to slightly higher than 8.0. A pH below 7 indicates acid urine and a pH above 7 alkaline urine.

Causes of acidic urine
- High protein intake leads to increase in acid phosphates and sulfates excretion, which in turn decreases the pH.
- Vegetarian diet

- At night because of mild respiratory acidosis.

Causes of alkaline urine

- On standing at room temperature, the urine turns alkaline due to loss of carbon dioxide and formation of ammonia by urea splitting bacteria.
- After a meal rich in milk and other dairy products.
- Medications, such as sodium carbonate, potassium citrate and acetazolamide.
- Urinary tract infection

For routine analysis, the urinary pH is measured using indicator paper strips and a color chart.

- *The traditional method includes the use of litmus paper.*

  Procedure: Dip the litmus paper strips in the urine, remove and read the color change immediately.

  Blue litmus turns red → Acid

  Red litmus turns blue → Alkaline

  Blue and red litmus turns purple → Neutral

  The pH can also be measured by the help of nitra zine paper which are sensitive and specific in the pH range of 4.5–8.0 range.
- *Colorimetric reagent strip test:* A variety of test papers impregnated with various chemicals are available for the easy and rapid colorimetric determination of pH. These reagent strips simultaneously measures pH and checks the urine for several other components. The pH portion of these strips is impregnated with two separate indicators, methyl red and bromothymol blue. These chemicals provide a wide range of spectrum of color changes, from orange to green to blue in the pH range of 5–8.5. The reagent strip is dipped into the urine specimen and the color change is compared to a standardized color chart on the bottle label.
- *pH meter*—is used for more accurate determinations and the reading is observed directly from the meter.

Specific gravity: The specific gravity of urine indicates the relative proportions of dissolved solid components to the total volume of the specimen. It reflects the degree of concentration or dilution of the specimen.

Under appropriate and standardized conditions of fluid restriction or increased intake, specific gravity measures the concentrating and diluting abilities of the kidney. The normal specific gravity is usually between 1.015 and 1.025 in a 24 hours specimen. It is highest in the first morning specimen and is generally greater than 1.020. The chief substances which affect the specific gravity of the urine are urea, sodium chloride and phosphates and abnormally albumin and sugar.

Causes of low specific gravity

- Diabetes insipidus
- Chronic glomerulonephritis
- Pyelonephritis

Causes of high specific gravity

- Diabetes mellitus: Increase concentration of glucose in the urine
- Adrenal insufficiency
- Excessive loss of water: Sweating, fever, vomiting and diarrhea

Fixed specific gravity: Urine with a fixed low specific gravity of 1.010, which varies little from specimen to specimen, is known as 'isosthenuric.' This is seen in severe renal damage with disturbance of both the concentrating and diluting abilities of the kidney.

Estimation of specific gravity: Specific gravity is a measurement that indicates the density of the urine. It is the ratio of the weight of a given volume of urine to the weight of the same volume of water, under standardized conditions.

- *Direct method:* The specific gravity of urine can be determined with a urinometer. This is a weighted bulb-shaped instrument with a cylindrical stem which contains a scale calibrated from 1.000 to 1.060 with divisions from 0.001 to 0.002 in specific gravity readings.

Procedure: Urine is poured into a cylinder or conical glass so that the vessel is nearly full. If there are bubbles of froth, they should be removed with a filter or blotting paper. The instrument is floated in the urine and care should be taken to see that it does not touch the sides. The depth to which it sinks in urine indicates the specific gravity of urine, which is red on the urinometer scale at the junction of the urine with the air. The reading is taken at eye level, the lowest part of the meniscus being taken. In case the urine is insufficient, it may be diluted with an equal volume of distilled water and the last two figures of the reading are then multiplied by 2.

Correction for temperature: The urinometer is calibrated to read 1.000 in distilled water at a specific temperature, indicated on each instrument, e.g., 15°C or 20°C. There is a change in the specific gravity of 0.001 for each 3°C above and below this temperature. Therefore add 0.001 to the reading for each 3°C above the temperature for which the urinometer is calibrated, subtract 0.001 for each 3°C, the temperature below the standard temperature.

Correction is also recommended when glucose or protein are present.

Solids in urine: An approximate estimate of the amount of solids in 1,000 mL of urine is obtained by multiplying the last two figures of the specific gravity of a 24 hours specimen at 15°C by 2.6 (This figure is called the 'Long's coefficient').

- *Indirect method-refractive index:* An indirect method of measuring specific gravity is refractometry using a refractometer, e.g., TS meter, which measures the refractive index of the solution. The refractive index varies with, but is not identical to the specific gravity of the urine. It has scale readings calibrated in terms of specific gravity, refractive index and total solids. It requires calibration daily and is temperature compensated between 60 and 100°F. The scale reads in increments of .001 from 1.001–1.035.

Chemical Examination of Urine

- Proteins
- Sugar
- Ketones
- Bile and bile salts
- Blood

Proteins in urine: Normally a very small amount of protein <30 mg/100 mL is present in the glomerular filtrate. However, most of it is reabsorbed in the tubules but a small amount is present in the urine (30–50 mg/24 hours). Approximately one-third of normal urinary protein is albumin. The majority of normal proteins in the urine are globulins. These globulins primarily consist of alpha-1 and alpha-2 globulins with smaller amounts of beta and gamma globulins. Trace quantities of other proteins may also be found in most urine. A high molecular weight mucoprotein, the Tamm-Horsfall protein occurs in normal urine in quantities up to 2.5 mg/dL. Excretion of increased amount of protein in the urine is referred to as 'proteinuria'. It is one of the single most important indicator of renal disease. Detection of protein in the urine combined with microscopic examination of the urinary sediment forms the basis of the differential laboratory diagnosis of renal disorders. The type of protein excreted in disease states is generally related to serum proteins. Smaller proteins, such as albumin and alpha-1 globulin are excreted more readily than larger ones. Certain disease are characterized by the excretion of specific globulins, e.g., in multiple myeloma, the urine of patients show increased excretion of a low molecular weight globulin called Bence-Jones proteins.

Marked proteinuria: It is characterized by the excretion of more than 4 g/day of proteins. It is seen in nephrotic syndrome, severe glomerulonephritis, renal vein thrombosis and congestive cardiac failure.

Moderate proteinuria: It refers to daily excretion of between 0.5 and 4 g of protein. It is seen in majority of the renal diseases, chronic glomerulonephritis, diabetic nephropathy, multiple myeloma, renal stones, and diseases of the lower urinary tract.

Minimal proteinuria—is excretion of proteins less than 0.5 g/day. It is seen in chronic glomerulonephritis, polycystic disease of the kidney and healing phase of acute glomerulonephritis **(Table 26.5)**.

There are three types of proteinuria:

1. *Accidental:* This is due to contamination of urine with blood, pus, vaginal discharge or seminal fluid. Protein is also present in the urine after prostatic massage.
2. *Functional:* It is also called as 'physiological proteinuria'. The causes include excessive exercise, exposure to heat cold, fever, emotional stress excessive ingestion of protein and in the late stages of pregnancy. The underlying mechanism that induces proteinuria in all these conditions is renal vasoconstriction. Excessive excretion of albumin related to posture is called ORTHOSTATIC or POSTURAL proteinuria. It is found when the subject is in an upright position and disappears when the individual lies down. The proteinuria is intermittent and found in 3–5% of normal healthy adults. It may be differentiated from other forms of proteinuria by testing for protein in urine specimens collected before and after the individual has been erect. The patient voids and discards his urine at bedtime. The urine specimen is collected immediately after awakening and before he is upright even for a moment. After 2 hours, another specimen is collected after being erect or walking. The first specimen should contain no protein and the second will be positive if the patient has postural proteinuria.
3. *Organic and renal albuminuria:* In this type of proteinuria, albumin passes from the blood into the urine through the walls of the kidney tubules and glomeruli. It is usually persistent and in greater quantity than functional albuminuria. It is found in inflammation, degenerative diseases, obstructive and irritation of the kidneys.

TABLE 26.5: Proteins in urine.

Type of protein	*Conditions*
Albumin	♦ Strenuous physical exercise ♦ Emotional stress ♦ Pregnancy ♦ Infections ♦ Glomerulonephritis ♦ Newborns (1st week)
Globulins	♦ Glomerulonephritis ♦ Tubular dysfunction
Hemoglobin	Hemoglobinuria
Nucleoproteins	WBC in urine, epithelial cells in the urine
Bence-Jones protein	Multiple myeloma

Test for detection of proteins

- *Semi-quantitative precipitation tests:* The heat and acetic acid method, sulfosalicylic acid method and the concentrated nitric acid protein precipitation method are the three methods for semi-quantitative method of detection of protein concentration in terms of one plus through four plus precipitation. The precipitation is red and interpreted as follows:

  Negative: No turbidity or cloudiness

  Trace: A faint precipitate visible against a black background, equivalent to about 5 mg/dL protein.

  1+ : Definite cloud without flocculation, equivalent to 10–30 mg/dL.

2+ : Heavy and granular cloud without flocculation equivalent to 40–100 mg/dL.
3+ : Dense cloud with marked flocculation equivalent to 200–500 mg/dL.
4+ : Cloudiness with precipitation equivalent to 500 mg/dL or more.

If the urine is alkaline, it is made slightly acidic by addition of a few drops of 3% acetic acid. The urine must be clear before testing for albumin. Turbid urine should be filtered. In case the turbidity is not easily removed, the urine can be mixed with kaolin and allowed to stand for some time and then filtered. Another method of clearing urine is to re-filter the filtrate through the same filter paper two or three times.

- *Heat and acetic acid method*
  Procedure
  - Take a long test tube and fill 3/4th the tube with clear urine.
  - Boil the upper portion over a flame. The lower portion serves as the control.
  - If proteins, phosphates or carbonates are present in the urine a white cloud develops. Add 1–3 drops of glacial acetic acid. Any turbidity due to phosphate precipitation will clear or if it is due to carbonates they disappear with effervescence. If it persists, it is due to albumin. Precipitates due to mucin or nucleoproteins will disappear on addition of 2 drops of nitric acid.

  If an alkaline urine containing protein is boiled, the protein is converted to alkaline meta-protein, which is not coagulated by heat. If acetic acid is added in excess before boiling, the protein may be converted to acid meta-protein, which is not coagulated by heat and this gives a false negative result.
- *Sulfosalicylic acid method*
  Procedure
  - Take 2 mL of clear urine in a test tube.
  - Add an equal volume of 3% sulfosalicylic acid.
  - Mix thoroughly, allow it to stand for 10 minutes and estimate the amount of turbidity.
- *Nitric acid method (Heller's test)*
  Procedure
  - Take 2–3 mL of concentrated nitric acid in a test tube.
  - Carefully pour about 5 mL of clear urine down the inner side of the inclined test tube so that the urine forms a layer over the nitric acid.
  - A ring of white precipitated protein will form at the interface. Estimate the amount of precipitate.
- *Colorimetric reagent strip test*
  Principle: The colorimetric reagent strip test is based upon the ability of proteins to alter the color of some acid-base indicators without altering the pH. When an indicator, such as tetrabromophenol blue is buffered at pH 3, it is yellow in solutions without protein. But in the presence of protein the color will change to green and then to blue with increasing protein concentrations.
  Procedure: Protein is determined by dipping the strip into well-mixed, uncentrifuged urine and immediately comparing the resultant color with the chart provided on the reagent strip bottle.
  Results: The results are reported as negative (yellow color), trace, 1+ to 4+. Trace readings may detect 5–20 mg of protein/dL. Albumin reacts more strongly than the other proteins.
- *Quantitative 24 hours protein determination:* Two methods are commonly used for 24 hours protein estimation, i.e., Esbach's and Aufrecht's method. Both these methods will precipitate proteins with the help of picric acid.
- *Bence-Jones proteinuria:* Bence-Jones protein is soluble at room and body temperatures. It precipitates upon heating between 45 and 60°C and then redissolves

when the urine is further heated to the boiling point. Gradual heating of a urine sample to the boiling point is the simplest screening method for Bence-Jones protein. When present, a precipitate will first appear and then dissolves again as the urine is further heated.

- *Acetic acid test:*
  - Place 4.0 mL of clear urine in a test tube (centrifuge if necessary)
  - Add 1.0 mL acetate buffer (add 17.5 g sodium acetate trihydrate and 4.1 mL glacial acetic acid to distilled water, dilute to 100 mL with distilled water).
  - Place in a 56°C water bath and heat for 15 minutes.
  - Precipitation indicates the presence of Bence-Jones proteins.
  - If precipitation occurs, heat the tube in boiling water for 3 minutes and observe. Bence-Jones proteins will dissolve again.
  - Cool the tube. Precipitation will recur as solution cools to 45–60°C and dissolves as the solution cools below 40°C.
- *Toluene sulfonic acid test:*
  - Add 1 mL of Toluenesulfonic acid (TSA) acid reagent slowly by the side of the test tube, to 2 mL urine.
  - A precipitate appears within 5 minutes if Bence-Jones protein is present.
- *Protein electrophoresis:* When only small amounts of Bence-Jones protein are present, electrophoresis is useful.

Sugars in urine

Glucose: Glucose is the sugar most commonly found in urine; although other sugars, such as lactose, fructose, galactose and pentose may also be found in certain conditions.

The presence of detectable amounts of glucose in the urine is known as glycosuria or glycosuria. It occurs whenever the blood glucose exceeds the reabsorption capacity of the renal tubules, i.e., when the glomerular filtrate contains more glucose than the tubules are able to reabsorb (renal threshold = 180 mg%). The condition may be either benign or pathological.

Renal glycosuria occurs with the normal blood glucose levels because tubular reabsorption of glucose is below normal, thus allowing certain glucose to spill into the urine. This is a benign condition as is the occurrence of glycosuria after eating a heavy meal or associated with emotional stress.

Diabetes mellitus, a pathological state, is the chief cause of glycosuria. This condition is associated with a marked elevation of blood sugar levels and usually an increase in urine volume. The urine is usually light in color with increased specific gravity due to the extra loads of dissolved solids.

Qualitative tests for sugar in the urine

Reduction tests: The reduction of metallic ions, such as Cu^{++} is non-specific for glucose since the reaction may be brought about by any reducing substance that may be present in the urine, such as creatinine, uric acid, ascorbic acid or other reducing sugar. Non-carbohydrate components seldom interfere, but occasionally in concentrated urines, some interference may occur. As little as 0.1% (100 mg/dL) glucose is capable of giving a positive reaction with Benedict's reagent.

- **Benedict's qualitative test:** This test is not specific for sugars and is affected by most of the reducing substances.

  Principle

Cupric ions ($CuSO_4$) Blue + Glucose (Reducing Substances)	heat → alkali	Cuprous ions (Cu_2O) + Oxidized glucose Orange-red

  Procedure

  - Take 5 mL Benedict's reagent and add to it 0.5 mL (8 drops) of protein free urine.

- Boil for 3–5 minutes
- Cool and note the color

Recording results:

The color varies from blue through green → Yellow → Orange → brick red negative - No change in color

Trace: Solution appears pale green to slightly cloudy

1+: Definite cloudy green (0.5% sugar)

2+: Yellow to orange precipitate, supernatant fluid pale blue (1% sugar)

3+: Orange to red precipitate, supernatant fluid pale blue (1.5% sugars)

4+: Brick red precipitate, supernatant fluid decolorizes (2% sugar)

False positive Benedict's test

- Reducing sugars: Lactose, fructose, pentose, galactose
- Non-reducing sugars: Dextrin's, homogentisic acid, glucoronates, chloroform, formaldehyde, indicant, rhubarb, ascorbic and creatinine.

❖ **Fehling's test:**

Fehling's reagent

Solution A:

- Copper sulfate: 34.65 g
- Distilled water: 500 mL

Solution B

- Sodium hydroxide: 125 g
- Sodium potassium tartrate: 173 g
- Distilled water: 500 mL

Procedure

- Take equal volumes of Fehling's Solution A and B, mix and boil.
- Add a few drops of urine and boil again.
- Note the color change similar to Benedict's test.

❖ **Colorimetric reagent strip test**

Principle: This test based on a double sequential enzyme reaction. One enzyme, glucose oxidase, catalyzes the formation of gluconic acid and hydrogen peroxide from the oxidation of glucose. A second enzyme, peroxidase catalyzes the reaction of hydrogen peroxide with potassium iodide chromogen to oxidize the chromogen to colors ranging from green to brown.

This test is specific for glucose and no other substance excreted in the urine other than glucose is known to give a positive result. Sugars, such as lactose, fructose, galactose, and pentose are not substrates for glucose oxidase and therefore do not react with this test. Ascorbic acid greater than 50 mg/dL and moderately high ketone levels may cause false negatives result.

Test for non-glucose reducing sugars

❖ **Lactose:** Lactose may appear in the urine of lactating women. It may also be found in the urine of 3–5 day old infants in trace amounts till the digestive system becomes mature and in children and adults who are deficient in intestinal lactase. It is differentiated from glucose by the following tests:

- **Rubner's test**

  Procedure

  » Add 3 g lead acetate to 10 mL undiluted urine and filter.

  » Boil the filtrate and add 1 mL concentrated ammonium hydroxide and boil.

  Result

  Lactose: Red solution + Red precipitate

  Glucose: Red solution + Yellow precipitate

- **Modified test**

  Procedure

  » Add 3 mL of liquor ammonia and 3 drops of 10% NaOH to 3 mL urine.

  » Heat in boiling water and note after 2, 3, 4 and 5 minutes.

  Result: A distinct but not brilliant red color indicates a positive reaction.

❖ **Fructose:** This sugar is found in the urine of patients consuming large quantities of fruit and in hepatic disorders.

It can be distinguished by the Seliwanoff's test.

Seliwanoff Reagent: It consists of 50 mg resorcin in 70 mL water and 30 mL of concentrated hydrochloric acid.

Procedure

To 2 mL of Seliwanoff's reagent add 0.3 mL urine and heat in boiling water bath for 5 minutes.

Result

A deep red color develops if fructose is present.

- **Pentose:** This is a rare sugar seen usually in a congenital disorder or associated with certain types of drug therapy. It is detected by the Bial's test.

  Bial's test for pentose

  Bial's reagent

  Dissolve 1.5 g of reagent orcinol and 20–30 drops of 10% ferric chloride in 500 mL of concentrated HCl.

  Procedure

  To 5 mL of Bial's reagent add 2–3 mL of urine and heat gently till the first few bubbles rise to the surface.

  Result

  If pentose is present, the solution becomes green and a flocculent precipitate of the same color may from.
- **Galactose:** Galactose is found in the urine of infants with galactosemia. These children are deficient in the enzyme necessary for conversion of galactose to glucose. It is occasionally found in the adults who consume large quantities of milk or other lactose containing foods.

Other tests for reducing sugars

- **Tablet test:** This consists of a self-heating tablet which determines the presence of reducing sugar by reduction of copper.

  Procedure: Place 5 drops of urine and add 10 drops of water in a test tube. Add one clinitest tablet and observe the reaction.

  Results: If the solution passes through orange to shades of brown, it indicates than 2% sugar is present. If there is no change wait for 15 seconds after the boiling stops, shake gently and compare the color of the mixture with the color chart provided.
- **Osazone test**

  Procedure
  - Take 10 mL of acidified urine and add 1 g of phenyl hydrazine hydrochloride and 2 g of sodium acetate. Mix thoroughly.
  - Heat till the contents dissolve and filter.
  - Place the filtrate in a boiling water bath for ½ to 1 hour.
  - Remove and as the solution cools, crystals form and settle to the bottom.
  - Examine the precipitate under the microscope for morphology structure of the crystals.

  Results
  - Glucosazone: Fine straight needles arranged in fans or sheaves of spherical clusters.
  - Lactosazone: Finely curled crystals—puff ball appearance.

Ketones in urine (Ketonuria)

The body normally metabolizes fats completely to carbon dioxide and water. Whenever there is inadequate carbohydrate in the diet or a defect carbohydrate metabolism or absorption, the body metabolizes increasing amounts of fatty acids. When the fatty acid utilization is incomplete the intermediary products of fat metabolism appear in the blood and the urine. These intermediary products are the three ketone bodies—acetone, diacetic acid (acetoacetic acid) and β-hydroxybutyric acid. The excretion of these products is called 'ketonuria'. They are seen in conditions of altered fat metabolism, such as uncontrolled Diabetes mellitus, and in severe starvation.

Diabetes mellitus is a disorder where the glucose metabolism is sufficiently impaired and the fatty acid is metabolized, with the result that ketone bodies accumulate in the in blood (ketosis) and are excreted in the urine (ketonuria). Ketone bodies are excreted in combination with normal basic ions, leading to a reduction in the carbon dioxide combining power and causing systemic acidosis. Progressive diabetic ketosis is the cause of diabetic acidosis which eventually leads to coma and death. The term ketoacidosis is used to designate the combined ketosis and acidosis in diabetes.

Other causes of ketonuria

1. Fever
2. Anorexia
3. Gastrointestinal disturbances
4. Fasting
5. Starvation
6. Severe vomiting

Common tests used to detect ketone bodies

- **Rothera's test for acetone and acetoacetic acid**

  Procedure

  - Take 5 mL urine in a test tube and saturate it with ammonium sulfate.
  - Add 1 crystal of sodium nitroprusside.
  - Run liquor ammonia carefully at the side of the tube so as to form a layer on top of the saturated urine.

  Result: If acetone is present, a permanganate calomel red (pink–purple) ring forms at the junction of the two layers. Negative result shows no ring or a brown ring.

- **Ferric chloride test for diacetic acid: Gerhardt's test**

  Procedure: To 5 mL urine in a test tube add 10% aqueous solution of ferric chloride (10 g ferric chloride in 100 mL distilled water) drop by drop, agitating well, until the precipitate that develops has dissolved.

  Result: If diacetic acid is present, the filtrate will develop a brown red color.

- **Hart's test for β-hydroxybutyric acid**

  Procedure

  - Take 20 mL of urine in a beaker.
  - Add 20 mL distilled water and a few drops of glacial acetic acid.
  - Boil until the volume is reduced to 10 mL. This removes acetone and acetoacetic acid.
  - Dilute to 20 mL with distilled water and divide into two equal portions.
  - Add 1 mL hydrogen peroxide to one portion. Warm the mixture gently for 1 minute. Cool in air.
  - To both tubes add 10 drops of glacial acetic acid and 10 drops concentrated Sodium nitroprusside to test for acetone.
  - Mix thoroughly
  - Overlay with liquid ammonia fortis
  - Allow to stand

  Result: When β-hydroxybutyric acid is present, the tube containing the hydrogen peroxide will show a red ring at the interface.

- **Reagent tablet test: Ace test**

  Detection of acetone and acetoacetic acid

  Procedure

  - Place a tablet on a clean surface, preferably a piece of white paper.
  - Put one drop of urine on the tablet.
  - Compare urine ketone test results to color chart at 30 seconds.

- **Colorimetric reagent strip test**

  Principle: The reagent strip is impregnated with sodium nitroprusside buffers.

  It is based on the development of colors ranging from buff-pink, for negative reading to purple when acetoacetic acid reacts with nitroprusside.

  Procedure: The strip is dipped into fresh urine, tapped to remove excess urine and compared to the color chart after exactly 15 seconds.

  Results: The chart has six color blocks indicating negative, trace, small, moderate, large 80 and large 160 concentrations of ketones and ranging in color from buff to lavender and maroon. The rest is sensitive to acetoacetic acid. It does not react with β-hydroxybutyric acid or acetone.

Blood in urine

Blood may be found in urine in the form of red blood cells or blood pigments alone. Hemoglobin is the oxygen-carrying pigment of red blood cells. When hemolysis occurs (lysis of red blood cells), free hemoglobin is released. If hemolysis occurs in the circulation (e.g., in certain hemolytic anemia), free hemoglobin is present in the blood. When in sufficient quantities, significant amounts enter the glomerular filtrate and appear in the urine. When red blood cells enter the urine at any point in the urinary tract (as a result of disease or trauma), hemolysis may occur in the urine, with the release of detectable amounts of free hemoglobin.

Normally an occasional red cell may be found on microscopic examination of the urine sediment. In women during menstruation, the urine may get contaminated with menstrual blood and hence examination of urine should not be done during that period.

Hematuria—Denotes the presence of red blood cells in urine. It is seen in various renal disorders, infectious or neoplastic or trauma related to any part of the urinary tract.

Hemoglobinuria—is the presence of blood pigments in the urine without the presence of red blood cells. It is associated with certain hemolytic anemias that cause hemolytic anemia, transfusion reactions, malaria, and paroxysmal nocturnal hemoglobinuria.

Tests for detection of blood

- **Microscopic examination:** The urinary sediment is obtained by centrifuging urine. It is examined under the microscope and the number of red cells per microscopic high power field reported.
- **Benzedrine test**
  Principle: Heme acts as a catalyst when hydrogen peroxide is mixed with benzidine.
  Reagents:
  - Saturated solution of benzidine in glacial acetic acid
  - Hydrogen peroxide

  Procedure:
  - Mix equal parts of A and B in a test tube.
  - Place a few mL of urine in a test tube and an equal amount of the mixed reagent.

  Results: A blue color indicates the presence of hemoglobin.
- **Colorimetric reagent strip method**
  Principle: The reagent area is impregnated with tetramethylbenzidine and buffered organic peroxide. This forms a green to dark blue compound when hemoglobin catalyzes the oxidation reaction of tetramethylbenzidine with peroxide.
  Results: Development of green spots indicates erythrocytes. The color strip is compared with a color chart 40 seconds after the strip is dipped in urine. The color blocks indicate negative, nonhemolyzed trace, hemolyzed trace, small (+), moderate (++) and large amounts (+++) of hemoglobin and range in color from orange through green to blue. Myoglobin if present in large concentrations gives a positive reaction. This test is capable of detecting 0.015–0.060 mg/dL free hemoglobin or 5–20 intact RBC per microliter.

The other tests used in detection of blood are:

- Guaiacum test
- Orthotolidine test
- Spectroscopic method

Bile in the urine

The constituents of bile are excreted in the urine as bilirubin (bile pigment), bile salts, urobilin and urobilinogen. Bilirubin appears in the urine when it is an excess in blood. This condition is known as 'jaundice'.

Bilirubin in urine: Bilirubin in the urine indicates the presence of hepatocellular disease or intra- or extrahepatic biliary obstruction. It is an early sign of these disorders and therefore a useful diagnostic tool. It is formed in the reticuloendothelial cells of the spleen and the bone marrow from the breakdown of hemoglobin. It is linked to albumin in the blood stream and transported to the liver.

This albumin-bound form, which is also known as indirect bilirubin is insoluble in water and does not appear in the urine. In the liver cells, it is separated from albumin and conjugated with glucuronic and sulfuric acids to form water soluble conjugated bilirubin, also known as 'direct bilirubin'. It is secreted into the bile and then excreted into the intestinal tract through the bile duct. This conjugated bilirubin in the intestinal tract is converted bilirubin can be excreted by the kidneys although its level in the blood is not sufficiently high to cause significant amounts to appear in the urine. In certain liver diseases due to infectious or hepatotoxic agents, liver cells are unable to conjugate all the bilirubin in the bile which results in an increase in both conjugated and unconjugated bilirubin and are returned to the blood to elevate blood levels and cause bilirubinuria. In obstructive biliary tract disease, biliary stasis interferes with the normal excretion of conjugated bilirubin to the intestinal tract. This increases its levels in the blood resulting in bilirubinuria. Bilirubin excretion in the urine is not increased when there is an increase in the amount of unconjugated bilirubin in circulation. This is seen in hemolytic anemias where a large amount of hemoglobin is released leading to greater production of albumin-bound bilirubin.

Tests for detection for bilirubin

- **Foam test:** Shake urine in a test tube. If the foam on top is yellow, bile pigments are present.
- **Gmelin's test:**

  Procedure:
  - Place ½ inch column of yellow nitric acid in a test tube.
  - Overlay with equal amounts of urine.

  Result: A play of colored rings, the most distinct being green indicates the presence of bile pigments.
- **Fouchet's test:**

  Fouchet's reagent:

  Trichloroacetic acid: 25 g

  Distilled water: 100 mL

  10% ferric chloride solution: 10 mL

  Procedure:
  - Place 10 mL of acidified urine in a test tube.
  - Add 2.5 mL of 10% barium chloride.
  - Mix and filter.
  - Unfold the filter paper and spread it on a dry filter paper.
  - Add 1 drop of Fouchet's reagent to the residual precipitate.

  Result: A green or blue color indicates the presence of bilirubin.
- **Colorimetric strip reagent test:**

  Principle: This test is based on the coupling of bilirubin with diazotized 2, 4-dichloroaniline in a strong acid medium to form a brown purple azobilirubin compound. The color ranges through various shades of tan.

  Procedure: The reagent strip is dipped into fresh, urine, tapped to remove excess urine and after 20 seconds, compared to the color chart on the reagent strip bottle.

  Result: The results are interpreted as negative, small (+), moderate (++), and large (+++) amounts of bilirubin.

Urobilinogen in urine

Conjugated bilirubin, secreted by the liver into the bile is excreted into the intestinal tract through the bile duct. Bacterial action in the intestinal tract converts the bilirubin to a group of compounds known as urobilinogen. As much as 50% of the urobilinogen formed in the intestine is reabsorbed into the portal circulation and re-excreted by the liver. Small amounts are normally excreted in the urine but the major excretion is in the faces. Normally 1–4 mg of urobilinogen is excreted in the urine in a 24 hours period. The concentration of urobilinogen in random normal urine is 0.1–1.0 Ehrlich units/dL. Urinary urobilinogen is increased by any condition that causes an increase in the production of bilirubin, and by any disease that prevents the liver from normally removing the reabsorbed urobilinogen from the portal circulation.

TABLE 26.6: Status of urinary urobilinogen and biliruin in normal and disease conditions.

	In health	*In hemolytic disease*	*In hepatic disease*	*In biliary obstruction*
Urine urobilinogen	Normal	Increased	Increased	Low or absence
Urine bilirubin	Negative	Negative	Positive or negative	Positive

It is increased whenever there is excessive destruction of red blood cells, e.g., hemolytic anemia, pernicious anemia and malaria. It is also increased in infective hepatitis, cirrhosis, congestive cardiac failure and infectious mononucleosis **(Table 26.6)**.

It is decreased or absent when normal amounts of bilirubin is not excreted into the intestinal tract. Conditions in which urobilinogen is absent in urine:

1. Complete obstruction of the bile ducts as in cholelithiasis, inflammatory or in tumors.
2. *During antibiotic therapy:* Due to the suppression of the normal intestinal flora which prevents conversion of bilirubin to urobilinogen.

Tests for detection of urobilinogen

- **Qualitative Ehrlich's test:**
  Ehrlich's reagent
  Paradimethylaminobenzaldehyde: 2 g
  20% HCl: 100 mL
  Procedure
  - Place 10 mL of urine in a test tube
  - Add 2.5 mL of barium chloride (to remove bilirubin).
  - Mix well and filter.
  - Add 0.5 mL of Ehrlich's reagent to 2.3 mL of the filtrate.
  - Allow it stand for 3–5 minutes.

  Results: Urobilinogen when present in the urine sample will change the solution to pink color, observable when viewed from the top of the test tube against a white background placed beneath the bottom of the test tube. Repeat the test with 1:10, 1:20, 1:50, 1:100, 1:200 dilutions and report the terms of highest dilution giving a positive reaction. Normally 1:10 and 1:20 dilutions should give a positive. Abnormally high amounts of urobilinogen will change the solution to a clearly discernable cherry red color.

  This result must be done with fresh urine or else urobilinogen is oxidized on exposure to air to urobilin.
- **Qualitative Schlesinger test:**
  Procedure:
  - Place 10 mL urine in a test tube and add 6 drops of tincture iodine.
  - In another test tube take 1 g of powdered zinc acetate and 10 mL of 95% alcohol.
  - Mix both the solutions repeatedly by inversion till the solid zinc acetate has dissolved into the solution.
  - Filter
  - Examine the filtrate by (i) transmitted light and (ii) reflected light with back to the window or looking down the test tube.

  Result: Urobilinogen will procedure a green fluorescence.
- **Colorimetric reagent strip test:**
  Principle: This test is based on modified Ehrlich's test. P-diethyl amino-benzaldehyde in conjunction with a color enhancer reacts with urobilinogen and porphobilinogen, in a strongly acidic medium to produce a pink-red color.
  Procedure: A freshly voided specimen is necessary for the test, preferably a sample collected over a 2 hours period in the early afternoon when the urinary urobilinogen excretion is the highest for the day. The strip is dipped into fresh uncentrifuged urine collected without preservatives, removed and tapped free of excess urine.

The color reaction is compared to the color chart, after exactly 45 seconds.

Result: The six color blocks provided on the chart range in color from light yellow to brown-orange, representing 0.1, 1, 2, 4, 6 and 12 Ehrlich units/100 dL of urine. The first two color blocks, 0.1 and 1 Ehrlich units/dL are within the normal range of values for urobilinogen. The remaining four color blocks indicate high values.

Test for detection of bile salts

Hay's test

Procedure: When granules of sulfur are sprinkled on the surface of the urine, if bile salts are present they sink to the bottom. Otherwise, they float on the surface. This is due to the property of bile salts to lower surface tension.

Microscopic Examination of Urine Sediment

A qualitative or a semiquantitative evaluation of urine sediment generally provides adequate information for majority of diagnostic and clinical needs. Quantitative examination of the urine is most helpful in evaluating the course and progression of renal disease.

Microscopic examination of urine sediment can provide the following information:

- Evidenced of renal disease as opposed to lower urinary tract infection.
- Indicate the type and state of activity of a renal lesion or disease condition.

Qualitative technique: Examination of the sediment is more reliable when the urine is concentrated. If the specimen is too dilute, the cellular elements may not be representative. The urine must be freshly voided and examined without excessive delay in order to prevent cellular deterioration. Cellular debris from the urethral meatus and secretions from the vagina may contaminate the urine specimen.

To obtain the sediment, 10–15 mL of urine should be taken from freshly mixed urine specimen and centrifuged at a standard speed, usually 1,500–2,000 rpm for 5 minutes. This is sufficient to bring to the bottom casts, pus cells, blood and supernatant fluid is poured off and the sediment mixed well in 1 mL of the same fluid. If the specimen is sparse, it should be examined with little or no additional dilution.

A drop of resuspended sediment is placed directly on a microscope slide and covered with a coverslip. The slide is first examined under low power magnification to locate the casts and elements that are present in only a few fields. Casts tend to congregate at the edges of the coverslip. After the entire slide has been scanned, a further examination is done under high power magnification in order to identify specific types of cells, crystals and elements present in the urine and to differentiate the various types of casts. A minimum of 10–15 high power fields should be scanned for this examination.

Precautions

- Urine must be examined fresh. If a 24 hours specimen is to be examined it should be preserved in a refrigerator or a preservative should be added.
- Care should be taken to make a thin preparation without any air bubbles.
- The condenser should be lowered and light reduced while examining under low power or else structures, such as casts will be missed.
- Examination of the sediment should always be done in low power and high power is used for finer details.
- The urine should always be well mixed before centrifuging or else the cellular elements and deposits may settle to the bottom leaving the supernatant clear.

Red blood cells, leukocytes and epithelial cells are conventionally reported in terms of cells per high power field; casts are reported per low power fields. For each determination, the number of elements seen in at least 10 fields should be counted and the average of this number used for the reported value. Other elements, such as bacteria, parasites, crystals and spermatozoa are reported as well.

Normal Sediment

Normal sediment contains a limited number of formed elements. It can be classified into two classes:

1. Unorganized sediment
2. Organized sediment

Unorganized sediment: These are the crystals of various substances present in the urine and they vary with the pH of the urine. Crystals of normal urine is formed as the specimen cools.

Crystals in acidic urine

- **Uric acid and urates:** Crystals are seen when urine is allowed to stand for some time and are not seen in freshly passed urine. Amorphous urates appear as red granules and are dissolved by heat and sodium hydroxide but not acetic acid. Uric acid crystals vary in shape and are yellow brown in color and are not dissolved by heat, acetic acid or HCl but are soluble when heated with sodium hydroxide. Excessive deposits of uric acid and urates in fresh urine are seen in disturbances of uric acid metabolism and in fevers where the urine is concentrated.
- **Calcium oxalate:** Crystals are also seen in neutral or slightly alkaline urine. They are commonly found in diets rich in tomatoes, spinach, etc. They are typically envelope-shaped crystals but occasionally appear dumb-bell shaped. They are insoluble in strong HCl.
- **Cystine crystals:** These are rare crystals and are highly refractive, hexagonal plates and are soluble in HCl but insoluble in acetic acid. They are seen in cystinosis which is an inborn error or metabolism in which cystine crystals are found in the urine, reticuloendothelial system and eyes.
- **Leucine:** Crystals are slightly yellow, oily looking spheres with radial and concentric striations. They are not soluble in HCl or ether. They are found in liver disorders.
- **Tyrosine:** Crystals appear in the form of fine needles arranged in concentric sheaves, with a marked constriction at the middle. They are seen in patients with liver disorders.
- **Sulfa crystals:** These are seen in the urine of patients taking sulfonamides.

Crystals in alkaline urine

- **Ammonium magnesium phosphates:** These are also called as 'triple phosphate' crystals. They are colorless and appear as coffin lid, feathery or leaf like forms. In freshly passed urine, they indicate stones in the bladder or kidney. Phosphates may occur as amorphous deposits in alkaline urine and are dissolved in acetic acid.
- **Dicalcium phosphates:** They are also seen in slightly acid or neutral urine. They are colorless prisms arranged in stars and rosettes (stellar phosphate). These individual prisms are usually slender with one beveled, wedge-like end but sometimes needle-like. They can also be seen as large, thin, irregular usually granular or colorless plates. They are soluble in acetic acid.
- **Calcium carbonate:** They are seen as amorphous granules or colorless spheres and dumb-bells which are soluble in acetic acid with gas formation.
- **Ammonium biurates:** They are usually seen along with phosphates in decomposing urine, when free ammonia is present. It forms opaque, yellow spherical crystals which are often covered with fine or coarse spicules. They dissolve on addition of acetic acid and rhombic plates of uric acid appear.

Organized sediment: The components of organized sediment include casts, red blood cells, white blood cells, epithelial cells, bacteria, yeast, parasites, spermatozoa and artifacts.

Casts: Casts are formed in the tubules and is composed of proteinaceous material. They are washed out by the glomerular secretion into the collecting tubules and the bladder. They are cylindrical in shape with round or broken ends with uniform diameter but varying in length. They require acidic conditions, high salt concentration, reduced urine flow and protein to be formed. Practically all casts have a hyaline matrix, which may/may not contain inclusions, such as desquamated cells.

The casts are named according to the matrix of the inclusions contained in them, e.g., red blood cell casts.

Many different casts are present in the urine. They include:

- **Hyaline casts:** These are colorless, semi-transparent and occasionally refractive cylinders and are soluble in acetic acid. They are seen when there is damage to the glomerular filtrate. They are seen in fever, orthostatic proteinuria, emotional stress or strenuous exercise.
- **Granular casts:** These are casts containing large or fine granules embedded in coagulated protein. They are not found in normal urine and their presence indicates pyelonephritis. They are also seen in chronic lead poisoning.
- **Epithelial casts:** These are formed of fused desquamated tubular cells. They are coagulated protein in which are embedded desquamated epithelial cells from the renal tubules. They are seen in diseases where there is damage to the tubular epithelium as in nephrosis, eclampsia, amyloidosis and heavy metal poisoning.
- **Red blood cell casts:** These are casts with red blood cells embedded in the coagulated protein in the tubule. Their presence indicates acute inflammation or vascular disorder in the glomerulus causing hematuria. They are seen in pathological conditions, such as acute glomerulonephritis, renal infarction and collagen vascular disorder.
- **White blood cell casts (pus cell):** These are composed of pus cells embedded in coagulated protein. They are seen in the urine of patients with acute glomerulonephritis, nephritic syndrome or pyelonephritis.
- **Fatty casts:** These are casts embedded with numerous fat globules. They are stained by adding a few drops of Sudan III solution where they take a red color. They are not normally found in urine and are derived from degenerating cells.
- **Waxy casts:** These are broad, and is formed in the collecting tubules when the urine flow through them is reduced. They are composed of homogeneous, yellowish material and have a refractive outline and appear very brittle. They are seen in chronic renal disease.

Red blood cells: Normally 1–2 red blood cells are found per high power field in the urine. They appear pale, light refractive, biconcave discs when viewed under high power magnification. They have no nuclei. Red blood cells in fresh, unstained sediment appear pale in color; in urine that is not fresh, they are pale or colorless "shadow cells". In urine that is not fresh, they are pale crenated; and in dilute urine, they are large and swollen and sometimes rupture to produce "ghost cells". They must be differentiated from yeast cells, urate crystals and oil droplets. Yeast cells are usually ovoid and frequently show budding. Ammonium biurate crystals occur in large quantities with great range in the size of crystals. Mineral oil droplets also vary greatly in size and are more refractive and spherical. Presence of red blood cells indicates a variety of renal and systemic disease, including trauma to the kidney. It may also be found following violent exercise. It may follow traumatic catheterization, passage of stones, or contamination from menstrual blood. Hematuria occurs with pyelonephritis, tuberculosis of the genitourinary tract, cystitis, prostatitis, renal calculi, renal tumors and other malignancies of the urinary tract and hemorrhagic diseases, such as hemophilia. Red cells will lyse or dissolve if allowed to stand in urine which is alkaline or dilute.

White cells: Normal urine shows about 3-5 pus cells or polymorph nuclear leukocyte per field. They have segmented nuclei, granular and are 11/2 times as large as red blood cells. Certain neutrophils are larger than the normal leukocytes and their cytoplasmic granules have Brownian movements. These cells are called 'glitter cells'. They are seen in infection of the urinary tract.

Epithelial cells: Normally a few epithelial cells occur in the urine. A marked increase is these cells in the urine are seen destruction of the tissue in the urinary tract. The cells seen are:

- Renal tubular cells—are round and are slightly larger than leukocytes. Each contains a single large nucleus.
- Bladder epithelial cells—are larger than renal tubular epithelial cells. They range in shape from flat, to cuboidal and columnar.
- Squamous epithelial cells—are large flat cells with a single small nuclei and a large cytoplasm. The majority of these cells are contaminants from the vagina or vulva, but some originate in the urethra.

Quantitative evaluation of the urine sediment—addis count

The addis count is a quantitative measurement of the excretion of red blood cells, leukocytes and casts in the urine during a 12 hours period.

Procedure: A 12 hours urine specimen is taken to which formalin is added as a preservative. Mix the specimen well. Measure the total volume. Transfer 10-9 mL of the supernatant fluid and mix the sediment thoroughly. Transfer one drop of sediment to a blood counting chamber and count in a similar manner to WBC count. The number and the differential cast count are made under low power in all 9 squares. Similarly erythrocytes and leukocytes are counted.

Values in diseased states

Increased excretion of red blood cells, leukocytes and casts usually occurs in the urine of patients with glomerulonephritis.

Bacteria: Fresh urine in a normal person does not show bacteria. However when allowed to stand and in bacterial infection the urine shows bacteria. The finding of bacteria in a random urine sample can be considered indicative of a urinary tract infection only if the specimen is a clean-voided midstream sample collected under aseptic condition in a sterile container that is immediately closed with a sterile cap. Meticulous care must be exercised during collection and or potential pathogens from sources external to the urinary tract. Preferably, testing for bacteriuria should begin within an hour from the time of collection, but if this is not possible, the specimen should be refrigerated at 5°C immediately after collection and tested within 8 hours. No preservatives should be added to the urine for bacteriological culture test. The preferable type of specimen is the first morning urine or urine that has been incubated in the bladder at least 4 hours. Bacteriuria is considered significant when there is the presence of 100,000 (10^5) or more bacteria per mL of urine specimen. If contamination of an otherwise sterile specimen with bacteria from external sources has occurred, the count may be as low as 10,000 (10^4) or less per mL. When the count is between 10^3 and 10^5, the possibility of an incipient urinary tract infection is suggested. Low counts may occur in patients with frank urinary tract infections, if the urine specimen is dilute or has remained in the bladder only a short time. Such counts may also occur during early stages of treatment with antimicrobial agent. Significant urinary tract infection may be present in patients who have no symptoms. This condition is known as asymptomatic bacteriuria and is defined as the finding of 10^5 of more bacteria per mL of urine in the absence of clinical symptoms.

Gram negative bacteria normally present in the large intestine are commonly identified in urinary tract infections. They are *Escherichia coli,* Proteus species, *Klebsiella* and *Pseudomonas aeruginosa*. Gram positive organisms, such as *Streptococcus faecalis* and *Staphylococcus aureus* cause infections less frequently.

Detection of bacteria

- **Microscopic examination:** The centrifuged sediment when examined microscopically can reveal if bacteria are present. The finding of 20 or more bacteria per high power field may indicate a urinary tract infection. Fewer bacteria should be interpreted with caution.
- **Yeast and parasites:** Yeast cells (*Candida albicans*) may be indicative of urinary candidiasis especially in patients with diabetes mellitus. Frequently, yeast appears as a contaminant in the urine of patients with vaginal candidiasis. They are sometimes confused with red blood cells. They differ by being ovoid rather than round, colorless, variable in size and frequently show budding. Addition of acetic acid will lyse red blood cells but leave the yeast cells intact. Large amount of yeast with hyphae are suggestive of vaginitis.
  The majority of parasites observed in urine are contaminants from fecal or vaginal material. *Trichomonas vaginalis* is the most frequently seen parasite in the urine. It is a unicellular organism with anterior flagella and undulating membrane. *Schistosoma haematobium* is a urinary parasite associated with the presence of red blood cells.
- **Spermatozoa:** Spermatozoa are frequently seen in the urine following nocturnal emissions or sexual intercourse. They have oval bodies and long delicate tails. They may be motile or stationary.
- **Chyle:** In conditions such as filariasis, the lymphatics in the wall of the bladder or kidney may rupture and the lymph with its fat droplets escapes into the urine to give a milky appearance. The fat can be determined by staining with Sudan III or by adding ether which dissolves the fat and clears the urine.

Points to Ponder

- Examination of urine is a basic and an invaluable procedure, and should be carefully performed to obtain the maximum and best test results. Analysis of urine serves two purposes. One is to ascertain the existence of metabolic and endocrine disturbances in the body in which the kidneys function normally and therefore excrete abnormal amounts of metabolic end products specific for a particular disease. The second purpose is to detect intrinsic conditions that affect the kidney and the urinary tract.
- The main constituent of urine is water which accounts for 95% of the urine. The remaining 5% is composed of 2% urea and the balance 3% is divided between organic and inorganic substances.
- The concentration of urine varies throughout the day depending partly on the person's water intake and partly on his activities. So the type of sample plays a vital role.
- Examination of urine should be done immediately or within 1–2 hours on a fresh sample. When urine examination is delayed for periods longer than 1 hour, special precautions must be taken both to avoid deterioration of chemical and cellular elements and to prevent multiplication of bacteria that may be present in the collected urine with resultant alteration in urinary constituents.

Contd...

Contd...

- A qualitative or a semiquantitative evaluation of urine generally provides adequate information for majority of diagnostic and clinical needs. Quantitative examination of the urine is most helpful in evaluating the course and progression of renal disease.
- Microscopic examination of urine sediment can provide the following information:
  - Evidence of renal disease as opposed to lower urinary tract infection.
  - Indicate the type and state of activity of a renal lesion or disease condition.
- Unorganized sediment contains the crystals of various substances present in the urine and they vary with the pH of the urine. Crystals of normal urine is formed as the specimen cools.
- Organized sediment includes casts, red blood cells, white blood cells, epithelial cells, bacteria, yeast, parasites, spermatozoa and artifacts.

ASSESSMENT QUESTIONS

1. **What is the normal composition of urine?**
2. **Name the various methods of collection of urine sample.**
3. **Enlist the common preservatives used for urine sample.**
4. **Define oliguria. Mention the common causes.**
5. **Mention the common causes for polyuria.**
6. **What is nocturia ? In which disease you see it.**
7. **What is the normal color of urine? Give reason.**
8. **Name the condition in which you see cola-colored urine.**
9. **Give examples for various abnormal color in urine analysis.**
10. **In which condition urine gives a fruity odor.**
11. **What is the importance of measuring the pH of urine.**
12. **Define specific gravity.**
13. **What are the methods used to demonstrate the specific gravity**
14. **Name the conditions in which specific gravity in increased.**
15. **What is Tamm-Horsfall protein?**
16. **Name the tests used to detect proteins in urine.**
17. **What is Bence-Jones protein ? In which condition you see them.**
18. **Name the tests used to detect reducing substances in urine**
19. **Enumerate the composition of Benedict's reagent.**
20. **Enlist the causes for false-positive Benedict's test.-**
21. **What are ketone bodies?**
22. **Enlist the common causes for ketoacidosis.**
23. **Name the tests used to detect bile salts and bile pigments in urine.**
24. **What will be color of urine in obstructive jaundice?**
25. **Name the tests used to detect blood in urine.**
26. **What are the common causes for hematuria?**
27. **How will you classify the sediments seen in urine?**
28. **Give examples for organized and unorganized sediments.**
29. **What do you mean by significant bacteriuria?**
30. **Name the common type of crystals seen in an acidic urine.**

MULTIPLE CHOICE QUESTIONS

1. Urinary sediments are best studied in one of the following type of urine sample:
- A. Early morning
- B. Random
- C. Fasting
- D. Midstream catch

2. Polyuria occurs in all of the following, *except*:
- A. Diabetes mellitus
- B. Acute renal failure
- C. Diabetes insipidus
- D. Diuretics

3. In alkaptonuria the color of urine is:
- A. Yellow
- B. Red
- C. Black
- D. Colorless

4. All of the following gives low specific gravity to urine, *except*:
- A. Diabetes insipidus
- B. Chronic pyelonephritis
- C. Chronic renal failure
- D. Diabetes mellitus

5. Refractometer is used to measure:
- A. Specific gravity
- B. Viscosity
- C. pH
- D. Color

6. Sulfosalicylic acid test is done to detect one of the following in urine sample:
- A. Sugar
- B. Proteins
- C. Bile pigments
- D. Blood

7. Rothera's test is done to detect one of the following in urine sample:
- A. Sugar
- B. Proteins
- C. Ketone bodies
- D. Blood

8. Benzidine test is done to detect one of the following in urine sample:
- A. Sugar
- B. Proteins
- C. Ketone bodies
- D. Blood

9. Fouchet's test is done to detect one of the following in urine sample:
- A. Bilirubin
- B. Proteins
- C. Protein
- D. Blood

10. All of the following are organized sediments of urine, *except*:
- A. Hyaline casts
- B. Uric acid crystals
- C. Waxy Cast
- D. RBC cast

Answer Key for MCQs

1	2	3	4	5	6	7	8	9	10
A	B	C	D	A	B	C	D	A	B

Appendix 1: Table of average normal values for urine determinations.

Test	*Average normal value*	*Type of specimen*
Addis count	♦ WBC 1,800,000 ♦ RBC 500,000 ♦ Casts 0–5,000	12 hours
♦ Albumin ♦ Qualitative ♦ Quantitative ♦ Aldosterone ♦ Amino acid nitrogen	♦ Negative ♦ 10–100 mg /24 hr ♦ 2–23 μg /24 hr ♦ 100–290 mg/24 hr	♦ Random ♦ 24 hours ♦ 24 hours refrigerated ♦ 24 hour refrigerated ♦ Collected in thymol
♦ Ammonia ♦ Ammonia nitrogen	♦ 20–70 m Eq/24 hr ♦ 0.14–1.47 g/24 hr	♦ 24 hours ♦ 24 hours
♦ Bence-Jones protein ♦ Bilirubin ♦ Blood occult	♦ Negative ♦ Negative ♦ Negative	♦ First morning specimen ♦ Random ♦ Random
♦ Calcium ♦ Sulk witch ♦ Quantitative ♦ Catecholamines ♦ Chloride ♦ Concentration test ♦ Coproporphyrin ♦ Random ♦ 24 hours ♦ Creatine ♦ Creatinine	♦ Positive 1 + ♦ 100–250 mg/24 hr on an average diet ♦ 100–230 g/24 hr ♦ 110–250 m Eq/24 hr ♦ Specific gravity of 1.025 or higher ♦ 20 g/100 mL ♦ Adults: 50–200 μg/24 hr ♦ Children 0–80 μg /24 hr ♦ Male: 0–40 mg/24 hr ♦ Female 0–100 mg /24 hr ♦ Higher in children ♦ Male: 1.0–1.9 g/24 hr ♦ Female 0.8–1.7 g/24 hr	♦ Random ♦ 24 hours ♦ 24 hours preserve with 1 mL ♦ Concentrated H_2SO_4 ♦ 24 hours ♦ Withholding fluids for the day prior to the test ♦ Random ♦ 24 hours preserve with ♦ 5 g Na_2CO_3 ♦ 24 hours ♦ 24 hours

Dilution test	*Specific gravity of 1.001 to 1.003*	*After 1200 mL water load*
Estrogens	♦ Male: 4–25 μg/24 hr ♦ Female: 4–60 μg/24 hr	24 hours refrigerate
♦ Glucose ♦ Qualitative ♦ Quantitative	♦ Negative ♦ 130 mg/24 hr	♦ Random ♦ 24 hours
♦ Hemoglobin ♦ 17-hydroxy corticosteroids ♦ 17 ketosteroids	♦ Negative ♦ Males: 5.5–14.5 mg/24 hr ♦ Females: 5–13 mg/24 hr ♦ Males: 8–15 mg/24 hr ♦ Female: 6–11.5 mg/24 hr ♦ Children: 5 mg/24 hr	♦ Random ♦ 24 hour sample ♦ Interfere ♦ 24 hour sample ♦ Interfere
Ketenes	Negative	Random
Lead	100 μg/24 hr	24 hours, collect in lead-free bottle
♦ Osmolality ♦ Normal fluid intake full range	♦ 500–800 mOsm/kg water ♦ 39–1400 mOsm/kg water	♦ Random ♦ Random

Contd...

Contd...

Dilution test	*Specific gravity of 1.001 to 1.003*	*After 1200 mL water load*
♦ pH ♦ Phenylpyruvic acid ♦ Phosphorous ♦ Porphobilinogen ♦ Potassium ♦ Pregnanediol ♦ Protein ♦ Qualitative ♦ Quantitative ♦ Bence-Jones	♦ 4.6–8.0 ♦ Negative ♦ 0.9–1.3 g/24 hr ♦ Negative ♦ 25–100 mEq/24 hr ♦ Male: 0–1 mg/24 hr ♦ Female: 1–8 mg/24 hr ♦ Children: Negative ♦ Male: 1.0–2.0 mg/24 hr ♦ Female: 0.5–2.0 mg/24 hr ♦ Children: <0.5 mg/4 hr ♦ Negative ♦ 10–150 mg/24 hr ♦ Negative	♦ Random ♦ Random ♦ 24 hours ♦ Random ♦ 24 hours ♦ 24 hours, refrigerate ♦ 24 hours refrigerate ♦ Random ♦ 24 hours ♦ First morning specimen
♦ Sodium ♦ Specific gravity ♦ Random ♦ 24 hours ♦ Sugars	♦ 110–260 mEq/24 hr ♦ 1.002–1.030 ♦ 1.015–1.025 ♦ Negative	♦ 24 hours ♦ Random ♦ 24 hours random
Titratable acidity	♦ 200–500 mL of 0.1 N ♦ NaOH/24 hr	♦ 24 hours ♦ Preserve with toluene
♦ Urea nitrogen ♦ Uric acid ♦ Urobilinogen ♦ Semiquantitative ♦ Uroporphyrin	♦ 6–17 g/24 hr ♦ 250–750 mg/24 hr ♦ 0.3–1.0 Ehrlich units 2/hr ♦ 1.0–4.0 mg/24 hr ♦ 10–30 g/24 hr	♦ 24 hours ♦ 24 hours ♦ 2 hour afternoon specimen ♦ 24 hours collect in dark bottle with 5 g Na_2CO_3 refrigerate ♦ 24 hours collect in dark bottle with 5 g Na_2CO_3
♦ Vanillylmandelic acid (VMA) ♦ Volume adults	♦ 1–8 mg/24 hr ♦ 600–1500 mL/24 hr	24 hour preserve in 3 mL 25% H_2SO_4. No coffee or fruit for 2 days prior to test 24 hours

CHAPTER

Analysis of Cerebrospinal Fluid

Learning Objectives

At the end of reading this chapter, the student shall be able to:

- Describe in detail the mechanism of formation of cerebrospinal fluid and its composition.
- Enumerate the indications for analysis of cerebrospinal fluid.
- Enlist the methods of common macroscopic examination of CSF sample and interpret abnormalities.
- Perform a systematic chemical analysis of the given CSF sample using a battery of laboratory tests and to interpret each of them.

INTRODUCTION

Cerebrospinal fluid (CSF) is present within the subarachnoid space surrounding the brain in the skull and the spinal cord in the spinal column. Its main function is to protect the brain and the spinal cord from injury by acting as a fluid cushion. It is the medium through which nutrients and the waste products are transported between brain/spinal cord and the blood.

FORMATION AND COMPOSITION OF CSF

- Cerebrospinal fluid is derived by ultra-filtration (of plasma) and by secretion through the choroid plexus located in the ventricles of the brain. It leaves the ventricular system through the medial and lateral foramina to surround the brain and the spinal cord surfaces within the subarachnoid space.
- Reabsorption of CSF occurs at the arachnoid villi which projects into the venous sinuses in the dura mater.
- CSF is produced at the rate of 500 mL/day.
- Total CSF volume is 90–150 mL in adults and 10–60 mL in neonates.
- Blood brain barrier maintains the relative homeostasis of central nervous system (CNS) environment by tightly regulating the concentration of substances by specific transport systems for H^+, K^+, Ca^{++}, Mg^{++}, HCO^-_3.
- Glucose, urea and creatinine diffuse between blood and the CSF.
- Proteins cross freely by passive diffusion along the concentration gradient and is also influenced by molecular weight.

CHARACTERISTICS OF NORMAL CSF

- *Color:* Colorless
- *pH:* 7.28–7.32
- *Appearance:* Clear
- *Specific gravity:* 1.003–1.004
- No clot formation on standing
- *Total solids:* 0.85–1.70 g/dL
- *PO_2:* 40–44 mm Hg

COMPOSITION OF CSF

	Conventional units	*SI units*
Proteins	15–45 mg/dL	0.15–0.45 g/L
	(Albumin = 50–70%)	
	(Globulin = 30–50%)	
Glucose	50–80 mg/dL	2.8–4.4 mmol/L
Urea	6.0–16 mg/dL	2.0–5.7 mmol/L
Uric acid	0.5–3.0 mg/dL	30–180 µmol/L
Creatinine	0.6–1.2 mg/dL	45–92 µmol/L
Cholesterol	0.2–0.6 mg/dL	
Ammonia	10–35 µg/dL	6–20 µmol/L
Electrolytes		
Sodium	135–150 mEq/L	135–150 mmol/L
Potassium	2.6–3.0 mEq/L	2.6–3.0 mmol/L
Chloride	115–130 mEq/L (650–750 mEq/dL)	115–130 mmol/L
Magnesium	2.4–3.0 mEq/L	1.1–2.4 mmol/L
Cells: 0–8 lymphocytes/cumm(µL)		

INDICATIONS OF CSF EXAMINATION

Analysis of the CSF is useful in the diagnosis of

- Bacterial, viral or fungal meningitis.
- Encephalitis
- Malignant infiltrates like in acute leukemia, lymphoma
- Subarachnoid hemorrhage
- Disorders with local immunoglobulin production in the CNS-multiple sclerosis, sub-acute sclerosing pan encephalitis (SSPE).
- Spinal canal blockage leading to elevated intracranial tension.

COLLECTION AND HANDLING OF CSF

Cerebrospinal fluid is usually obtained by lumbar puncture (LP) using and LP needle.

The needle measures 10-12 cm in length and is made of platinum or German alloy. It has a needle and the stylet. The stylet of the needle has a pin which fits into the lot of the head of the needle. The stylet of the needle helps to keep the needle patent.

Specimen Collection

PROCEDURE

- Procedure for specimen collection by lumbar puncture
  - **Position:** The patient is place on his side at the edge of the bed with his knee drawn up and the head flexed.
  - **Site:** In the 3rd lumbar space. This space lies in the plane which joins the highest points on the iliac crest. The skin over the back from the lower thoracic vertebra to the coccyx is sterilized with cetavlon, ether, iodine and spirit.
  - **Local anesthesia:** The skin to be punctured is infiltrated with 5 mL of 2% lignocaine.
  - **Puncture:** The LP needle with stylet is introduced after 2–3 minutes into the anesthetized space, with the cutting edge of the bevel in the direction parallel to the fibers of the *Ligamentum flavum*. The needle is introduced (slightly upwards

Contd...

Contd...

and forwards at 5° to avoid injury to the disk) through the supraspinous ligament and interspinous ligament. At about 4–7 cm, the firmer resistance of the *Ligamentum flavum* gives way as the needle enters the dura mater.
- The stylet is then withdrawn and the fluid which trickles down is collected in sterile containers but only after recording the CSF pressure (by attaching a manometer to the LP needle).

- *CSF pressure:* The normal CSF pressure in an adult is 90–180 mm of water in the lateral position, while in infants and children it ranges from 10 to 100 mm of water reaching the adult level by 6–8 years.

Causes of Abnormal CSF Pressure

Causes for Elevated CSF Pressure

- *Meningitis*: Only finding in cryptococcal meningitis
- Congestive heart failure
- Cerebral edema
- Thrombosis of venous sinuses
- Mass lesion of the brain
- Superior vena cava syndrome

Causes for Decreased CSF Pressure

- Dehydration
- Circulatory collapse
- CSF leakage
- Spinal sub arachnoid block

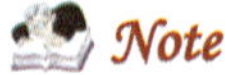

- If the opening CSF pressure in a relaxed patient is >200 mm of water, no >2 mL of fluid should be withdrawn.
- A sudden drop of CSF pressure after removal of 1–2 mL of CSF suggests herniation or spinal block above the site of puncture and in such situations the procedure should be abandoned.

Contd...

Contd...

- Collect about 6–8 mL of CSF (up to maximum of 20 mL can be collected) in 3 sterile test tubes, as suggested below:
  Tube 1: First several drops for microbiological examination and culture.
  Tube 2: About 2.5–3 mL for biochemical tests and immunologic studies.
  Tube 3: About 2 mL for cell count, differential count and cytological studies.

Handling of CSF Sample

- CSF sample should be examined immediately (within 30 minutes of collection). Delay causes inaccurate cell count and decrease in the glucose levels.
- CSF sample for bacterial cultures should be processed immediately. The sample should never be refrigerated as low temperature kills *Neisseria meningitides*.
- Specimen for biochemical tests can be stored at 2–8°C for a maximum of 2–3 hours.
- Careful pipetting and handling of CSF by the lab personnel is important, for it may contain contagious and virulent organisms.

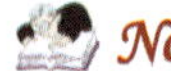

CSF sample is very precious, for it is collected by an invasive procedure. Hence, careful and economical handling of the sample is very important.

EXAMINATION OF CSF

Routine examination of CSF includes:
- Gross/physical examination
- Microscopic examination
- Chemical examination

Gross/Physical Examination

Observe the collected sample for color, appearance, clot/coagula formation on standing and presence of blood.

- pH determination (using pH paper)
- Color

  Hold the tube containing CSF against a sheet of white paper and compare it with a tube of distilled water. Normal CSF is clear and colorless.

  Causes for change in CSF color

  - **Yellow color (Xanthochromia):**
    - Following a subarachnoid bleed: Color changes from pale pink to orange and finally yellow. The yellow color develops by 12 hours and persists for 2–4 weeks. It is due to the formation of bilirubin following the breakdown of hemoglobin.
    - Severely jaundiced patient: Only conjugated bilirubin cross the blood—CSF barrier in adults, while in infants even the unconjugated bilirubin can cross over imparting a yellow color to CSF.
    - In cases of high protein content in the CSF (>150 mg/dL): Caused by complete spinal block by tumors and in meningitis.
    - Artefactual red cell lysis: Caused by detergent contamination of the needle or delay of more than 1 hour before examining the CSF sample.
  - **Orange color:** Dietary hypercarotenemia
  - **Brown color:** Meningeal metastatic melanoma
  - **Red to orange:** Patients on rifampicin therapy
  - **Pink to red:** Indicates the presence of blood in CSF.
- *Appearance:* Normal CSF is clear.

  Causes for change in CSF appearance

  - **Turbid/cloudiness:** Increase in the number of cells in the CSF (>400–500 cells/μL) or presence of numerous bacteria or both.
  - **Smoky/opalescence:** Smaller number of cells (RBCs and/or leukocytes).
- *Clot/coagulum formation*: Allow the specimen of CSF to stand overnight and examine the sample for fibrin clot, which is formed if the sample contains fibrinogen. Also note the nature of the clot.
  - Delicate clot, which resembles a cobweb, is characteristically seen in tubercular meningitis due to marked increase in CSF proteins. The clot may have entrapped tubercle bacilli, which could be demonstrated microscopically by staining for acid-fast bacilli.
  - Coarse clot is formed in pyogenic meningitis, traumatic tap and in case of complete spinal block, (due to spinal tumors, or chronic meningitis).
- *Blood tinged CSF*: Blood in CSF may be due to traumatic tap, subarachnoid hemorrhage, intracerebral hemorrhage or brain infarct.

For the CSF to be grossly bloody, the RBC count should be greater than 6,000/μL. It is very important to differentiate traumatic tap from subarachnoid hemorrhage (**Table 27.1**). The following features helps in the differentiation.

Microscopic Examination (Table 27.2)

- *Total leukocyte count*: Normal CSF contains no red blood cells and 0–8 WBC/μL (only lymphocytes).

  Requirements:

  - Glass slides
  - **Counting chamber:** Fuchs Rosenthal (preferable) or Levy's chamber with improved Neubauer ruling
  - Coverslip of uniform thickness with size of 22 × 23 mm
  - CSF diluting fluid
  - **1% toluidine blue or 1% crystal violet:** Stains the WBC without lysing the RBC, thus enabling to count both RBC and WBC in the same chamber. The stain is mixed with CSF in the ratio 1:9.
  - **Dilute acetic acid:** 0.1 g crystal violet is added to 1 mL of glacial acetic acid which is made up to 50 mL by adding

TABLE 27.1: Comparative features of traumatic and subarachnoid hemorrhage.

Features	*Traumatic tap*	*Subarachnoid hemorrhage*
CSF pressure	Normal	Elevated
Blood staining	Varies between the tubes	Same in all the tubes Usually clears between first and third tubes
Xanthochromia	Absent (present in a jaundiced/or protein >100 mg/dL	Present (2–12 hours after bleeding)
Microscopy		
♦ RBCs	RBCs are not crenated	RBCs are crenated
♦ Hemosiderin laden macrophages	Absent	Present
♦ Erythrophagocytosis	Absent	Present
Coagulum	May occur	Absent

TABLE 27.2: Reference values for CSF differential counts by cytocentrifuge.

Cell type	*Adults*	*Neonates*
Lymphocytes	40–90%	10–30%
Monocytes	20–40%	60–90%
Neutrophils	0–4%	0–6%

distilled water. Few drops of phenol are also added to this. As this fluid lyses the red cells, it is useful in cases of blood tinged CSF. In such cases the RBC count is estimated separately, using undiluted CSF sample.

- Microscope

Procedure

- **Dilution:** Mix the CSF sample carefully.
  - » If CSF is clear, there is no need for dilution and both RBC and WBC can be counted simultaneously in the same chamber.
  - » If CSF is cloudy then make a dilution of 1:10. Using the WBC pipette, draw CSF sample up to mark 1 and the diluting fluid up to mark 11 to get the desired dilution. One can also pipette out 10 mL of CSF diluting fluid in a tube and add 1 mL of CSF to it. 9:10 dilution may be used instead of 1:10 dilution.
- Charging the counting chamber and counting of cells:
  - » Charge the counting chamber properly
  - » Wait for 5 minutes before counting, to allow the cells in CSF to settle down.
  - » Count the cells in all 9 squares in case of Neubauer chamber or in all 16 squares in case of Fuchs Rosenthal chamber by using low power objective.

❖ *Differential leukocyte count:*

- **Chamber differential:** It is possible to identify the leukocytes as polymorphs (neutrophils) and mononuclear cells (lymphocytes and monocytes) in the counting chamber while estimating the total leukocyte count. 100 leukocytes are examined and the chamber differential reported.

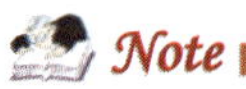

Note

A differential count performed in a counting chamber is unsatisfactory because of low cell numbers and identification of the cell type beyond granulocyte and mononuclear cells is difficult in wet preparation.

- Differential leukocyte count on Leishman stained smear
  - » If the cell count is low (<200 WBC/µL) centrifuge the CSF sample, prepare a thin smear of the sediment and allow it to dry before staining with Leishman's stain.
  - » If the cell count is <500 WBC/µL prepare a thin smear of the uncentrifuged CSF and dry it before staining.
  - » Direct smear of centrifuged CSF sediment show cellular distortion and fragmentation. Hence, better and more accurate methods are employed in many laboratories.

❖ *Cytocentrifuge/cytospin*: Recommended for all body fluids. The advantages are good cell yield and better cell preservation than simple centrifugation. About 30–50 cells are obtained from 0.5 mL of normal CSF sample.
To further minimize cell distortion use a fresh sample or add 2 drops of 22 bovine serum albumin to the CSF sample before centrifugation.

❖ *Filtration methods*: The advantages of this method are good cell recovery, excellent cell preservation and ability to concentrate large volumes of CSF for cytological studies.
The main drawback is that it is costly, time consuming and needs technical expertise.

❖ *Sedimentation methods*: Cell morphology is well preserved but the yield is low and the procedure is very cumbersome.

PROCEDURE

Staining procedure: Place the slide horizontally on a slide rack and add 10–15 drops of Leishman's stain on the smear and wait for 1 minute. Then add equal volume of buffer solution (pH 7.0) and keep it for 10 minutes. Wash the smear gently under running tap water, then air dry the smear and observe under the microscope to determine the differential leukocyte count.

Diagnosis of Abnormal CSF Differential Count

Causes for increase neutrophils in CSF

❖ Bacterial meningitis
❖ Amoebic encephalomyelitis
❖ Cerebral abscess
❖ Subdural empyema

Causes for increased lymphocytes in CSF

❖ Viral meningitis
❖ Tuberculous meningitis
❖ Syphilitic meningoencephalitis
❖ Leptospiral meningitis
❖ Fungal meningitis
❖ Degenerative disorders: Multiple sclerosis, SSPE

Causes for increased eosinophils in CSF

❖ Parasitic infections
❖ Fungal infections
❖ Reaction to foreign body in CSF
❖ Idiopathic eosinophilic meningitis
❖ Idiopathic hyper eosinophilic syndrome

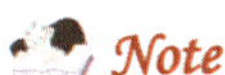

While doing the differential count observe for the presence of lymphoblast as leukemic involvement of meninges is common in ALL.
A WBC count of >5 cells/µL with unequivocal lymphoblast on a centrifuged preparation indicates meningeal involvement in a case of leukemia.

Biochemical Examination

Protein Estimation

Normal CSF protein content is 15–45 mg/dL.

Cerebrospinal fluid protein increases with increase in permeability of blood vessels in the choroids plexus and the meninges.

Causes for increased CSF protein

❖ *Inflammatory conditions*: Bacterial, viral, fungal and tubercular meningitis.
❖ *Hemorrhage*: Subarachnoid, intracerebral.
❖ *Drug toxicity*: Ethanol, phenothiazine's.
❖ *Disorders causing obstruction to CSF flow*: CNS tumors and abscess.

- *Increased immunoglobulin synthesis*: Neurosyphilis, multiple sclerosis.

Sulfosalicylic acid test

Principle: Proteins are precipitated by sulfosalicylic acid. The turbidity thus formed is measured by a spectrophotometer of a colorimeter against a standard curve or a single standard. If spectrophotometer is not available then turbidity is measured by visual comparison against a series of standards.

Reagents: 3% sulfosalicylic acid—30 g of sulfosalicylic acid is dissolved in distilled water to make up to 1 liter.

Procedure:

- Pipette 0.5 mL of CSF into a small test tube (100 × 75 mm)
- Add 1.5 mL of 3% sulfosalicylic acid reagent and mix gently.
- Allow to stand for 5 minutes. Then invert and mix.
- The turbidity thus formed is compared with the set of turbidity standards, matching the test with that concentration of the standard which shows the same or closest turbidity. It is best compared by viewing against a white paper bearing black lines or print.

It can also be more accurately measured by a spectrophotometer or a colorimeter against a standard.

Pandy's test for determining the globulin: It is a simple, poorly quantitated screening test to detect the globulins in the CSF. It is based on the fact that when protein increases in the CSF the majority of that protein is globulin, which precipitates and causes turbidity in this test.

Principle: Globulins are precipitated by a saturated solution of phenol in water.

Reagents: Pandy's reagent—10 g of phenol in 100 mL of distilled water, shake well and place it in an incubator at 37°C for 3 days. Allow it to settle and use only the supernatant.

Procedure:

- Pipette 2 mL of Pandy's reagent into a small test tube (100 × 75 mm)
- Add 2–3 drops of clear CSF specimen, do not mix
- Observe for the formation of turbidity

Observations:

- No turbidity: Normal globulin
- Formation of a precipitate ring: Increased globulin
- The result can be graded as traces, 1+, 2+, 3+ and 4+.

Glucose Estimation

Cerebrospinal fluid glucose is derived from blood glucose hence, ideally CSF glucose levels should be compared with fasting plasma glucose level (after 4 hours fasting) for adequate clinical interpretation.

Normal CSF glucose is 50–80 mg/dL (2.8–4.4 mmol/L) in adults and 60–90 mg/dL in children up to 10 years of age, which amounts to 60% of the plasma glucose. The normal CSF/plasma glucose ratio may vary from 0.3 to 0.9.

Clinical significance: CSF glucose <40 mg/dL (2.2 mmol/L) or CSF/plasma glucose ratio <0.3 are considered abnormal.

Increased CSF glucose is of no clinical significance.

Causes for decreased CSF glucose:

- *Meningitis*: Bacterial, fungal, tubercular and syphilitic meningitis
- Tumors involving the meninges
- Subarachnoid hemorrhage
- Cerebral amoebiasis

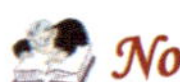

Note

The cause for decreased CSF glucose in the above conditions is due to increased glucose utilization via anaerobic glycolysis by the bacteria (in case of meningitis), brain tissue and leukocytes.

Qualitative test for glucose

Procedure

- Take 0.5 mL of benedicts qualitative reagent and to this add 4.5 mL of distilled water to get a dilution of 1:10.
- Add 0.5 mL of CSF to the above solution.
- Boil for 2 minutes on a flame and then allow it to cool.

Observations:

- *No color change:* Very low or absent glucose.
- Color change to turbid greenish yellow: Normal glucose level in CSF.
- Color change from blue to purple (due to biuret reaction with alkaline copper reagent) indicates elevated CSF glucose.

 *Note*

Ideally one has to do a quantitative test for glucose estimation and the above test should be discouraged.

Quantitative test for glucose: Modified Folin—Wu method

Principle: CSF sample when heated with alkaline cupric tartrate solution, the glucose in the sample reduces cupric ion in the soluble cupric tartrate to cuprous ions which gets precipitated as insoluble cuprous oxide. The amount of cuprous oxide produced is measured by the reduction of phosphomolybdate to molybdenum blue. The intensity of blue color produced is proportional to the glucose in the sample and is compared with the color given by the standard solution of glucose.

Chloride Estimation

The chloride level in the CSF is higher than the level in the serum.

The normal CSF chloride level is 115-130 mEq/L (650-750 mg/dL) CSF. Lately chloride estimation is omitted in the examination of CSF as good bacteriological examinations are available.

Clinical significance: Causes for reduced CSF chloride level:

- The CSF chloride level is decreased in case of bacterial and tubercular meningitis.
- Severe electrolyte imbalance with reduced serum chloride levels after a prolonged vomiting due to increased intracranial tension.

Cerebrospinal fluid chloride estimation can be done in the same way as that done for serum chloride. The estimation can be done by automated instruments or manually.

Microbiological Examination

Microbiological examination helps in finding the specific etiological agent in cases of meningitis. This information is of a great value in treating the patient with appropriate drugs, as the delay in the therapy causes significant morbidity and mortality. Most common agents causing bacterial meningitis are group B *Streptococcus*, *Haemophilus influenzae* (in children), Neisseria meningitides (in adolescents) and *Streptococcus pneumonia* (in adults).

- *Microscopic examination:* Take the CSF sample and centrifuge it at 1,500 g for 15 minutes. Make a smear out of the sediment, which is obtained after centrifugation. Cytospin concentration is a better alternative.

  Dry and fix the smear, stain and AFB stains. In addition, examine a wet preparation with Indian ink to demonstrate Cryptococcus neoformans (encapsulated yeast form) which is a common fungal infection of the CNS.
- *Culture:* CSF culture is mandatory in cases of suspected meningitis and is done with CSF collected in the first tube.

Serological examination

The usual serological examination relates to testing for syphilis.

Cerebrospinal fluid VDRL is inappropriate as a screening test for neurosyphilis for it has a low sensitivity (50-50%) but high specificity. It should be performed on a CSF sample only if the serum fluorescent Treponema antibody absorption (FTA-ABS) test is positive. This test is virtually diagnostic of neurosyphilis.

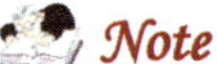

Dark ground microscope for the identification of spirochete in CSF sample in a suspected case of neurosyphilis is unpopular, for it demands technical expertise and experience.

Normal value of CSF fluid and in meningitis

Test	*Appearance*	*Pressure*	*WBC cells/μL*	*Protein (mg/dL)*	*Glucose (mg/dL)*	*Chloride*
Normal CSF	Clear	90–180 mm of water	0–8 lymphocytes	15–45	50–80	650–750 mg/d 115–130 mEq/L
Acute bacterial meningitis	Turbid	Increased	1,000–10,000 (Mainly neutrophils)	100–500	<40	Decreased
Viral meningitis	Clear	Normal to moderate increase	5–300 rarely >1,000 (Mainly lymphocytes)	Normal to mild increased	Normal	Normal
Tubercular meningitis	Slightly opaque with cobweb formation	Increased/ decreased with spinal block	100–600 (mixed for lymphocytic)	50–300 marked increase in spinal block	Decreased	Decreased
Fungal meningitis	Clear	Increased	40–400 lymphocytes and or neutrophils	50–300 (average about 100)	Decreased	Decreased
Acute syphilitic	Clear	Increased	About 500 (lymphocytic)	Increased but <100	Normal	Normal

Points to Ponder

- Analysis of the CSF is useful in the diagnosis of bacterial, viral or fungal meningitis. Encephalitis malignant infiltrates, such as in acute leukemia, lymphoma and subarachnoid hemorrhage.
- Routine examination of CSF include gross/physical examination, microscopic examination and biochemical examination.

ASSESSMENT QUESTIONS

1. **Enumerate the common indications for examination of cerebrospinal fluid.**
2. **What are the abnormal cells seen in cerebrospinal fluid?**

MULTIPLE CHOICE QUESTIONS

1. **Fuchs-Rosenthal counting chamber is used to count the cells in ____________ sample.**
   A. Blood C. Cerebrospinal fluid
   B. Urine D. Semen
2. **Cobweb formation in CSF occurs in which of the following type of meningitis?**
   A. Pneumococcal C. Candidal
   B. Cryptococcal D. Tuberculous
3. **What is the primary function of cerebrospinal fluid (CSF) in the central nervous system?**
   A. Nutrient transport to brain cells C. Protection and cushioning for the brain
   B. Temperature regulation in the brain D. Electrolyte balance in neural tissues
4. **Which of the following is the main site for the production of cerebrospinal fluid?**
   A. Pineal gland C. Choroid plexus
   B. Hypothalamus D. Cerebral cortex
5. **What is the primary method for collecting cerebrospinal fluid for diagnostic purposes?**
   A. Lumbar puncture (spinal tap) C. Magnetic resonance imaging (MRI)
   B. Blood test D. Electroencephalogram (EEG)

Answer Key for MCQs

1	2	3	4	5
C	D	C	C	A

CHAPTER 28 Analysis of Effusion Fluids

Learning Objectives

At the end of reading this chapter, the student shall be able to:

- Enlist the methods of common macroscopic examination of body fluid sample and interpret abnormalities.
- Perform a systematic chemical analysis of the given body fluid sample using a battery of laboratory tests and to interpret each of them.

INTRODUCTION

The commonly examined body fluids in the laboratory are:

- Pleural fluid in the pleural space surrounding the lungs
- Pericardial fluid—around the heart
- Peritoneal fluid—in the peritoneal cavity of the abdomen and pelvis
- Synovial fluid—in the joint space

Normally a small amount of fluid is present in these cavities to keep the surfaces moist and lubricated so that the movement of the adjacent or the opposing membrane surfaces occur with minimal frication. When there is an increase in the volume of the fluid in any of these cavities, the condition is called as effusion.

Aspiration of the excess fluid from the cavity is necessary for the following reasons:

- Effusion if in excess may interfere with the normal functioning of the organ.
- Examination of the fluid helps in determining the causes of the effusion and thus guide appropriate therapy for the condition.

PATHOPHYSIOLOGY OF EFFUSION

The plasma component of blood contains water, organic substances, such as glucose, urea etc., along with large molecular weight proteins.

Normally, there is exchange of fluid between intravascular compartment (capillaries) and extravascular space. Most of the fluid which moves back and forth through the capillary membrane is water containing salts, and low molecular organic substances, such as glucose, urea, etc. This movement is possible because of the pressure exerted by the blood on the capillary wall and is called the hydrostatic pressure.

The large molecular weight proteins stay within the capillaries and are responsible for drawing the fluid from the extravascular space and is called the colloidal osmotic pressure.

Lymphatics (lymph vessels) also removes the residual fluid from the extravascular space.

The amount of fluid entering the extravascular space and the body cavities is equal to the amount of fluid which leave these spaces and as a result, there is no accumulation of excess fluid in these spaces.

The mechanism which causes the accumulation of fluid in the tissue and the cavities are:

- *Increased venous pressure*: Causes increased movement of fluid from the vascular system than that can be absorbed. The capillary permeability does not alter and hence the fluid which accumulates in the extracellular space or the body cavity resembles the normal tissue fluid. It contains few cells and very low concentration of proteins and is called transudate.
- *Increased capillary permeability*: Caused due to inflammation or damage to the capillaries by the toxins. The accumulated fluid contains high concentration of proteins. Often fibrin along with cells are present and this fluid is called exudate.
- *Interference with the lymphatic flow*: Caused by filariasis, cancer or scar tissue in the lymphatics. This results in the accumulation of fluid with high proteins and lipids giving a milky appearance.
- *Decreased colloidal osmotic pressure*: Results from hypoproteinemia caused by nephritic syndrome (increased loss of proteins in urine), and decreases protein synthesis caused by extensive liver damage (e.g., cirrhosis). The protein content is less than 1 g/dL.

TRANSUDATE AND EXUDATE (TABLE 28.1)

The evaluation of serous body fluids (pleural, pericardial, peritoneal) is directed towards.

- Differentiating transudative from exudative effusion.
- Identifying malignancy or infection in exudative effusion, and
- Establishing a specific diagnosis.

EXAMINATION OF PLEURAL FLUID

Introduction

Accumulation of pleural fluid in the pleural space is called as pleural effusion.

TABLE 28.1: Difference between transudate and exudate.

Characteristics	*Transudate*	*Exudate*
Appearance	Clear, serous	Cloudy/ purulent/ hemorrhagic/ chylous
Color	Straw yellow	Yellow to red
Specific gravity	<1.018	>1.018
Protein	<2 g/dL	>2 g/dL
Clot	Absent	Clots spontaneously
Cells	Low count—few lymphocytes and endothelial cells	High count—neutrophils in acute, lymphocytes in chronic inflammation
Bacteria	Absent	Usually, present
Mechanism	Due to non-inflammatory process—(increased hydrostatic pressure)	Due to inflammation

The causes for pleural effusion are:

- Infection and inflammation of the pleura (increased capillary permeability),
- Mitral stenosis, pulmonary embolism, congestive cardiac failure (increased pulmonary hydrostatic pressure), and
- Cirrhosis of the liver and nephrotic syndrome (decreased colloidal osmotic pressure).

Specimen Collection

The pleural fluid is collected under aseptic precautions by percutaneous puncture (thoracocentesis). The specimen should be examined as early as possible to prevent chemical changes, growth of bacteria and disintegration of cells. The pleural tap should be done atraumatically to avoid mixing of fresh blood with the pleural fluid.

The pleural fluid is collected in the following three sterile test tubes:

1. *Tube containing 15 mg fluoride*: Oxalate (one part of sodium fluoride and three parts of potassium oxalate): Collect 5 mL of pleural fluid for sugar and protein estimation.
2. *Tube containing 15 mg EDTA*: Collect 5 mL of pleural fluid in this tube for microscopic examination.
3. *A plain tube (without anticoagulant)*: Collect 5 mL of pleural fluid in this tube for observation of clot and for bacteriological examination.

Physical Examination

Appearance and Color

Normal pleural fluid is pale and straw colored.

Causes for altered color/appearance

- Increased turbidity—increase in cells and cell debris.
- Cloudy appearance—bacterial or viral infection.
- Blood-tinged fluid—traumatic tap, pulmonary infraction, pleural malignancy.
- Milky fluid—tuberculosis, rheumatoid pleuritis (pseudochylous effusion), leakage from thoracic duct by lymphatic obstruction due to lymphoma or carcinoma (chylous effusion).

Ability of Pleural Fluid to Clot

Normal pleural fluid does not clot. Formation of a clot in the plain tube indicates inflammatory cause for effusion. The fibrin clot is a result of capillary wall damage.

Specific Gravity

Specific gravity helps to differentiate the transudate from specific gravity <1.018 indicates that the fluid is transudate specific gravity >1.018 indicates that the fluid is exudates.

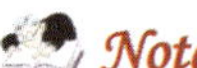

Increased specific gravity is due to protein content of >2 g/dL.

Microscopic Examination

Includes RBC counts, WBC counts, differential WBC counts and cytological examination for tumor cells.

Clinical Significance

- WBC counts of 1000 cells/μL has been used a cut-off point between a transudate (<1000 cells/μL) and exudates (>1000 cells/μL).
- WBC count of >1000 cells/μL and > 50% of neutrophils suggest bacterial infection.
- RBC count of >100,000 cells/μL is highly suggestive of malignancy, trauma or pulmonary infarction.
- High percentage of lymphocytes suggests tuberculosis, viral infection of lymphoma.

Estimation of WBC Count

If the specimen is clear, do not dilute it. Charge the Neubauer chamber directly with the pleural fluid.

If the specimen is turbid then dilute it with saline, the dilution being 1:20 (using a WBC pipette).

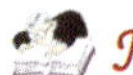

For dilution, do not use WBC diluting fluid as it contains acetic acid which may cause turbidity by reacting with the high protein content of the fluid. The procedure is exactly the same as described for determining the WBC count in blood sample.

Differential WBC Count (Table 28.2)

Centrifuge the specimen. Use the sediment for preparing the smears (at least 2 smears). One smear is stained with Leishman's stain and the other with Gram's stain. Make a count of 100 cells in the smear and it is expressed as a differential WBC count.

TABLE 28.2: Etiology and types of effusion.

Types of effusion	*Causes*
♦ Neutrophilic effusion (Neutrophils >50%)	♦ Bacterial pneumonia, pulmonary infarction, subphrenic abscess, pancreatitis
♦ Eosinophilic effusion (Eosinophils >10%)	♦ Drug reaction, asthma, pulmonary infarction, pneumothorax, parasitic disease
♦ Lymphocytic effusion (Lymphocytes)	♦ Tuberculosis, viral infection, rheumatoid pleuritis, infectious mononucleosis, SLE

Cytological Examination for Tumor Cells

The pleural fluid specimen is centrifuged, smears are made of the sediment, fixed immediately in absolute alcohol and stained by Papanicolaou stain. Cytospin concentration is a better alternative. Hematoxylin and eosin stain can also be used.

Chemical Examination

The following tests are performed:

- *Protein estimation:* Use Biuret method for protein estimation. The procedure is the same as for serum total protein estimation
- *Glucose estimation:* Use Folin-Wu's method, glucose oxidase method or orthotolidine method. Normal value is 70–110 mg/dL.

Clinical Significance

Value <40 mg/dL usually suggests bacterial infection including tuberculosis, malignancy or non-specific inflammation.

Immunologic Studies

Pleural effusion is seen in patients with systemic lupus erythematosus (50%) and rheumatoid arthritis. ANA (anti-neutrophilic antibody) titers may be useful in diagnosing effusion due to SLE, as it has a sensitivity of 85% using a cut-off titer of 1:160 (the specificity is low).

Rheumatoid factor (RF) is commonly present in pleural effusion associated with seropositive rheumatoid arthritis (cut-off titer employed is 1:320). It can also be positive in a few cases of bacterial pneumonia, malignant effusion and tuberculosis.

Low complement levels are seen in most patients of rheumatoid arthritis and SLE.

EXAMINATION OF PERICARDIAL FLUID

Introduction

About 10–50 mL of fluid is normally present in the pericardial space and this fluid is clear and straw colored. Accumulation of excess fluid in this space is called **pericardial effusion**.

Fluid is obtained by aspiration using a sterile needle under aseptic condition, a procedure called as **pericardiocentesis**.

Gross/Physical Examination

Observe the color and clot formation; Determine the specific gravity.

- Increased amount of normally appearing pericardial fluid—seen in congestive cardiac failure, early stages of inflammation and idiopathic pericarditis.
- Cloudy/turbid pericardial effusion—chronic effusions of any etiology (post-myocardial infarction, myxedema, etc.), septic conditions (bacterial inflammation), rhematic or rheumatoid pericarditis.
- Blood-tinged fluid—traumatic tap.
- Grossly bloody effusion—bacterial pericarditis, post-myocardial infarction syndrome, tuberculosis, systemic lupus erythematosus, damage to the aorta during any procedure.
- Milky effusion—tuberculosis, rheumatoid pleuritis (pseudochylous effusion), leakage from thoracic duct due to lymphatic obstruction caused by lymphoma or carcinoma (chylous effusion).

Microscopic Examination

This includes WBC count, RBC count, differential WBC count and cytologic examination for malignant cells.

The procedure for these tests is as described under the section on pleural fluid.

Clinical Significance

- Total leukocyte count of >10,000 cells/cu mm suggests—bacterial, tuberculous or malignant pericarditis.
- Leukocyte differential count adds a little diagnostic information; however, a stained smear should be examined.
- Cytological identification of malignant cells has a sensitivity of 87%, specificity of 100% and diagnostic accuracy of 94%. Metastasis from the lungs and breast are the most frequent causes for malignant pleural effusion.

Chemical Examination

Includes estimation of glucose and protein.

Microbiological Examination

The sensitivity of grams stain and culture of pericardial fluid for bacterial pericarditis is 50% and 80% respectively. Sensitivity for acid fast stain and culture in case of tuberculosis is just 50%.

EXAMINATION OF PERITONEAL FLUID (ASCITIC FLUID)

Introduction

Peritoneal cavity is lined by mesothelial cells and it normally contains up to 50 mL of clear straw-colored fluid. Peritoneal fluid is produced as an ultrafiltrate of plasma and its production is dependent on vascular permeability, hydrostatic pressure and oncotic pressure.

The patient with peritoneal effusion is said to have ascites and the fluid is called **ascetic fluid**. The procedure of collection the ascetic fluid is called as **abdominal paracentesis**.

Indications for Abdominal Paracentesis

- Possible ruptured viscus or intra-abdominal hemorrhage due to trauma.
- Acute abdominal pain of unknown etiology.
- Postoperative hypotension
- Ascites of unknown etiology
- Instillation of therapeutic drugs in case of malignant ascites.

Physical Examination

Color

Normal ascitic fluid is clear and colorless.

Causes for altered color of ascitic fluid

- Turbid—appendicitis, pancreatitis, intestinal perforation due to trauma
- Pale yellow/amber—hepatic vein obstruction, cirrhosis of the liver, nephritic syndrome, congestive cardiac failure
- Green—intestinal perforation, cholecystitis, gallbladder perforation gangrenous appendicitis, perforated duodenal ulcer
- Milky—nephritic syndrome, parasitic infections, carcinoma and lymphoma
- Bloody ascites—hemorrhagic pancreatitis, ruptured spleen, ruptured liver traumatic rupture of mesenteric vessels

Microscopic Examination

Includes RBC count, WBC count, differential WBC count and cytologic examination for malignant cells. The procedure is the same as that for the CSF.

Clinical Significance

Total leukocyte count helps to distinguish ascites due to uncomplicated cirrhosis from spontaneous bacterial peritonitis (high count with numerous neutrophils).

Points to Ponder

The commonly examined body fluids in the laboratory are:
- Pleural fluid—in the pleural space surrounding the lungs.
- Pericardial fluid—around the heart.
- Peritoneal fluid—in the peritoneal cavity of the abdomen and pelvis.
- Synovial fluid—in the joint space.

ASSESSMENT QUESTIONS

1. **Enlist the common causes for pleural effusion.**
2. **Enlist the common causes for peritoneal effusion.**
3. **Enlist the common causes for pericardial effusion.**
4. **Enlist the differences between a transudate and an exudates.**

MULTIPLE CHOICE QUESTIONS

1. **The most common cause for hemorrhagic pleural effusion is:**
   A. Tuberculous
   B. Malignancy
   C. Traumatic
   D. Pneumonia
2. **Which of the following conditions is commonly associated with transudative pleural effusion?**
   A. Congestive cardiac failure
   B. Bacterial pneumonia
   C. Lung cancer
   D. Pulmonary embolism
3. **What is the normal function of pericardial fluid?**
   A. Lubrication to reduce friction between the pericardial layers
   B. Oxygen transport to the heart muscle
   C. Immune defense against infections
   D. Regulation of blood pressure
4. **What is the most common symptom of pleural effusion?**
   A. Chest pain
   B. Shortness of breath
   C. Coughing up blood
   D. Wheezing
5. **What condition is characterized by an abnormal accumulation of fluid in the pericardial sac, leading to compression of the heart?**
   A. Pericarditis
   B. Pericardial effusion
   C. Aortic stenosis
   D. Myocardial infarction

Answer Key for MCQs

1	2	3	4	5
A	A	A	B	B

Analysis of Synovial Fluid

Learning Objectives

At the end of reading this chapter, the student shall be able to:

- Enlist the methods of common macroscopic examination of synovial fluid sample and interpret abnormalities.
- Perform a systematic chemical analysis of the given synovial fluid sample using a battery of laboratory tests and to interpret each of them.

INTRODUCTION

Synovial fluid is found around the joints such as knee, ankle, hip, elbow, wrist and shoulder. The chemical composition of synovial fluid resembles that of the other serous body fluids and CSF. In addition, it also contains mucopolysaccharide and hyaluronic acid, which are seen in any connective tissues.

CLINICAL SIGNIFICANCE

The laboratory examination of synovial fluid is useful in the diagnosis of a variety of joint disorders, such as infective arthritis (septic arthritis, rheumatic), gouty arthritis (metabolic disorder), rheumatoid arthritis (connective tissue disorder) and degenerative arthritis, which guide the clinician in the proper management of the patient.

SPECIMEN COLLECTION

The specimen is collected in the following three sterile tubes:

1. Tube with EDTA—used for cell counts and microscopic examination.
2. Tube with fluoride—oxalate mixture—used for glucose estimation.
3. Plain tube—used for physical, chemical, microbiological and serological examinations.

PHYSICAL EXAMINATION

- *Color and appearance:*
  - Normal synovial fluid is clear, straw colored and viscous. It does not clot.
  - Turbid appearance is seen in infection and inflammation of the joint space. If the fluid is highly purulent, it indicates septic arthritis. The turbidity may also be due to the presence of crystals, amyloid and cartilage fragments (These can be confirmed by microscopic examination).
  - A grossly red or a brown supernatant is seen in hemarthrosis (joint bleed) or in a traumatic tap.

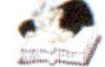

Note

In case of traumatic tap, the intensity of color will decrease in the second and the third tubes.

- *Viscosity test:* Synovial fluid is viscous and the viscosity is due to the presence of hyaluronic acid. The viscosity of the synovial fluid decreases in cases of inflammatory joint disorders due to the breakdown of hyaluronic acid by the enzyme hyaluronidase.

PROCEDURE

Draw the synovial fluid in a syringe and expel the fluid slowly and note the length of the string/strand that is formed. Use a scale to measure the length of the strand.

The normal synovial fluid forms a strand of at least 4 cm long. If the strand breaks before reaching 3 cm length, the viscosity is lower than normal.

- *Mucin clot test:* Hyaluronic acid forms a compact clot in the presence of acetic acid. Low concentration of hyaluronic acid does not allow the formation of a firm clot.

PROCEDURE

- Take 20 mL of 5% (v/v) acetic acid in beaker
- Add 1.0 mL of synovial fluid.
- Observe the nature of the clot that is formed and categorize it as firm clot, friable clot, soft clot and no clot.
- Agitate the solution and observe the following:
  - Clot does not break down.
  - Clot breaks into small shreds (poorly formed clot).

Clinical Importance

A poorly formed fibrin clot is seen in tuberculous arthritis and other severe inflammatory joint disorders. Fair to poorly formed fibrin clot is seen in rheumatoid arthritis, gout and pseudogout.

MICROSCOPIC EXAMINATION

- *Total leukocyte count*: Normal WBC count of synovial fluid is 50 cells/mm^3. The procedure is same as that of the blood count.
- *Differential leukocyte count:* Prepare a thin smear of the sediment (after centrifugation of synovial fluid) and stain with Leishman's stain in the same way as we do for blood smear. Normally, synovial fluid contains 25% of polymorphs. If polymorphs are >70%, it indicates bacterial arthritis.
  Moderate increase of polymorphs (40 - 60%) is seen in rheumatic fever, gout, tubercular arthritis and rheumatoid arthritis.

Note

- Normal clear synovial fluid should be used undiluted.
- If the synovial fluid is turbid, then use saline containing methylene blue as the diluent.

- *Wet smear examination:* Centrifuge the synovial fluid and take the sediment thus obtained on a glass slide and cover it with a coverslip.
  Observe the slide first under low power objective, than under high power objective with reduced light and carefully note for the presence of following crystals:
  - Urate crystals—seen in gouty arthritis.
  - Rhomboid calcium pyrophosphate crystals—seen in pseudogout.
  - Cholesterol crystals—seen in rheumatoid arthritis.

CHEMICAL EXAMINATION

- Glucose estimation by any of the conventional methods.
- Protein estimation by Biuret method.

MICROBIOLOGICAL EXAMINATION

- *Microscopic examination*: Make smears from the sediment and stain it with gram's stain or acid-fast stain in suspected cases of infective/tubercular arthritis.
- *Culture studies*: Synovial fluid culture is recommended in suspected cases of infective/tubercular arthritis.
  Table 29.1 highlights the salient findings on synovial fluid analysis in various diseases.

TABLE 29.1: CSF fluid analysis results in common disease conditions.

	Rheumatic fever	*Rheumatoid arthritis*	*Gout*	*Pseudogout*	*Tuberculous arthritis*
Appearance	Slightly turbid	Turbid, yellow, milky	Turbid, yellow, milky	Clear or slightly turbid yellow	Turbid
Mucin clot	Good–fair	Fair–poor	Fair–poor	Fair–poor	Poor
Viscosity	Variable	Decreased	Decreased	Decreased	Decreased
Leukocyte Count per mm^3	50–50,000	200–80,000	100–1,00,000	50–75,000	2,000–1,00,000
Neutrophils %	0–60	0–90	0–90	0–90	20–95
Glucose, mg/dL	50–70	10–70	0–80	50–70	0–70

Points to Ponder

The laboratory examination of synovial fluid is useful in the diagnosis of a variety of joint disorders, such as infective arthritis (septic arthritis, rheumatic), gouty arthritis (metabolic disorder), rheumatoid arthritis (connective tissue disorder) and degenerative arthritis, which guide the clinician in the proper management of the patient. Arthroscopy is a common method for obtaining a sample of synovial fluid for diagnostic purposes.

ASSESSMENT QUESTION

1. **Enumerate the common indications for examination of synovial fluid.**

MULTIPLE CHOICE QUESTIONS

1. **The type of crystals seen in gouty arthritis is made up of:**
   A. Phosphates
   B. Urates
   C. Calcium
   D. Oxalates
2. **What is the primary function of synovial fluid in joints?**
   A. Nutrient transport to joint cartilage
   B. Lubrication and reducing friction between joint surfaces
   C. Production of antibodies for joint protection
   D. Regulation of blood pressure in the joint capsule
3. **Which of the following conditions is often associated with an abnormal increase in synovial fluid within a joint?**
   A. Osteoarthritis
   B. Rheumatoid arthritis
   C. Gout
   D. Osteoporosis

4. What is the main component responsible for the viscosity and lubricating properties of synovial fluid?

A. White blood cells
B. Hyaluronic acid
C. Cholesterol
D. Red blood cells

5. Which of the following is a common method for obtaining a sample of synovial fluid for diagnostic purposes?

A. Arthroscopy
B. Blood test
C. Electrocardiogram (ECG)
D. Bronchoscopy

Answer Key for MCQs

1	2	3	4	5
B	B	B	B	A

CHAPTER

Sputum Analysis

Learning Objectives

At the end of reading this chapter, the student shall be able to:
- Enlist the methods of collection, common macroscopic examination of sputum sample and interpret abnormalities.
- Perform a systematic chemical analysis of the given sputum sample using a battery of laboratory tests and to interpret each of them.

INTRODUCTION

Sputum is colorless watery and odorless tracheobronchial secretion which is altered in a variety of conditions affecting the lungs and the tracheobronchial tree. Sputum collection and its examination is simple cost-effective and provides vital information which helps in diagnosis of a variety of lung diseases.

PRODUCTION AND NORMAL COMPOSITION OF SPUTUM

Normal sputum is a mixture plasma, mucin electrolytes and water and is produced in the tracheobronchial tree. As this secretion passes through the upper and the lower respiratory tract. It gets contaminated with cellular exfoliations nasal and salivary gland secretions and the normal bacterial flora of the oral cavity. The principal source of the tracheobronchial secretions is the goblet cells and submucous glands. The goblet cells of the surface epithelium produce thick mucin which is diluted by the secretions of the submucous glands (contain acid glycoproteins and sulfoproteins).

Composition of Sputum

About 95% water and 5%—solids—carbohydrates, proteins, lipids and DNA

The lysozymes and the secretory immunoglobulins (IgA) present in the sputum contribute to the antimicrobial activity).

The consistency of the sputum is determined by the glycoprotein content (especially sialic acid) and the degree of hydration.

Sputum Collection

The patient is instructed to rinse his mouth with water before collecting the sample.

The sputum must be coughed up from the lungs or the bronchi and should be collected carefully in a wide mouthed sterile, glass/plastic container of about 50 mL capacity with screw cap.

Types of specimen collected:
1. Early morning sputum sample for routine examination.
2. 24 hours sample for the demonstration of tubercle bacilli by concentrating the sputum sample.

Concentration Method for Tubercle Bacilli in the Sputum

Collected 24 hours sputum sample in a wide mouthed sterile bottle. Add equal volume of 6% sulfuric acid to the sample and allow it to stand for 20 minutes. Centrifuge at 3000 rpm. for 30 minutes. Decent the supernatant and carefully wash the sediment with distilled water, repeating this for three times make the smear from the sediment. Dry fix the smear and then stain it which Ziehl-Neelson stain. The sediment may also be used for culture if desired.

EXAMINATION OF THE SPUTUM

Physical Examination

Observe the following:

- *Quantity*: Measure the quantity of the sample. Normal morning specimen—2.5 mL and amount of 24 hours sample—about 100 mL
  - The amount of sputum coughed up in 24 hours varies in different lung diseases.
  - 24 hours collection >500 mL is seen in amoebic lung abscess (due to rupture of amoebic liver abscess into the lungs). In this case, the color of the sputum will resemble anchovy sauce (chocolate brown).
- *Color*: Normal sputum is clear and colorless. Causes for altered sputum color:
  - *Greenish color*: *Pseudomonas* infection and rupture of the liver abscess into the lungs.
  - *Rust color*: Pneumonia and pulmonary infarction. This color results from the decomposition of the hemoglobin.
  - *Bright red*: Pulmonary tuberculosis, lung tumors pulmonary infarction. This is due to the presence of fresh blood in sputum.
  - *Black*: Inhalation of coal dust (coal workers) or in heavy smokers.
  - *Yellowish*: Pulmonary infections (presence of pus).
- *Consistency and appearance:* Normal sputum is colorless opalescent with slightly uneven consistency (due to mucus).

Causes for Altered Sputum Consistency and Appearance

- Serous, frothy, colorless or yellow sputum—pulmonary edema
- Mucoid, glassy, tenacious sputum— acute bronchitis, asthma lobar pneumonia
- Purulent and foul smelling sputum—ruptured empyema and *bronchiectasis*
- Mucopurulent sputum—lung cavitation (admixture of mucus and pus.
- Blood tinged sputum—mitral stenosis pulmonary infarction, carcinoma of the lungs pulmonary tuberculosis.
- *Odor:* Normal sputum is odorless. Causes for altered sputum odor
  - Four smelling odor (putrid—lung abscess, bronchiectasis, pulmonary infarction.
  - Cheesy odor—malignant tumor with necrosis perforating empyema.
- *Layer formation*: Place the specimen in a test tube for 2-3 hours and the observe. Normally, there is no layer formation. Formation of 2-3 layers with the top layer composed of frothy mucus, middle layer consisting of opaque watery material and the sediment formed by pus cells and bacteria is seen in bronchiectasis infraction and lung abscess.
- *Other macroscopic finding*: Pour a portion of the specimen in a Petri-dish and closely observe for the following:
  - Cheesy masses (fragments of necrotic tissue)—present in tuberculosis).
  - Bronchial casts—present as white branching tree like casts and is made of fibrin
  - Sulfur granules—present as yellow granular structure in the sputum. They are made up of colonies of fungus. They are seen in infection of the lungs by *Actinomyces* species
  - Foreign bodies—includes a variety of objects, such as pins, beads of ground

nuts, coins, etc., usually in a young children who have aspirated them.

Microscopic Examination

Unstained Specimen

Place a drop of well mixed sputum on a glass slide and place a coverslip over it. Observe first under low power objective and then high power objective. Note the following:

- *Pus cells (neutrophils):* Normally, a few pus cells are seen. Numerous pus cells indicates inflammation of the respiratory tract.
- *Red blood cells:* Normally a few red cells may be present.
- *Heart failure cells (hemosiderin—laden macrophages):* They are present in chronic venous congestion (CVC) of the lung's secondary to mitral valve stenosis (valve between the left atrium and the left ventricle of the heart). Pulmonary infraction and pulmonary hemorrhage. They are absent in the normal sputum.
- *Anthracotic laden cells (carbon piment laden):* Few cells are seen in normal individual increased numbers are seen in anthracosis coal workers pneumoconiosis and those who live in smoky polluted atmosphere.
- *Curschmann's spiral:* These appear as spiral structures with a central thread. Their exact nature is not known but are present in the sputum of patients with bronchial asthma.
- *Elastic fibers:* They are seen as wavy refractile fibers in bundles. Their presence indicates breakdown of lung parenchyma.

Crystals

- *Charcot laden crystals*: These are fine needle shaped or hexagons colorless crystals, usually about 20-30 µm in length. They are generally not present in the freshly collected sputum, but are formed as the sputum stands for some time. They are thought to arise from the disintegration of eosinophils in a case of bronchial asthma.
- *Fatty acid crystals*: They are not seen in a normal patient but are seen in patients with chronic tuberculosis, bronchitis and gangrene of the lungs.
- *Cholesterol crystals*: They are seen in empyema and chronic lung abscess.
- *Hematoidin crystals*: Seen in cases of hemorrhage into the lungs.

Parasites

- *Entamoeba histolytica*: Cysts or the trophozoites of the parasite may be found in cases of rupture of the amoebic liver abscess into the lungs.
- *Echinococcus granulose*: Scolices and hooklets of the larval form of this parasite may be seen in cases of rupture of the hydatid cyst of the lungs into the bronchus.
- *Paragonimus westermani*: Ova are found in cases of infection by liver fluke, which is common in Japan and other Asian countries.
- Larvae of *Strongyloides stercoralis* and roundworm may be found in sputum of those individuals who harbor the parasite.

Stained Sputum Smear

This is an important part of the sputum examination. 3–4 smears are made on clean, dry, glass-slides, allowed to dry at the room temperature and then fixed by gently heating over a flame. Stain one of the smears with Leishman's stain or Wright's stain for differential leukocyte count.

The other smears are stained with—Gram's stain, Ziehl-Neelson stain/acid fast stain for tubercle bacilli, special stains for fungi, and Papanicolaou stain for detailed cytomorphologic study for malignant cells.

Differential leukocyte count: A normal sputum consists of a few neutrophils few lymphocytes and occasional eosinophils.

- Increased neutrophils indicates pyogenic infection.
- Increased eosinophils are seen in asthma and parasitic infections of the lings.
- Increased lymphocytes are seen in early or mild cased of tuberculosis.
- Erythrocytes are not normally seen. If increased indicates hemorrhage (bleeding) into the lungs or the bronchi.
- Culture studies in the diagnosis of various infections of the lungs and the tracheobronchial tree, culture is often done to find the etiological agent.

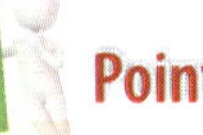

Points to Ponder

Sputum is colorless watery and odorless tracheobronchial secretion which is altered in a variety of conditions affecting the lungs and the tracheobronchial tree. Sputum collection and its examination is simple cost effective and provides vital information which helps in diagnosis of a variety of lung diseases.

ASSESSMENT QUESTIONS

1. **Enumerate the common indications for examination of sputum.**
2. **What are Curschmann's spiral? In which condition you see them?**
3. **What are Charcot-Leyden crystals?**

MULTIPLE CHOICE QUESTIONS

1. **Layer formation of sputum is pathognomonic of:**
   A. Bronchiectasis
   B. Emphysema
   C. Chronic bronchitis
   D. Lung abscess
2. **Presence of Curschmann's spiral in sputum is pathognomonic of:**
   A. Bronchiectasis
   B. Bronchial asthma
   C. Chronic bronchitis
   D. Lung abscess
3. **What is the primary purpose of analyzing sputum in a clinical setting?**
   A. Determining blood glucose levels
   B. Assessing lung function
   C. Identifying gastrointestinal disorders
   D. Monitoring kidney function
4. **In sputum analysis, what does the presence of eosinophils indicate?**
   A. Bacterial infection
   B. Fungal infection
   C. Viral infection
   D. Allergic or inflammatory conditions
5. **Which condition is characterized by the presence of "Charcot-Leyden crystals" in sputum?**
   A. Tuberculosis
   B. Chronic obstructive pulmonary disease (COPD)
   C. Asthma
   D. Pneumonia

Answer Key for MCQs

1	2	3	4	5
A	B	B	D	C

CHAPTER 31

Semen Analysis

Learning Objectives

At the end of reading this chapter, the student shall be able to:

- Enlist the methods of common macroscopic examination of semen sample and interpret abnormalities.
- Perform a systematic chemical analysis of the given seminal fluid sample using a battery of laboratory tests and to interpret each of them.

INTRODUCTION

Problems with male semen account for 40% of all infertility. Another 40% relate to female reproductive and hormone problems. The remaining 20% is related to problems with both the partners. Semen analysis is the cornerstone of testing for male infertility. This test provides important information about the quality and quantity of the sperm. A properly performed semen analysis provides the physician with clinically relevant data which gives an indication to the causes for male infertility.

COMPOSITION AND PRODUCTION OF SEMEN

Semen consists of four fractions contributed by the testis, bulbourethral glands, the seminal vesicle, and the prostate. Spermatozoa or sperms, are produced in the testis and mature in the epididymis, where they are stored until ejaculation.

Sperms account for roughly 1–2% of the total volume of an ejaculate.

The secretory product of the bulbourethral glands (also known as Cowper's glands) functions to lubricate the urethra and is also thought to neutralize any residual urine.

The majority of the semen is contributed by the seminal vesicles in the form of an alkaline, viscous coagulum, which contains prostaglandins and fructose.

The prostatic fluid in semen is acidic, contain acid phosphatase and proteolytic enzymes which acts on the coagulum of the seminal vesicles, thus resulting in the liquefaction of the semen. Problems with these fluids may therefore interfere with natural fertilization.

Since, the spermatozoa are the cells which fertilize the egg, they are the main focus when performing a semen analysis.

CLINICAL APPLICATIONS OF SEMEN ANALYSIS

- Evaluation of infertility
- Pre- and postoperative semen analysis are done for evaluation of various medical and surgical therapies for infertility.
- To select the appropriate donor for therapeutic insemination.
- Screening for exposure to reproductive toxins and to set the exposure limit for these toxins.
- To evaluate the effectiveness of vasectomy.
- In suspected cases of rape, denial of paternity on the grounds of infertility (medicolegal cases), etc.

SPECIMEN COLLECTION AND TRANSPORTATION

- The person has to abstain from sex for a period of at least 3 days but not more than 5 days. It has been shown that shorter abstinence periods may result in lower sperm counts but possibly higher quality sperm. Whereas longer periods may yield lower percentage of motile sperms and overall poor-quality sperms.
- The patient has to evacuate the bladder before ejaculation.
- The sample should be collected by masturbation only, ideally in privacy of a room adjacent to the laboratory. If proper facilities are not available, he may collect the sample at home, but should ensure that it is transported to the laboratory within 1 hour.
- The sample should be transported to the laboratory within 30 minutes to 1 hour collection.

A minimum of two semen samples analysis, 2–3 weeks apart and collected in a similar manner is recommended because the sperm counts tend to fluctuate. If the results of the tests vary significantly then an additional specimen should be collected.

Storage of the semen sample—the sample should not be stored in refrigerators. It should be evaluated within 1 hour of collection (i.e., after liquefaction is complete) during this time the sample should be kept at room temperature (20°C–30°C).

Name of the patient, date and time of collection, length of abstinence and the time interval between collection and analysis should be recorded in the semen analysis report.

ROUTINE EXAMINATION OF SEMEN

Thoroughly mix the sample before examination. The examination includes physical examination chemical examination and microscopic examination.

Physical Examination

It is performed after a maximum of 60 min by which time the liquefaction complete.

Record the following observation:

- *Color and appearance:* Normal semen is gray white viscid and opaque.
  Causes for altered semen color:
  Yellowish color—pyospermia (inflammatory process)
  Rust (blood tinged) color—minor bleeding in the seminal vesicle
- *Volume:* Normal volume is 2–5 mL
  Decreased volume is seen due to reduced secretions from seminal vesicle/prostatic glands, blockage of the ejaculatory duct vas deferens and retrograde ejaculation.
  Semen volume >5.5 mL is called as hyperspermia.
  If no semen is produced, the condition is called as **aspermia**.
- *Viscosity:* Take the specimen in a pasture pipette and expel it. The specimen with normal viscosity can be poured drop by drop. Increased viscosity results in poor invasion of the cervical mucus as demonstrated by post-coital studies.
- *Liquefaction time:* Normally, a sample of semen takes <60 minutes to liquefy. Failure to liquefy 60 minutes indicates inadequate prostatic secretions.

Note

In instances where liquefaction is not progressing as anticipated, incorporating proteolytic enzymes, such as plasmin or chymotrypsin can be instrumental. These enzymes specialize in breaking down proteins, which can effectively address any impediments to liquefaction.

Chemical Examination

- *Determination of pH (using a pH* Paper strip):
  Normal pH = 7.2 to 7.8
  Causes for alteration in the pH
  pH <7—obstruction to ejaculatory duct and congenital absence of seminal vesicle.

Such specimen contains mainly prostatic secretions and hence an acidic pH
pH 8—acute infection of the prostate (acute prostatitis), seminal vesicle and epididymis.

- *Quantization of the semen fructose:*
This is based on the principle that the fructose reacts with resorcinol in a strong acidic medium to give a red colored complex which is compared with a known fructose standard at 490 nm.

Microscopic Examination

- *Motility of the sperms:*
  - Place a small drop of liquefied semen on a glass slide and cover it with a 22 × 22 mm glass coverslip
  - Examine the preparation under the high power objective with reduced illumination

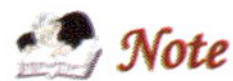

Note

As the motility and the velocity of the spermatozoa are dependent on temperature, assessment of motility is performed using a microscope with a warm stage.

  - Count at least 200 sperms and grade the motility
  - **Grade 0:** No motility
  - **Grade 1:** No forward progression but mild lateral movement
  - **Grade 2:** Slow forward progression with substantial yaw
  - **Grade 3:** Slightly faster forward progression with little yaw
  - **Grade 4:** Spermatozoa moving rapidly in a straight with little yaw and no lateral movement
  - Express as percentage the number of sperms belonging to each grade normally at the end of 1 hour the individual should have.
    » >25% of sperms belonging to grade 4 and or 3
    » <50% sperms belonging to grade 2.3. or 4

  Causes for asthenozoospermia (decreased motility of sperms)
    » Abnormal spermatogenesis
    » Abnormal maturation of sperms in the epididymis
    » Abnormalities in the transportation
    » Varicocele
- *Sperm count*
  - Mix the specimen after it undergoes liquefaction
  Draw the semen up to 0.5 in a WBC pipette
  - Draw the semen diluting fluid up to mark 11 and mix it well semen diluting fluid
  Sodium diluting fluid:
    » Sodium bicarbonate—5 g
    » Formalin—1 g
    » Distilled water—99 mL

  It should be stored in plain bottle room temperature.
  - Charge the improved Neubauer chamber and allow the sperms to settle for 5 minutes
  - Count the sperms in the four large corner

Calculation:
Sperms/mL of semen

$$= \frac{\text{sperms counted in 4 squares}}{\text{Area} \times \text{depth} \times \text{dilution}}$$

= (sperms counted × 10 × 20 × 1) × 1000
Normal count is 40-300 millions/mL
Sperm count <20 million/mL is called as **oligozoospermia**.
Absence of sperms is called as **azoospermia**.

Causes for low sperm count
- Infections—mumps orchitis, prostatitis
- Obstruction—occlusion or absence of efferent ducts

- Endocrinopathies—hypopituitarism, hypogonadism, hypo- and hyper-thyroidism and estrogen secreting tumors

❖ *Sperm morphology:*

- After liquefaction make a thin smear of the semen on a glass slide (similar to the blood smear).
- Allow the smear to dry in the air and then heat the slide very gently to fix the smear. If necessary remove the mucus which would interfere in the microscopic examination by dipping the smear in semen diluting fluid and then in buffer distilled water (pH 7.0).
- Stain the smear using Leishman's stain (Method is similar to the staining of blood smear). 0.25% aqueous basic fuchsin (w/v) can also be used for staining (timing is 5 minutes).
  - » ***Normal sperm:*** It has a head 4μ in length and 3 μ in diameter. It has a cap called **acrosomal cap (head cap)** which stains blue and the nucleus stains dark blue.

    Middle piece (body)—measures 7 μ in length, 1 μ in diameter,

    Neck—measures 0.3 μ; situated between the head and the middle piece,

    Tail—measures 45 to 50 μ in length and stains red or pink.
  - » ***Abnormal sperm forms:*** Morphological abnormalities can be found in the head, middle piece or the tail.
- **Abnormalities of the head:** Too large (macrocephaly) or too small heads (microcephaly), double heads, pointed heads, ragged heads and vacuoles in the chromatin.

  A sperm with an acrosomal cap <1/3rd of the head surface is considered abnormal. In a normal semen sample, the sperms with head defects will be <35%. It is pathological if the head defects are >60%.
- **Abnormalities of the middle piece:** Includes absent, bifurcated or swollen middle piece. In a normal semen sample, the sperms with mid-piece defects will be < or = 20%.

  It is pathological if the middle piece defects are >25%.
- **Abnormalities of the tail:** Includes double, triple, quadruple tails, rudimentary or absent tails. A tail less than 45μ in length is considered abnormal. Cytoplasmic vacuoles along the tail indicate an immature sperm. In a normal semen sample, the sperms with tail piece defects will be < or = 20%. It is pathological if the sperms with tail piece defects is >25%.

Note

- Abnormal spermatozoa has normally multiple defects. >70% of abnormal forms are associated with infertility.
- *Teratozoospermic index:* It is the average number of defects per spermatozoa and is a significant predictor of sperm function.
- *Kruger morphology:* Slides are especially stained and a detailed evaluation of sperm morphology is made based on a set of stringent criteria in order to consider the sperm as normal. This test helps to determine which of the available advanced reproductive techniques may be most appropriate and successful in a particular case of male infertility.

❖ *Agglutination of spermatozoa:* In the presence of the anti-sperm antibody, the motile spermatozoa stick to each other in various orientations, such as head-to-head, tail to tail, mid piece to mid piece depending on the specificity of the sperm antibodies directed against these structures.

- *Other findings:*
  - Neutrophils/plus cells—(normal—1 to 2 cells/hpf). An increase indicates infection and inflammation in some part of the male reproductive system.
  - Epithelial cells—(normal—1 to 2 cells/hpf). Increase in number is of no significance.
  - Red blood cells—these are generally absent and may be present in conditions like tuberculosis of the seminal vesicle, prostatitis and rupture of the blood vessels.
  - *Trichomonas*—it is a motile flagellate and their presence indicates *Trichomonas* infection.
  - Immature germ cells (IGC's)—they are round cells (larger than a polymorph) with single or double, highly condensed nucleus surrounded by large amount of cytoplasm. They can be often mistaken for leukocytes.
  - Bacteria—it generally indicates contamination of the sample and such sample should be discarded.

Sperm Functional Tests

These tests are done only in specialized Andrology laboratories. Defective sperm function may adversely affect the various fertilizing activities, such as transportation of the sperms in the male and female reproductive tracts, binding of the sperm to the zona pellucida of the egg, penetration into the egg and formation of the male pronucleus. One should be aware of various tests done to ascertain the sperm function.

- *Sperm penetration assay (SPA):* This test measures the fertilizing capacity of the sperm. In this test, zona denuded golden hamster egg is exposed to the human sperms. If the sperm successfully penetrates the egg, then there is a high likelihood that the sperm will be able to fertilize the human egg if exposed.
- *Hemi-zona assay:* In this test, the unfertilized human egg obtained through donation is exposed to the sperms. Then the egg is bisected and the number of sperms tightly bound to the outer surface is counted. The results of this test show a good correlation with the success rate of in vitro fertilization (IVF).
- *Cervical mucus penetration assay:* This test measures the relative ability of motile sperm to penetrate the cervical mucus (human/bovine mucus) at the mid-cycle. This assay quantitates penetration, by counting the number motile sperm at different travel distance from the point of entry.
- *Hypo-osmotic swelling (HOS) test:* This test measures the membrane integrity of the sperm. The normal, viable sperm when placed in hypo-osmotic solution allows the water to enter into the cells resulting in the swelling and curling of the tail. This test correlates well with the results of the sperm penetration assay (SPA).
- *Tests for anti-sperm antibodies/immunobead test:* The presence of sperm antibodies is a cause for male infertility. These antibodies are detected by immunobead test. In this test, the semen is mixed with latex beads coated with human IgG and a monospecific antiserum to human IgG is added and observed under the light microscope. If the antibodies are present in the semen then the beads will bind to the specific sperm structure.

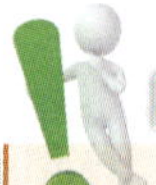

Points to Ponder

Semen analysis is the cornerstone of testing for male infertility. This test provides important information about the quality and quantity of the sperm. A properly performed semen analysis provides the physician with clinically relevant data which gives an indication to the causes for male infertility.

ASSESSMENT QUESTIONS

1. **Enumerate the common indications for semen analysis.**
2. **Mention the common causes for decreased motility of spermatozoa.**
3. **Enumerate the different types of sperm functional tests.**

MULTIPLE CHOICE QUESTIONS

1. **Estimation of fructose levels are very significant in the analysis of:**
   A. Sputum
   B. Synovial fluid
   C. Semen
   D. Urine
2. **What parameter is primarily assessed in semen analysis to evaluate male fertility?**
   A. Sperm count
   B. Testosterone levels
   C. Prostate-specific antigen (PSA)
   D. Seminal vesicle function
3. **What is the normal pH range of semen?**
   A. 4.0–5.0
   B. 6.0–7.5
   C. 8.0–9.0
   D. 10.0–11.0
4. **Which parameter in semen analysis assesses the motility and forward progression of sperm?**
   A. Sperm morphology
   B. Sperm concentration
   C. Sperm viability
   D. Sperm motility
5. **What is the term for the absence of sperm in the ejaculate?**
   A. Azoospermia
   B. Oligospermia
   C. Asthenospermia
   D. Teratospermia

Answer Key for MCQs

1	2	3	4	5
C	A	B	D	A

32

CHAPTER

Stool Examination

Learning Objectives

At the end of reading this chapter, the student shall be able to:

- Enlist the methods of common macroscopic examination of stool sample and interpret abnormalities.
- Perform a systematic chemical analysis of the given stool sample using a battery of laboratory tests and to interpret each of them.

INTRODUCTION

Many diagnostic tests can be easily done on a sample of stool (feces). Stool examination is very useful in the evaluation of colorectal carcinoma, malabsorption, diarrheal diseases and parasitic infestations. Its unpleasant odor and appearance should not be hindrance to a trained technician in doing a systematic examination. This would provide useful information about the patient and his disease.

COLLECTION

The patient should be properly instructed about the manner of stool collection. The sample is transferred from a clean bed pan or the toilet to suitable collection containers. The containers may be of disposable wide mouthed, glass or preferably plastic jars with screw caps.

Precautions in Collection

- Preferably a morning sample is to be collected.
- The sample is to properly labeled and the time of collection is to be mentioned.
- The sample should always be covered to avoid a drying effect.
- The specimen should not be contaminated with urine has a harmful effect on protozoa.
- The container should not be overfilled. This is to release the gas which accumulates, carefully. If this is not done there can be an explosive release of contents.
- The specimen is to be examined within 1 hour of collection.
- Warm stool is best for detecting ova and parasites. Do not refrigerate the stool.
- The sample of stool required is small. If blood and mucus is present that area is to be included in the study.
- It is preferable to collect the stool sample before antibiotic treatment.
- Certain interfering substance, such as meat, barium, oil, bismuth and antibiotics can interfere with tests.

Preservation: The fecal specimen can be done using formalin saline regent. It is prepared by mixing 25 mL of 40% commercial formaldehyde with 75 mL of normal saline. This helps to preserve protozoan morphology and further development of some helminth eggs.

ROUTINE TESTS FOR STOOL

The various laboratory investigations done on the feces include.

Physical Examination

The following are noted on gross examination of the feces.

Quantity

The quantity of stool varies depending on the dietary habits of the individual. Persons on strict vegetarian diets have bulkier stools. The normal amount excreted is about 100–250 g/day.

Consistency and Form

Normally feces when passed is well formed.

- When feces are extensively hard indicates constipation.
- Passages of large, bulky pale frothy stool which floats on water is characteristic of steatorrhea (poor fat digestion).
- Flattened and ribbon like stool indicates obstruction in the lumen of the bowel.
- Semi-solid stool is seen in mild diarrhea, digestive upsets and after taking a laxative.
- Watery stool is seen in bacterial infections use of purgatives (drugs used to induce diarrhea)
- Rice water stool is typical of 'cholera' where the stool is thin, watery and colorless.

Color

The normal color of feces is brown. It is caused by stercobilin, a pigment derived from bilirubin after conversion to urobilin. The formation of normal color requires bacterial oxidation to take place in the colon. The abnormal colors of feces include.

- Black and tarry stool due to bleeding from the upper gastro-intestinal tract (GIT) this is called as **melena**. It is altered blood. Iron administration in iron deficiency anemia, bismuth and charcoal also give a black color to stool
- Bright red color due to bleeding from the lower GIT, e.g., bleeding piles.
- Clay color as seen in obstructive jaundice due to obstruction to the flow of bile to the intestine.
- White color after barium meal studies.

Odor

Normal odor is due to indole and skatole formed by intestinal fermentation and putrefaction. The odor varies with pH of the stool.

Blood and Mucus in Stool

The most common condition associated with blood and mucus in the stool is termed dysentery. Dysentery may be of 2 types—(a) amoebic dysentery (protozoa), (b) bacillary dysentery. It is very important to different amoebic and bacillary dysentery as the disease course and treatment is different. The main difference between the two are given in **Table 32.1**. Other conditions associated with

TABLE 32.1: Difference between amoebic and bacillary dysentery.

	Amoebic dysentery	*Bacillary dysentery*
Reaction	Acidic	Alkaline
Consistency	No adherence to container	Adherence to container
Nature	Blood, mucus with feces	Blood, water and mucus may be present. No fecal matter
Odor	Offensive	Odorless
Red blood cells	In clumps	Discrete
Pus cells	Scanty	Plenty
Macrophages	Scanty	Plenty
Parasites	Trophozoites	Nil
Charcot-Leyden crystals	Present	Nil

blood mucus are ulcerative colitis, neoplasms or intestinal tuberculosis.

Parasites: Stool may contain adult worms or segments of worms. For example, round-worm, pin-worm, whip-worm, hood-worm or tape-worm. These have to be carefully looked for.

Chemical Examination

Chemical examination of stool is usually conducted to study either or both the below mentioned elements.

- *Reaction and pH:* The pH of normal stool sample could be acidic, alkaline or neutral. The pH ranges between 5.8-7.5.
  The pH becomes strongly acidic in the following conditions:
  1. Excess carbohydrate diet
  2. Lactose intolerance

  It is strongly alkaline with intake of excess dietary proteins.
- *Occult blood:* Blood in the stool should never be ignored however slight the quantity. Bleeding from the upper GIT in significant amounts produces black tarry appearance wile lower GIT bleeding give a red color to stool.

Principle

The peroxides activity of hemoglobin molecule convents hydrogen peroxide to nascent oxygen. The released oxygen oxidizes the regent in an acidic pH to colored oxidation products which are blue or green in color.

The reagents commonly used are:

- Benzidine
- Gum Guaiacum
- Ortho-toluidine
- Phenolphthalein

The referents vary in their sensitivity. The gun guaiacum is the most reliable indicator.

The chemical examination of stool includes.

- *Benzidine test:* It is extremely sensitive test and can give false positive in people on abundant meat diet. Only 1-2% people with significant bleeding will shows a negative. False positive can be overcome in some cases by boiling the emulsion with 1 mL of reagent in a test tube and add several drops of 3% hydrogen peroxide.
  Method: The benzidine regent consists of 4 gm benzidine base in 10 mL glacial acetic acid. It is stable for 2 to 4 months. Emulsify a bit of feces in 5 mL water. Mix 1 mL of emulsion with 1 mL of reagent in a test and add several drops of 3% hydrogen peroxide.
  Positive reaction: Blue color
  Disadvantage: Benzidine reagent is carcinogenic
- *Guaiacum test:* This is less sensitive. It gives 5% false positive in patients on non-vegetarian diet and 3-5% false negatives. It is the best screening test. With loss of 20-30 mL blood all tests will be positive.

Method: Guaiacum reagent consists of 1 g guaiacum in 5 mL of 95% ethanol. To an emulsion of feces on a piece of filter paper add 2-3 drops of guaiacum reagent, 2-3 drops of glacial acetic and 2-3 drops of 3% hydrogen peroxide.

Positive reaction: Blue color

Various commercial tests are available using guaiacum reagent for occult blood. Hemoccult is a commonly used slide test using this method.

- Tests using ortho-toluidine and phenol-phthalein—these however are less commonly or not commonly used.

False Positive Reactions in Occult Blood Examination

- Presence of interfering substance in diet like myoglobin and hemoglobin in red meat
- Presence of vegetable peroxidases as in horse radish, bananas, black grapes, pears, plums, melons
- White blood cells and bacteria
- The use of drugs, such as boric acid, bromides, iodine and oxidizing agents.

False Negative Reactions in Occult Blood Examination

Use of vitamin C and other oxidants.

Clinical significance: Detection of occult blood in the feces is important in determining the cause of hypochromic microcytic anemia due to chronic blood loss. These include neoplastic and ulcerative diseases of the GIT. Hookworm infection is another important and common causes of chronic blood loss. Drugs such as aspirin, iron containing compounds, steroids and indomethacin can be associated with increased GI bleeding and hence a positive occult blood test.

Other Chemical Tests

- Quantitative fecal fat estimation. Increase in fecal fat of >6 g per day is seen in pancreatic diseases, malabsorption syndromes or after surgical removal of intestine
- Presence of reducing substance in stool like lactose is seen in infants with diarrhea.

Microscopic Examination (Table 32.2)

A fresh sample of stool which is not contaminated with disinfectants is ideal for microscopic examination. It is useful to detect the presence of leukocytes (pus cells), red blood cells, muscle fibers fat globules, crystals cysts and yeast cells.

TABLE 32.2: Listing the common findings in the microscopic examination of stool.

Cells	*Nature of the substance*	*Normal finding*	*Abnormal finding*	*Pathological condition*
1	Pus cells	Few	Many	Bacillary dysentery ulcerative colitis
	Epithelial cells	Few	Many	Inflammation of the bowel
	Macrophages	Occasional	Many	Bacillary dysentery ulcerative colitis
	Erythrocytes	Absent	Present	Lesion in the colon, rectum or anus. They clump in amoebiasis
2	Crystals	Present due to ingestion of certain food, i.e., spinach berries tomatoes, etc.	-	-
	Charcot-Leyden crystals	Absent	Present	Ulcerative conditions amoebiasis
	Hematoidin	-	Present	Intestinal hemorrhage
3	Vegetable matter vegetable, cells, spirals, fibers, hairs, etc.	Present	-	-
4	Animal matter connective tissue, muscle fibers and elastic tissue	Present	-	-
5	Undigested ingredients	Absent	Present in high proportion	Indigestion
	Fat	Absent	Present in high proportion	Indigestion

The cells are usually reported as number seen per high-power field.

Parasitic amoebae, flagellates, collates, eggs, larvae and cysts. They are reported as the number seen in the entire preparation that is scanty, few, moderate or many.

The methods for the preparation of stool for microscopy include:

- *Saline preparation:* Take a little fecal material on a slide, mix with normal saline (0.85%) to make a thin emulsion. Cover it with a cover slip. The thickness should be such that one should be able to see fine print through it.
- *Iodine preparation:* This is done as above using Gram's iodine instead of saline. Iodine is used to examine the nuclear structure of cysts. It stains the chromatin granules of amoebic cysts brown. But, the chromatin bars are unstained. As iodine kills living material, motility of parasites will not be detected. In routine use, iodine preparation is complementary to the saline preparation.
- *Stool concentration methods:* These methods are used to identify ova and cysts which are few in number and not detached by routine methods. The methods used are:
    - *Floatation method:* The stool is mixed with zinc sulfate or magnesium sulfate which has a high specific gravity so that the parasite floats in the solution. It is useful to concentrate cysts larvae and most helminth eggs.
    - *Sedimentation methods:* In this method, the parasites are not floated but deposited by centrifugation. It can be done by simple sedimentation method or by formal—saline ether sedimentation method.
    - *Simple sedimentation method:* A small piece of stool is mixed with saline in a tube or bottle and sieved through a strainer. The sieved contents are centrifuged and the supernatant fluid poured off. The deposit is resuspended in more saline, mixed and centrifuged. This is repeated until the supernatant fluid clear. The deposit is examined directly on a slide.
    - *Formol-saline ether sedimentation method:* This method gives a good concentration of parasitic contents and is recommended for routine work. This method, however cannot be used to concentrate free-living forms as formalin kills the parasites.

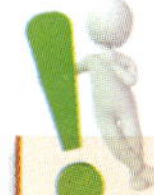

Points to Ponder

Stool examination is very useful in the evaluation of colorectal carcinoma, malabsorption, diarrheal diseases and parasitic infestations. Its unpleasant odor and appearance should not be hindrance to a trained technician in doing a systematic examination. This would provide useful information about the patient and his disease.

ASSESSMENT QUESTIONS

1. **Enumerate the common indications for stool analysis.**
2. **Enlist the common causes for presence of blood in stools.**
3. **Name the tests used to detect presence of occult blood in stools**
4. **What is steatorrhea? What are the causes?**
5. **What is Addis count? What is its significance?**
6. **Name the various methods of stool preparation for microscopy.**
7. **Mention the importance of biomedical waste in a clinical pathology laboratory.**

MULTIPLE CHOICE QUESTIONS

1. **One of the following is NOT a stool concentration method:**
   A. Floatation
   B. Sedimentation
   C. Filtration
   D. None of the above
2. **Which test is commonly used to detect the presence of blood in stool, indicating gastrointestinal bleeding?**
   A. Occult blood test
   B. Ova and parasite examination
   C. Stool culture
   D. *Clostridium difficile* toxin test

Answer Key for MCQs

1	2
C	A

UNIT 5

Genetics

Section Outline

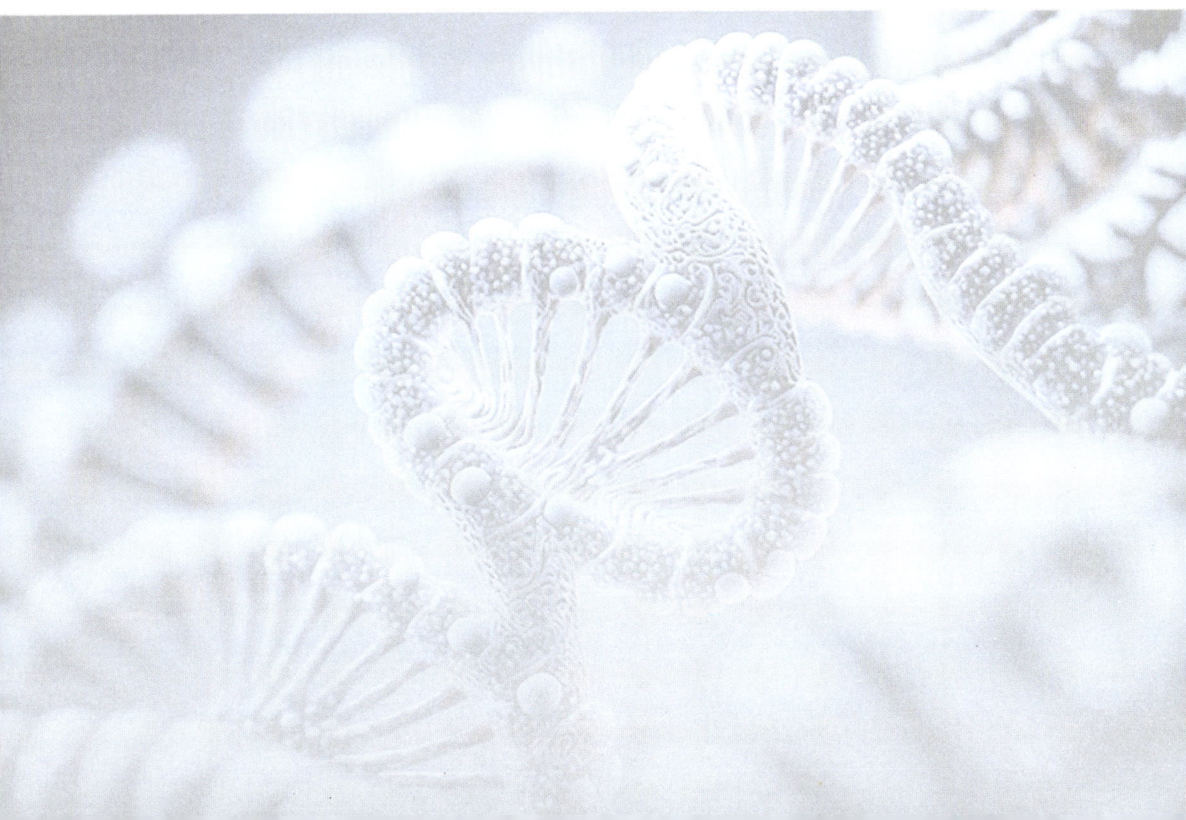

CHAPTER

Introduction and Practical Application of Genetics in Nursing

Learning Objectives

At the end of reading this chapter, the student shall be able to:

- Enlist the practical application of genetics in the practice of nursing.

INTRODUCTION

Practical Application of Genetics in Nursing

Genetics is of increasing importance in health care, as more is now known about the basic facts of inheritance. As genetics gains greater predictive power and becomes increasingly incorporated in daily health care, it will be more imperative that all nurses have a strong knowledge on genetic basis. Nearly most of all diseases are now recognized to have a genetic component. The recent development of commercial testing for susceptibility genes has had a great impact of nursing role in the identification and management of individuals at risk for developing many diseases. This development has led to tremendous changes in genetic nursing practice. As a result of this, the scope of genetic knowledge application in nursing is limitless.

In 1865, Johann Gregor Mendel was the first scientist, to describe the elements of hereditary genes. Scientific discoveries during the last several decades have provided more information about how genes function and how they contribute to human health and disease. Currently more than 10,371 identified genetic disorders are known to be inherited in a predictable pattern in families.

The term "Genetics" was first introduced by Bateson in 1906. It has been derived from the Greek word "Gene" which means "to become" or "to grow into". Genetics is that branch of biological sciences which deals with the transmission of characteristics from parents to offspring. Medical genetics has focused on the inheritance of hereditary disorders affecting only a small portion of the population

Genetic services have been primarily associated with prenatal genetic counseling, identification of pediatric disorders associated with birth defects and dysmorphology, and in some cases rare adult onset single gene disorder. Recent genetic and technological advances are helping us to better understand how genetic changes impact human variation as well as the development of cancer, Alzheimer's disease, diabetes and other multifactorial diseases that are prevalent in adults.

According to Forsman, "Nursing can ignore genetics no longer. The time for meaningful action is now." With the knowledge of genetics, nurses can collect appropriate family information, provide current and appropriate information and support patients, families and communities as they integrate this new information and technology into their daily lives.

Genetic disease and congenital malformations occur in approximately 3–5% of all live births. There is an increasing knowledge of the role of genetic factors in common illness such as cancer, diabetes, neuropsychiatric disorders, cardiovascular disease, and atherosclerosis.

Genetic knowledge now has implications for all areas of health and disease management and nursing practice. This creates a challenge for change in nursing education to meet changing needs in health care delivery. Thus, all licensed nurses, regardless of their work setting, have a role in the delivery of genetics services and the management of genetic information. Nurses require genetic knowledge to support and care for patient affected by genetic disease. In addition, nurses will be counselors to explain the benefits of gene therapy versus traditional therapy for a specific disease. Nurses can also function as teachers to explain the rationale behind screening for numerous genetic diseases.

The majority of disease risk, health conditions, and the therapies used to treat those conditions have a genetic and/or genomic element influenced by environmental, lifestyle, and other factors, therefore impacting the entire nursing profession.

Nurses have intimate knowledge of the patient's, family, and community's perspectives; an understanding of biologic underpinnings; experience with genetic/genomic technologies and information will be ideal to disseminate the information to the needy patients.

Nurses are expected to have a significant role in caring for patients with genetic predispositions or disorders. To carry out this role effectively and efficiently, they must be able to:

- Identify hereditary, familial, environmental and lifestyle characteristics that increase individual and family members' risk for disease.
- Facilitate informed decision making.
- Promote behaviors that facilitate surveillance and reduce disease risks.
- Identify, refer and/or prescribe appropriate disease management strategies.
- Advocate publicly and politically promotion of optimal health care, including genetic health care for all.

In short, by carrying the roles of a counselor, technician, care manager, and teacher for patients and their families, nurses will have an opportunity to expand as well as to create new leadership roles in health care.

As early as in 1962, Brantal and Esslinger, two nursing educators, recommended that human genetics be included in the content of basic nursing education. They said that knowledge of genetics was needed by nurses "to enhance and enrich the care of patients and their families".

Effects of the human genome project have raised awareness among health care providers about the necessity of providing appropriate information on genetics and consulting skills.

The progress in genetics and genomics is applicable to the entire spectrum of health care and all health professionals.

Across the lifespan, nursing focuses on health promotion and disease prevention, which is an integral component of genetic/genomic healthcare practices.

The nursing profession is a pivotal provider of quality health care services and is essential to closing the gap between research discoveries that are efficacious to health care and their successful adoption to optimize health.

For people to benefit from widespread genetic/genomic discoveries, nurses must be competent:

- To obtain comprehensive family histories

- To identify family members at risk for developing a genomic influenced condition
- For genomic influenced drug reactions
- Help people make informed decisions about and understand the results of their genetic/genomic tests and therapies, and
- Refer at-risk people to appropriate healthcare professionals and agencies for specialized care.

Nurses knowledgeable about genetics/genomics and skilled at obtaining and assessing risk in a family history have the potential to help people avert adult-onset disorders and consequential morbidity and mortality.

In preconception and prenatal settings, nurses have an opportunity to help families prepare for a child with a genetic condition.

The goal of nursing research in clinical genetics and genomics is to improve the quality of health care for patients and families.

Education is required for nurses and all health professionals to assure that the revolutionary advances in genetics and genomics reach the patients and families for whom they were developed.

IMPACT OF GENETIC CONDITIONS ON FAMILIES

Genetic disorders are unique in the fact that every individual diagnosis becomes a family diagnosis. After the diagnosis of a genetic disorder in one individual, family members may discover that they themselves are mildly affected by the disorder, are at risk of developing it, and/or may potentially pass it to their offspring. The family diagnosis can have a significant impact on family relationships and communication. One parent may blame the other for carrying a gene that has adversely affected their children.

Another familial unique issue to genetic disease involves the transmission of information about the condition between family members. Not only is there biological inheritance of a genetic condition, there is also a kind of psychological inheritance attached to it. Just as a disease-related gene may be passed from parent to child, representations of the disease and its consequences may be inherited too. Because family attitudes toward the genetic condition play a critical role in psychological adjustment, clinicians should always explore and discuss these beliefs with their clients.

Since more than one individual in a family is often affected with a given condition, the burden of care for the rest of the family becomes greater than usual.

Currently, there are about 4,000 known genetic diseases, with new ones being discovered every year. The vast majority of such diseases are extremely rare, only affecting one in several thousand or million people worldwide per year. A high number of these individuals are young adults who are faced and diagnosed with, a range of genetically transmitted medical conditions that are associated with progressive and often severe acquired disability.

Clinical genetics is concerned with the diagnosis and management of the medical, social, and psychological aspects of hereditary disease. As in all other areas of medicine, it is essential to make a correct diagnosis and to provide appropriate treatment, which must include helping the affected person and family members understand and come to terms with the nature and consequences of the disorder.

The confirmation of the presence, or absence, of a genetic diagnosis can, as in all areas of medical practice, produce both positive and negative responses. Genetic diagnoses have the added dimension that most results may not only affect the individual concerned, but potentially their siblings, their children, and their unborn children.

Fear

Individuals may be fearful at every stage like:

1. Awaiting the initial contact with genetic counselor

2. Deciding whether or not to have genetic tests
3. Awaiting relevant results
4. Discussing the diagnosis with family and friends
5. Deciding whether to have (more) children.

Practitioners need to be gentle, supportive, clear, and concise in their explanations, checking back that those explanations are understood. They will need to allow time, may be over several consultations, for patients' fears to be explored as much as they require them to be. However, nurses must ensure that family members, for whom they care, have their fears dealt with in a way that does not compromise confidentiality.

Depression

The knowledge that an individual has a genetic problem and may have passed it on to the next generation, the decision to not have children, the decision to opt for the termination of an affected fetus all have the potential to trigger a depressive response of varying severity. Warning signs may include a patient's description of their sense of hopelessness or inevitability. The primary care nurses must help in the diagnosis of depression, and use the services of the local mental health available and support the patients.

Relationship Jeopardy

People in any relationship occasionally have to deal with the discovery of secrets from their past or present, difficulties in communication, differences of opinion over whether to have children or not. The diagnosis of a genetic problem in the family may precipitate tension.

Stigmatization

Intolerant attitudes may cause distress to those with obvious genetic conditions, such as achondroplasia. Better education on genetic issues in schools and the media may help to replace stigmatization with understanding. Support groups for genetic disorders can:

- Provide peer and family support
- Provide information and advice
- Help affected individuals and their families
- Feel less isolated.

Financial

Affected individuals may have fears about the impact of their genetic diagnosis on both their income and the affordability of insurance. The primary care nurses can provide some information about the financial support system to the affected individuals and their families.

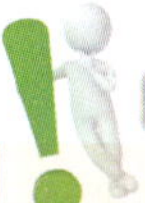

Points to Ponder

- Genetic disease and congenital malformations occur in approximately 3–5% of all live births. There is an increasing knowledge of the role of genetic factors in common illness, such as cancer, diabetes, neuropsychiatric disorders, cardiovascular disease, and atherosclerosis.
- Genetic knowledge now has implications for all areas of health and disease management and nursing practice.

ASSESSMENT QUESTION

1. **Discuss in detail the practical role of nurses in the field of biomedical genetics.**

MULTIPLE CHOICE QUESTIONS

1. **How can the principles of genetics be applied in nursing practice?**
   A. By understanding the genetic basis of diseases and providing appropriate patient education and counseling
   B. By administering genetic engineering therapies to patients to treat genetic disorders
   C. By performing gene editing procedures to modify patients' genetic makeup
   D. By utilizing genetic testing solely for diagnostic purposes
2. **Which of the following is NOT a potential application of genetics in nursing practice?**
   A. Predicting the risk of developing genetic disorders in patients and their families
   B. Offering genetic counseling and education to patients and their families about inherited conditions
   C. Administering gene therapy to patients to treat genetic disorders
   D. Analyzing genetic data solely for research purposes without clinical application

Answer Key for MCQs

1	2
A	D

CHAPTER 34 Historical Highlights

Learning Objectives

At the end of reading this chapter, the student shall be able to:

- Enumerate the historical changes happened in the evolution of genetics.
- Describe the basic principles of laws of genetics.

INTRODUCTION

Our present knowledge in genetics dates back to the Johann Gregor Mendel (1822-1884) in the latter half of the nineteenth century who found out that both the parents contributed equally to their offspring's which he substantiated with his experiments on garden pea plants. This was akin to the observations made a century earlier by a French naturalist, Pierre Louis Moreau de Maupertuis who said that certain hereditary particles are responsible for the formation of a particular body part, and each body part has two particles one from the father and one from the mother.

This was followed by a series of observations by various workers worldwide which led to the development of a science specialty called **Genetics**. The milestones include:

- Discovery of the blood groups and its pattern of inheritance by Karl Landsteiner in 1900.
- In 1902, William Bateson coined the term "Genetics" for the science that deals with Heredity.
- In 1903, Walter Sutton and Theodor Boveri proposed Chromosomal Theory of Hereditary.
- The term "gene" was coined by Johannsen in 1909.
- In 1927, Bridges demonstrated that genes are sequences of nucleotides which are oriented in a linear fashion on the chromosomes. This led to a branch of genetics called **cytogenetics**.
- In 1927, Muller found that exposure of X-rays leads to subtle damages in the gene, which are called **mutations**.
- In 1949, Barr and Bertram found out that in female genotypes only one of the X chromosomes is activated. The other X chromosome gets inactivated in the 14th day of the embryo. The inactivated X chromosome is identified in the buccal smears as Barr body. Presence of the Barr body is indicative of a female genotype. The concept of inactivation was coined by Mary F Lyon (1961) and it is called as **Lyon's hypothesis**. The process of inactivation is called as **Lyonization**.
- One of the major milestones in the development of genetics came after the discovery of the double helix model for **DNA by Watson and Crick in 1953**. They were awarded the Nobel Prize.
- In 1956, Tijo and Levan demonstrated the actual number of chromosomes in human as 46.
- Various chromosomal defects were analyzed by several workers worldwide and in

1959, Lejune described the chromosomal defect in Down's syndrome. During the same period, Nowell and Hungerford associated chromosomal changes with cancer (Philadelphia chromosome in chronic myeloid leukemia).

- In 1976, an eminent Indian Genetic scientist Hargobind Khorana and his colleagues synthesized a functional artificial gene.

MENDELIAN LAW OF GENETICS

With the experiments on the various characters of the garden pea plant, Mendel proposed certain laws which were later called as the **Mendelian law of Genetics**. They include:

- *Law of unit inheritance:* Mendel observed that in the offspring the characters of the parents do not blend. The characters may be expressed in the first generation or they may be reappear without change in the subsequent generations. This is referred to as the law of unit inheritance.
- *Law of segregation:* This law states that the numbers of the gene pair segregate and pass into different gametes. They are never found in the same gamete. An error in this pattern of segregation is called as **nondisjunction**.
- *Law of independent assortment:* This law states that the members of the different gene pairs assort independently of one another during gametogenesis. Random assortment of the maternal and paternal chromosome forms a physical basis of the law of independent assortment.

Points to Ponder

- Historical highlights on the evolution of medical genetics
- The common Mendelian laws of inheritance are:
  - Law of unit inheritance
  - Law of segregation
  - Law of independent assortment

ASSESSMENT QUESTION

1. **Mendelian laws of inheritance.**

MULTIPLE CHOICE QUESTIONS

1. **The common laws of inheritance was coined by:**
   A. William Boyd
   B. John Gregor Mendel
   C. Rudolph Virchow
   D. Walton Sutton
2. **According to Mendelian law of genetics, which of the following statements is true about the inheritance of traits?**
   A. Traits are always inherited in a continuous spectrum
   B. Offspring inherit traits from only one parent
   C. Traits are determined by the blending of parental characteristics
   D. Traits are inherited as discrete units, with each parent contributing one allele

Answer Key for MCQs

1	2
B	D

CHAPTER

Principles of Cytogenetics

Learning Objectives

At the end of reading this chapter, the student shall be able to:

- Describe the mechanisms and principles of cytogenetics.

INTRODUCTION

Cytogenetics mainly deals with the study of chromosomes within a cell.

In human beings, the chromosome is located within the nucleus of the cell. In a normal cell, the chromosome has a coiled dark staining portion called the *heterochromatin* and an extended pale staining portion called *euchromatin.*

The number of chromosomes in human cell is 46. They are arranged as 23 pairs. This pattern is called *diploid*. Out of the 46 chromosomes, 44 chromosomes are called *autosomes* and the rest 2 are called *sex chromosomes*.

In men, the pattern of sex chromosome is XY and in women, it is XX. Every species has a fixed number of chromosomes.

The literal meaning of chromosome is a colored body (chrome—color and some—body). Each chromosome is made up of a pair of identical double helix of chromosomal DNA called *chromatids*. The point at which both the chromatids cross is called *centromere*. The distal portion of each chromosome is called *telomere*. The chromosomes are divided into three groups based on the location of the centromere (**Table 35.1**).

The chromosomes have small units located in specific portions called **genes**. The location of the genes is called a **genetic locus**.

TABLE 35.1: Classifications of chromosomes.

Type	*Location of centromere*	*Numbers*
Metacentric	Central	1, 3, 16, 19, 20
Sub-metacentric	Divides the chromosome into short and Long arm	1, 3
Acrocentric	Eccentrical with satellites	13, 14, 15, 21, 22
Telocentric	Centromere at one end with a single arm	

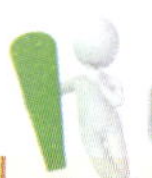

Points to Ponder

- Cytogenetics mainly deals with the study of chromosomes within a cell.
- In human beings, the chromosome is located within the nucleus of the cell. In a normal cell, the chromosome has a coiled dark staining portion called the **heterochromatin** and a extended pale staining portion called **euchromatin**.
- The number of chromosomes in human cell is 46. They are arranged as 23 pairs. This pattern is called *diploid*. Out of the 46 chromosomes, 44 chromosomes are called **autosomes** and the rest 2 are called sex **chromosomes**.

MULTIPLE CHOICE QUESTION

1. **Which of the following best describes the role of cytogenetics?**
   A. Studying the structure and function of cells
   B. Analyzing the chemical composition of cells
   C. Investigating the genetic material within cells
   D. Examining the metabolic processes of cells

Answer Key for MCQ

1
C

CHAPTER

Cell Cycle and Cell Division

Learning Objectives

At the end of reading this chapter, the student shall be able to:
- Describe in detail the mechanism of cell division methods.

CELL CYCLE

Any cell capable of undergoing division, the events occur in a cyclical pattern called the **cell cycle** (**Fig. 36.1**)

The cell cycle has got the following phases:

1. **G1 phase**—resting phase, this occurs following mitotic phase.
2. **S phase**—synthetic phase, in which the DNA is synthesized.
3. **G2 phase**—premitotic phase.
4. **Mitotic**—the actual replication occurs in this phase.

CELL DIVISION

Mitosis

This occurs only in somatic cells. From each cell two daughter cells are produced. There is both division of cytoplasm and nucleus. The mitosis is divided into four stages—prophase, metaphase, anaphase and telophase. The events are depicted in **Figure 36.2.**

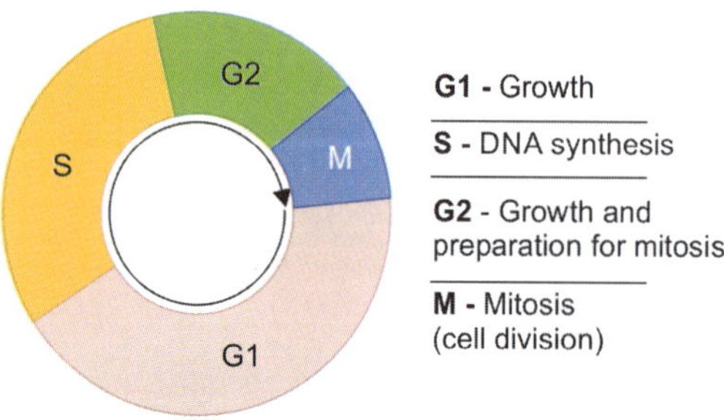

Fig. 36.1: Phases of cell cycle.

Prophase

In this phase, the chromosomes arrange themselves as rod-shaped strands joined by centromere. There will be gradual disappearance of the nuclear membrane with duplication of the centrioles.

Metaphase

The centrioles move to the opposite poles of the cell. The chromosomes condense further and arrange in the central portion of the nucleus. Microtubules radiate from the centriole to the centromere of the chromosome. These microtubules are called **the spindle fibers**.

Anaphase

The centromere divided vertically and two daughter chromosomes are formed. The new chromosomes move to the pole of the cell by the action of the spindle fibers. The onset of cytoplasmic division occurs by the formation of a furrow in the equatorial plane of the cell.

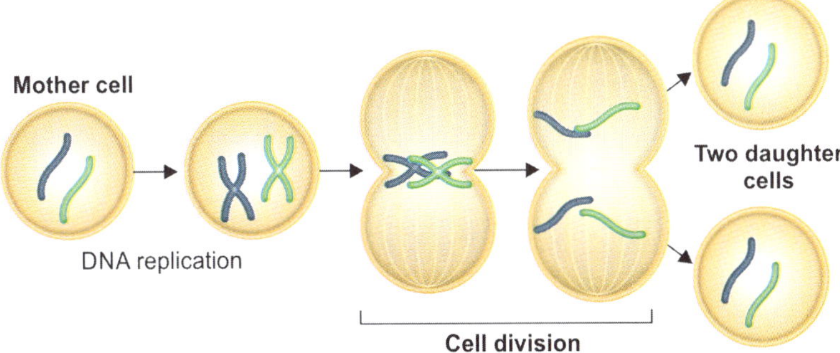

Fig. 36.2: Phases of mitosis.

Telophase

In this phase, the furrow in the equatorial plane further deepens to form two daughter cells with two individual copies of the chromosome. The chromosomes appear as chromatin network with reconstitution of the nuclear membrane. Thus two individual daughter cells are produced.

Meiosis I

This is a special type of cell division seen in the gametes. It consists of two divisions—meiosis I and II. Each daughter cell at the completion of meiosis I contains half the number of chromosomes (23 chromosomes). This is called **haploid number**. This haploid number is maintained in the cell in meiosis II.

The meiotic cell division also has similar phases like that of mitotic division with some differences. The events are depicted in **Figure 36.3**.

Prophase

The prophase of a meiotic division is prolonged and it consists of the following phases—leptotene, zygotene, pachytene, diplotene and diakinesis.

Leptotene: The chromosomes appear as thin thread-like structures with alternate thin and thick portions. This gives a beaded appearance, called **chromomeres**.

Zygotene: Pairing of the homologous chromosomes occurs during this phase. In sex chromosomes, the pairing occurs only at the tip of the short arm.

Pachytene: The chromosomes become tightly coiled and stain deeply. Each chromosome now appears to be made up of two chromatids.

Diplotene: This stage is characterized by the longitudinal separation of chromosomes without split in the centromere. The two chromatids of each chromosome remain together.

Diakinesis: The chromosomes condense further and take up a deeper staining.

Metaphase

There will be gradual disappearance of the nuclear membrane with the movement of the chromosomes to the equatorial plane of the cell.

Anaphase

In this phase, two members of the homologous chromosome disjoin

There is a random assortment of maternal and paternal chromosomes. One chromosome from each bivalent pair goes to each pole.

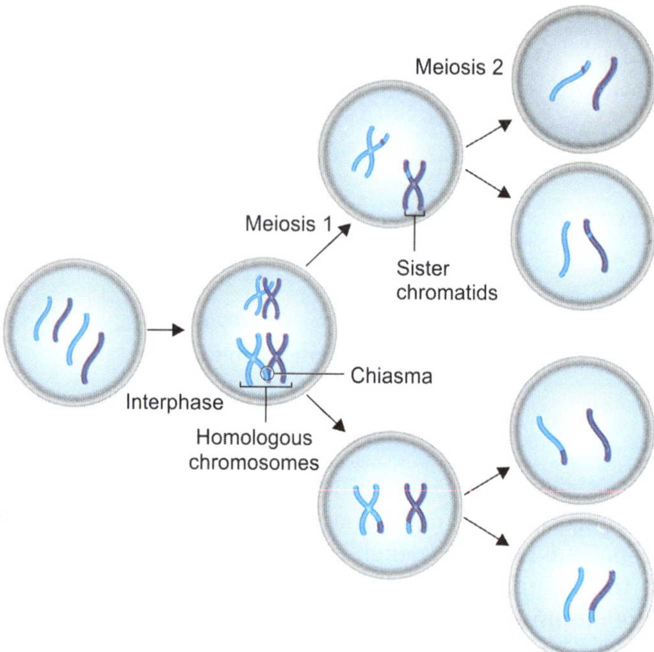

Fig. 36.3: Stages in meiosis.

Telophase

Cytoplasmic division occurs during this phase.

Meiosis II

This resembles mitotic division with two main differences. There is no DNA replication in this pattern of cell division and this phase of cell division immediately follows Meiosis I without any interphase. The Meiosis II is also divided into phases similar to mitosis—prophase II, metaphase II, anaphase II and telophase II.

CELL DIVISION IN HUMAN BODY

Spermatogenesis

The process of gametogenesis in males is referred to as spermatogenesis.

It occurs within the seminiferous tubules of the testis. The primary germ cell that lines the tubules is called **stem cells**. There are two forms of the stem cells—Type A and B. These cells undergo further division to produce primary spermatocytes. The primary spermatocytes undergo a meiotic pattern of cell division producing two secondary spermatocytes with haploid number of chromosomes. The secondary spermatocytes undergo Meiotic II division to form two spermatids. Thus four spermatids are formed from each primary spermatocyte. These spermatids undergo further division to form mature spermatozoa. This process is called as **spermiogenesis**. The total time taken for the formation of a mature spermatozoon is 64 days. About 200 to 300 million sperms are produced per ejaculate.

Oogenesis

The process of gametogenesis in women is referred to as oogenesis. This differs from spermatogenesis in the following aspects:

- Oogonia divides to from primary oocyte in the prenatal life and no primary oocyte is formed after birth. This primary oocyte remains in a suspended prophase from birth to puberty. Certain primary oocyte completes their first meiotic division very late around 30–40 years. This is the reason for higher incidence of genetic errors in elderly prime mothers.

- The primary oocyte divides unequally producing a large secondary oocyte and a smaller first polar body.
- The second meiotic division starts when the oocyte travels in the uterine tube and is completed only after fertilization. The secondary oocyte completes its second meiotic division and extrudes the second polar body.

Points to Ponder

- There are two forms of cell division: Mitosis and meiosis.
- There are four phases in cell cycle of mitosis.
- The germinal epithelium usually undergoes meiotic cell division.

ASSESSMENT QUESTION

1. **Phases of cell cycle.**

MULTIPLE CHOICE QUESTIONS

1. **The word S in a cell cycle usually indicates:**
   A. Growth
   B. Cell division
   C. Synthesis
   D. Survival
2. **What is the primary function of mitosis in multicellular organisms?**
   A. Production of gametes
   B. Growth and repair of tissues
   C. Genetic diversity
   D. DNA replication
3. **During which phase of the cell cycle does DNA replication occur?**
   A. G1 phase
   B. S phase
   C. G2 phase
   D. M phase
4. **Which of the following is NOT a phase of mitosis?**
   A. Prophase
   B. Metaphase
   C. Interphase
   D. Telophase
5. **What is the end result of meiosis?**
   A. Two identical daughter cells
   B. Four genetically unique daughter cells
   C. Two genetically identical daughter cells
   D. One genetically identical daughter cell

Answer Key for MCQs

1	2	3	4	5
C	B	B	C	B

CHAPTER

Morphology of Chromosome and Karyotyping

Learning Objectives

At the end of reading this chapter, the student shall be able to:

- Describe in detail the morphology of a chromosome and enlist the methods of banding techniques.

INTRODUCTION

There are **46 chromosomes** in human being arranged in **23 pairs**. Of this, there are **22 pairs** of autosomes and one pair of sex chromosome. The normal arrangement of chromosome in a female is depicted in **Figure 37.1** and of male is shown in **Figure 37.2**.

They are rod-shaped structures made up of two chromatids. These are held together with a narrowed portion called the **centromere**. Based on the location of the centromere the chromosomes are classified as—metacentric, submetacentric, acrocentric and telocentric chromosomes.

The submetacentric chromosomes have a short arm and a longer arm. **The short arm is called as p and long arm is referred to as q**.

The acrocentric chromosomes have tiny structures called **satellites** attached to the short arm. These contain genes coding for ribosomal RNA.

KARYOTYPING (FIG. 37.3)

This is a process to study the structural patterns of the chromosomes. The cell division is arrested at the level of metaphase, stained with specific dyes and then photographed for morphological identification. This picture is called **ideogram**.

Classification

There are various systems used to study the morphology of the chromosomes.

Denver System of Classification

According to this system, the chromosomes were grouped from A to G according to the length and position of the centromere of the chromosomes (**Table 37.1**).

Paris System of Classification

This included identification of the chromosomes based on the various banding patterns. This is an accepted classification worldwide. According to this the p and q arm are numbered as 1, 2, 3 from the centromere. These regions are further divided into subregions for precise localization of the gene.

Banding Technique

It is a staining methodology done on a chromosomal preparation to bring about finer details by alternate dark and light staining patterns. There are various types of banding procedures which include:

- G—banding (Giemsa stain)
- Q—banding (Quinacrine fluorescent stain)
- R—banding (Reverse banding)

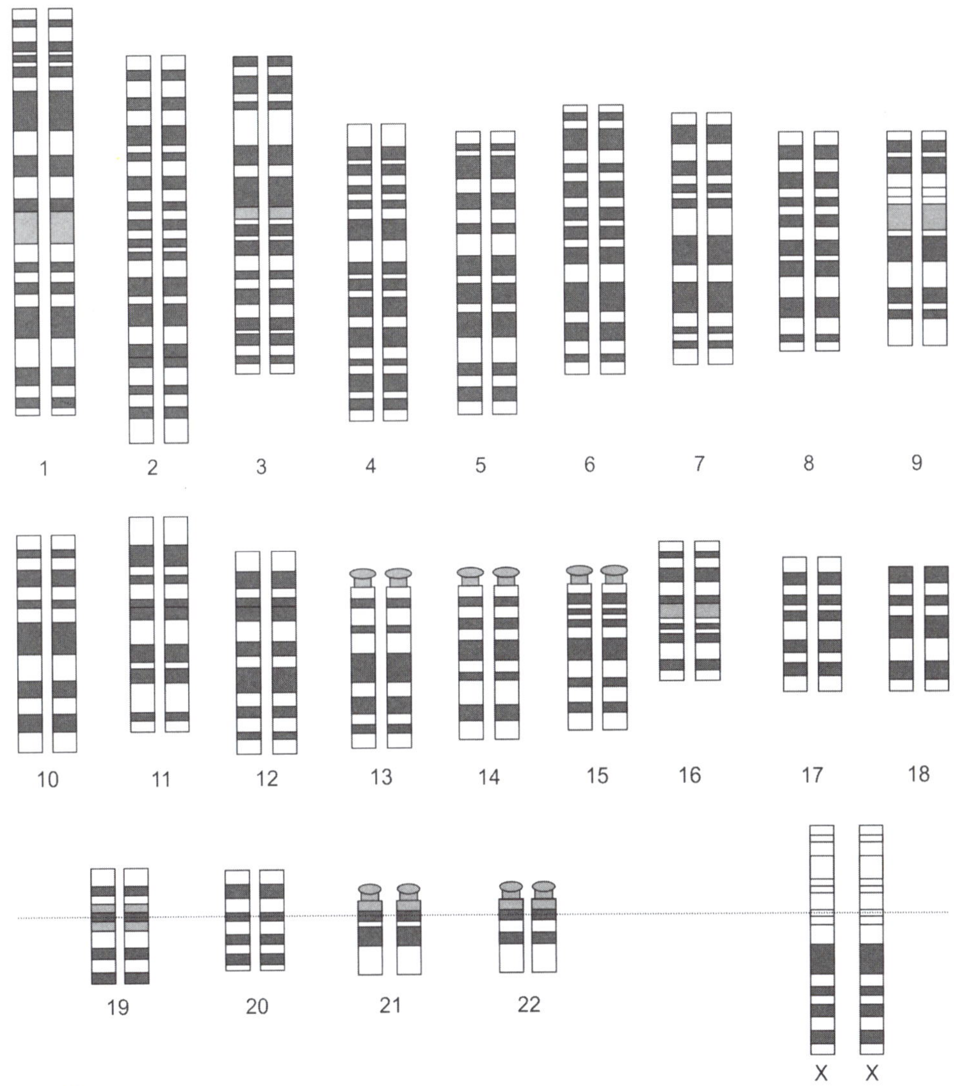

Fig. 37.1: Normal chromosomal spread in a female.

- C—banding (Constitutive heterochromatin demonstration)
- High resolution banding

Chromosome Preparation Techniques

Chromosomes can be studied from any somatic cell in culture like the fibroblastic cells and amniotic fluid cells or they can be studied directly from bone marrow cells and chorion villous samples without culture. The more common method is preparation of chromosomes from peripheral blood culture.

The blood sample is collected and cultured in media, such as **HAM F10, TC 199, and RPMI**, etc. Fetal calf serum is added to nourish the cells. The cells are also treated with phytoagglutinin which acts as a mitogenic agent. Antibiotics are added to the culture media to prevent bacterial overgrowth. They are incubated for three days at 37°C. They are then treated with

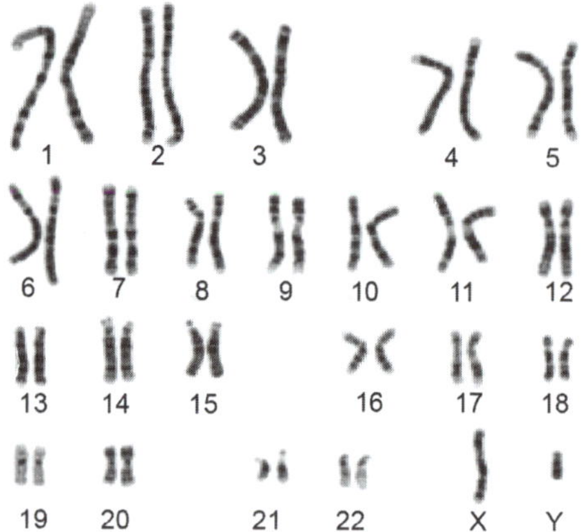

Fig. 37.2: Normal karyotype of a male.

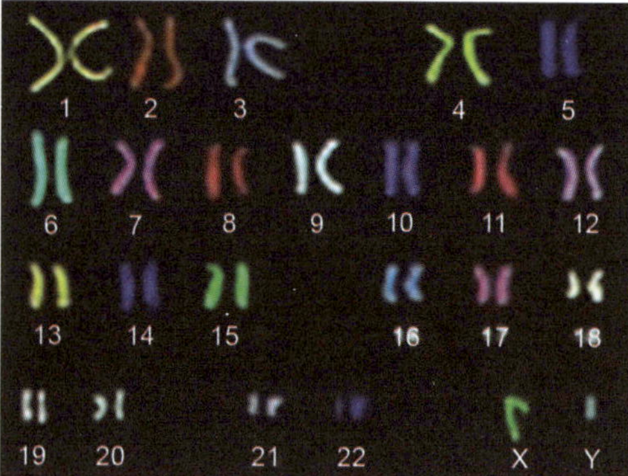

Fig. 37.3: Normal karyotype.

TABLE 37.1: Classification of human chromosomes (Denver system).

Group	Chromosome numbers
A	1, 2, 3
B	4, 5
C	6, 7, 8, 9, 10, 11, 12 & X
D	13, 14, 15
E	16, 17, 18
F	19, 20
G	21, 22, Y

colchicine which will arrest the cell division at metaphase, preventing the formation of spindle tubules. This allows proper visualization of the chromosomes. They are then stained with Giemsa or any other fluorescent dyes for proper evaluation of the morphology.

Other Recent Methods to Study Chromosomes

Flow Cytometry

It is a highly rewarding recent technique to study the morphology of the chromosomes. In this method, the cells are first separated to make single cell suspension and are stained with selective DNA dye. They are allowed to pass through a narrow jet of laser in a flow chamber. The laser beam excites the chromosome to fluoresce and the emitted fluorescence can be measured by a detector. This depends upon the size of the chromosome. This method allows a rapid analysis of the chromosomes.

Fluorescent In Situ Hybridization (FISH) (Fig. 37.4)

This is a very useful recent method for chromosomal analysis. This uses specific single stranded DNA probes conjugated with a fluorescent label. This probe will hybridize with its complementary pair and produce a fluorescent signal which can be directly visualized with an ultraviolet light (**Fig. 37.5**).

Whole Chromosome Paint (WCP)

This is a modification of FISH technique in which a probe for the whole chromosome is prepared and applied to the metaphase spread. This is very useful in detecting chromosomal rearrangements, translocations, deletions and other errors.

Clinical Applications for Karyotyping

- *Clinical diagnosis:* It is useful in establishing the genetic basis for congenital malformations, mental retardation and other conditions.

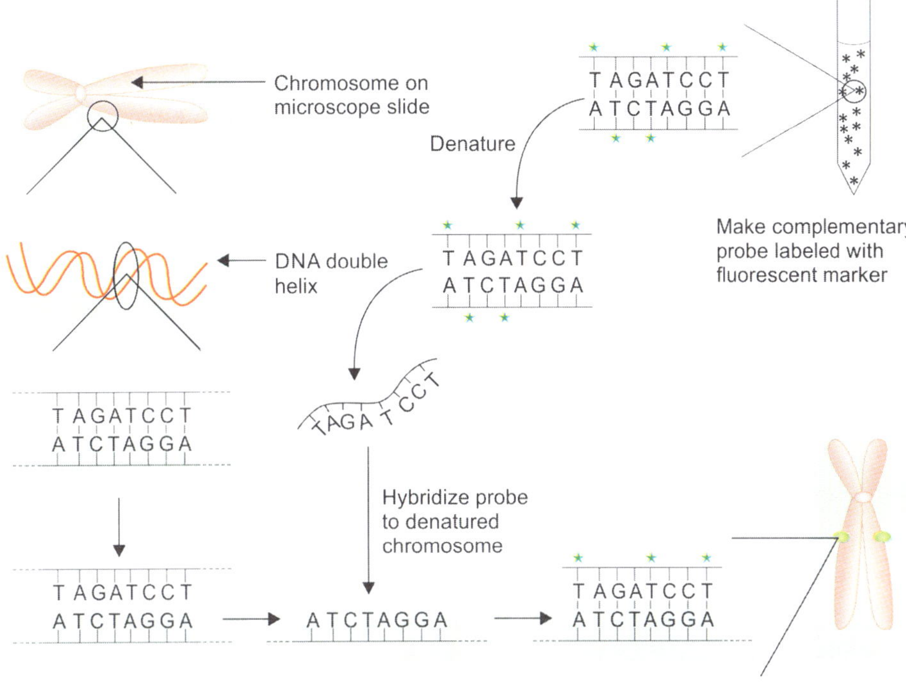

Fig. 37.4: Technique for FISH.

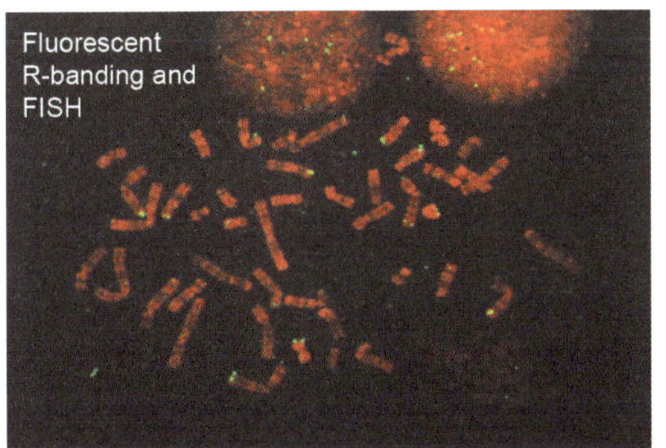

Fig. 37.5: A FISH preparation showing fluorescent signals.

- *Repeated fetal loss:* Many chromosomal aberrations can induce spontaneous abortions. The nature and type of the error can be detected with karyotyping.
- *Prenatal diagnosis:* Karyotyping is very helpful in prenatal diagnosis of disorders, such as hemophilia, muscular dystrophy which may warrant a medical termination of pregnancy.
- *Neoplasia:* Identification of specific chromosomal anomalies may be helpful in the diagnosis of certain neoplastic condition and also to predict the course and prognosis. For example, presence of Philadelphia chromosome in chronic myeloid leukemia (CML).

DETECTION OF SEX CHROMATIN

The sex chromatin can be demonstrated by two common methods:

1. Detection of the Barr body (sex chromatin) in the buccal smears
2. Detection of drumstick appendage attached to one of the nuclear lobe of the neutrophils.

The Barr body is an inactivated X chromosome present within the nucleus of the somatic cell as a clump of chromatin.

This is ideally studied from the buccal smears. The number of Barr bodies in a cell depends upon the number of X chromosomes. Presence of Barr bodies indicates female genotype. Since men have only one active X chromosome, they do not show Barr body.

This pattern of random inactivation of one of the X chromosome either paternal or maternal occurs during the 16th day of embryogenesis. This is called **Lyon's hypothesis** after Mary F Lyon who described this in 1962. The inactivation occurs by DNA methylation.

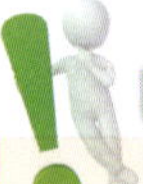

Points to Ponder

- Humans possess a total of 46 chromosomes, organized into 23 pairs. Among these pairs, 22 are autosomes, while one pair comprises the sex chromosomes. They are rod-shaped structures made up of two chromatids. These are held together with a narrowed portion called the centromere. They are rod-shaped structures made up of two chromatids.
- Banding technique is a staining methodology done on a chromosomal preparation to bring about finer details by alternate dark and light staining patterns.

ASSESSMENT QUESTION

1. **Banding techniques.**

MULTIPLE CHOICE QUESTIONS

1. **What is karyotyping primarily used for?**
   A. Determining the genetic code of an individual
   B. Identifying specific genes responsible for diseases
   C. Analyzing the structure and number of chromosomes in a cell
   D. Studying the biochemical pathways within cells
2. **What is the typical source of cells used for karyotyping?**
   A. Blood samples
   B. Skin tissue
   C. Muscle tissue
   D. Hair follicles

Answer Key for MCQs

1	2
C	A

CHAPTER

Structure of DNA and Gene

Learning Objectives

At the end of reading this chapter, the student shall be able to:

- Describe in detail the structure of a genome.

INTRODUCTION

The genetic information of the human cell is stored within the nucleus of the cell. This is stored in the form of nucleic acids. Every nucleic acid is composed of long chains of molecules called the **nucleotides**.

Each nucleotide is made up of a nitrogenous base, sugar moiety and phosphorus molecule. There are two types of nitrogenous bases—purines and pyrimidines:

1. The purine bases are adenine and guanine.
2. The pyrimidine bases are thymine, cytosine and uracil.

There are two types of nucleic acids—the deoxyribonucleic acid (DNA) and ribonucleic acid (RNA). The DNA contains a deoxyribose sugar and RNA contains ribose sugar. The pyrimidine base present in DNA is thymine. The pyrimidine base present in RNA is uracil. Rest of the nitrogenous bases are common for both.

The DNA is mostly located within the chromosomes and a minor component within the mitochondria. The RNA is chiefly present within the ribosomes and nucleolus.

DNA is a macromolecule that carries genetic information from generation to generation. It is responsible to preserve the identity of the species over millions of years. DNA may be regarded as the reserve bank of genetic information.

STRUCTURE OF DNA (FIG. 38.1)

The structure of DNA was first described by Watson and Crick. They received Nobel Prize for their discovery. They suggested that the DNA contains two nucleotide chains arranged in the form of a double helix. Each chain has a backbone of sugar and phosphate molecule. The chains are held together by hydrogen bonds.

The bases in DNA molecule pair with specificity. Adenine always pairs with thymine and guanine pairs with cytosine. The two chains of the DNA molecule get separated during the nuclear division and create its own complement. This process is called **replication**.

There are three types of DNA:

1. **Unique sequences:** They constitute 60% of the total DNA. They usually code for proteins.
2. **Highly repetitive sequences**: They constitute 10% of the total DNA. They are found in chromosomes 1, 9, 16 and long arm of chromosome Y.
3. **Moderately repetitive sequences:** They constitute 30% of the total DNA. They usually code for functional genes—ribosomal RNA, histones, immunoglobulins.

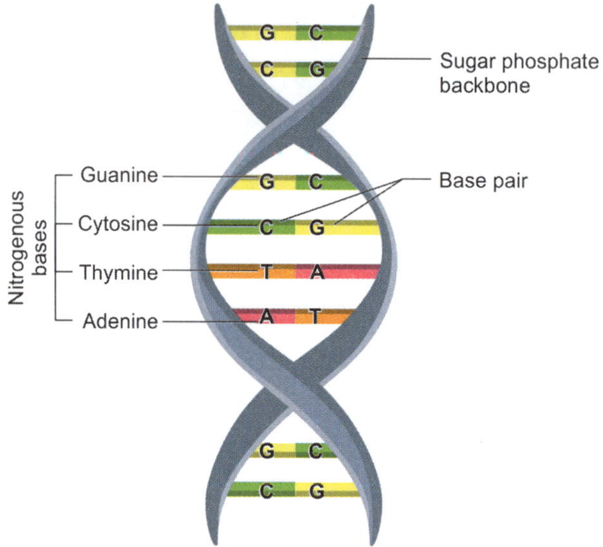

Fig. 38.1: Structure of DNA.

Mitochondrial DNA

Many mitochondria possess their own DNA. It is in circular form and called as **mtDNA**. It codes for two specific enzymes—cytochrome B and Cytochrome oxidase which are involved in oxidative phosphorylation. The mitochondrial DNA is purely maternal in origin. Since they are involved in cell metabolism, mutations in the mitochondrial DNA are seen in disorders of central nervous system, heart and skeletal muscle tissues. Example for disease transmitted through mitochondrial DNA is Leber's optic atrophy.

Ribonucleic Acid (RNA)

The RNA molecule is single stranded and it contains a ribose sugar. It contains a specific pyrimidine base, uracil. There are three types of RNA:

1. Messenger RNA (mRNA)
2. Transfer RNA (tRNA)
3. Ribosomal RNA (rRNA)

Messenger RNA (mRNA)

It is the type of RNA that carries the message from the DNA. This is derived from a heterogeneous nuclear RNA (hnRNA). It contains both coding and non-coding sequences. The coding sequences are called the **exons** and noncoding sequences are called the **introns**. The noncoding sequences of the hnRNA are cut and removed and it then forms a mRNA. This mRNA undergoes a variety of modifications before they mature. They acquire a methylated cap and a poly(A) tail. This poly(A) tail helps in transporting the mRNA from the nucleus to the ribosomes of the cytoplasm.

Transfer RNA (t RNA)

This is an intermediate RNA molecule that conveys the message carried by the mRNA to the ribosomes. This intermediate RNA molecule is called as tRNA. It is a single stranded molecule with a molecular weight of 25,000 daltons. Each amino acid has its own specific tRNA.

Ribosomes

The ribosomes are tiny particles rich in ribonucleoprotein within the cytoplasm. They occur is two sizes 60S and 80S. The 60S ribosomes are located within the mitochondria and 80S within the cytoplasm. They may lie free in the cytoplasm or found coupled to endoplasmic reticulum called **rough endoplasmic reticulum**. They are also present within the nucleus in the form of nucleolus. When they are arranged in a string like manner it is called **polyribosomes**.

Ribosomal RNA

It is predominantly double stranded and is involved in protein synthesis.

The biological information flows from the DNA to RNA and from there to proteins. This is the central dogma of life. The DNA ultimately controls every cell function through protein synthesis.

As a carrier of genetic information, DNA must be duplicated, maintained and passed accurately to the daughter cells. DNA is the genetic material. When the cell divides, the daughter cells receive an identical copy of the genetic information from the parent cell.

REPLICATION

It is a process in which the DNA copies itself to produce two identical daughter molecules of DNA. The parent DNA has two strands complementary to each other. Both the strands undergo simultaneous replication to produce two daughter molecules. Each of the newly synthesized DNA has one half of the parental DNA and one half of new DNA.

TRANSCRIPTION

It is a process in which the information is transmitted from the DNA to the mRNA. The two strands of the DNA get separated and against a single strand of DNA a new mRNA molecule is synthesized. The mRNA thus formed migrates from the nucleus to the cytoplasm due to presence of poly(A) tail.

TRANSLATION

The genetic information stored in the DNA is passed on to the RNA through transcription and ultimately expressed in the language of proteins. The biosynthesis of a protein or a polypeptide in a living cell is referred to as translation. The term translation is used to represent the biochemical translation of a four letter language information from the nucleic acid into a 20-letter language of proteins. It is a process of translating the information carried by the mRNA into protein synthesis. The mRNA gets associated with the ribosomes and it acts like a template to stimulate the synthesis of amino acid and there by proteins.

GENOME

The total DNA contained in an organism or a cell is regarded as the genome. It is storehouse of biological information; it includes the chromosomes in the nucleus and the DNA in the mitochondria.

The study of structure and function of genome is called the **genomics**.

Gene

It is regarded as the functional unit of the DNA that can be transcribed. It is a segment/ sequence of DNA molecule possessing a code for a specific amino acid. There are about 50 to 100 thousand DNA sequences that code for various proteins in human beings. These are called the **structural genes**.

Every gene will have coding sequences called the **exons** interrupted by non-coding sequences called the **introns**.

Code

This is defined as a sum of signals by which new information can be formulated and transmitted to the recipient.

Triplet Codon

The basic function of gene is to direct protein synthesis. The genetic information for the synthesis of proteins is stored within the DNA in the form of a triplet code. Each triplet code has three bases that code for one amino acid. As there are four bases, 64 such combinations can occur. This sequence of three bases coding for an amino acid is called a **triplet codon**. There may be mutations occurring within these codons. Two different types of mutations can occur:

1. **Nonsense mutations:** This leads to a significant error in the base sequences leading to complete shutdown of the amino acid.
2. **Missense mutations:** This leads to an erroneous base sequence, which codes for a different amino acid instead of the original one.

Control of Gene Action

Apart from the major structural genes, there are another set of genes that regulate the expression and function of the structural genes. These are called the **regulatory genes and operator genes**.

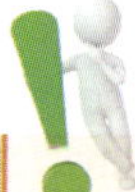

Points to Ponder

- The genetic information of the human cell is stored within the nucleus of the cell. This is stored in the form of nucleic acids. Every nucleic acid is composed of long chains of molecules called the **nucleotides**.
- Gene is regarded as the functional unit of the DNA that can be transcribed. It is a segment/sequence of DNA molecule possessing a code for a specific amino acid. There are about 50 to 100 thousand DNA sequences that code for various proteins in human beings. These are called the structural genes. Every gene will have coding sequences called the exons interrupted by non-coding sequences called the introns.

ASSESSMENT QUESTIONS

1. **Define a genome.**
2. **What is a codon?**

MULTIPLE CHOICE QUESTIONS

1. **The normal number of base pairs in human DNA is:**
   A. 1 billion B. 3 billion
   C. 5 billion D. 10 billion
2. **Which of the following accurately describes DNA replication?**
   A. It is a process where RNA is synthesized from a DNA template
   B. It involves the synthesis of two identical DNA molecules from one original DNA molecule
   C. It occurs during mitosis but not during meiosis
   D. It involves the formation of gametes from diploid cells
3. **What is the primary outcome of transcription?**
   A. Production of a complementary DNA molecule from an RNA template
   B. Synthesis of mRNA from a DNA template
   C. Formation of amino acids from mRNA
   D. Assembly of nucleotides to form a DNA molecule
4. **During translation, what is the role of transfer RNA (tRNA)?**
   A. To carry amino acids to the ribosome and match them with the appropriate codons on mRNA
   B. To transcribe DNA into mRNA

C. To unzip the DNA double helix during the initiation of translation
D. To catalyze the formation of peptide bonds between amino acids

5. **Which of the following best defines a genome?**
A. The complete set of proteins synthesized by an organism
B. The entire collection of DNA sequences found within an organism's chromosomes
C. The process by which cells divide and reproduce
D. The total number of cells in an organism's body

Answer Key for MCQs

1	2	3	4	5
B	B	B	A	B

CHAPTER 39

Mutations

Learning Objectives

At the end of reading this chapter, the student shall be able to:

- Describe in detail the various methods of genetic mutations.
- Describe the methodology of gene mapping.

It is defined as a permanent change in the structure of DNA. Mutations of the germ cells are transmitted to the progeny and give rise of inherited diseases and that of the somatic cells can induce carcinogenesis and malformations.

There are three categories of mutation:

1. *Genome mutations*—loss or gain of whole chromosome (monosomy/trisomy)
2. *Chromosome mutation*—rearrangement of genetic material with structural change in the chromosome
3. *Submicroscopic gene mutations*—may result in partial or complete deletion of a gene or often a single base.

The gene mutations are further categorized as:

- *Point mutations*—substitution of a single base for the other
- *Frame shift mutation*—due to insertion or deletion of a base pair
- *Trinucleotide repeat mutation*—amplification of a sequence of three nucleotides.

Point mutation: In this, there is a single base exchange in DNA sequence. This alters the triplet code and causes replacement of one amino acid, with the other. Due to the change in the amino acid, there is an alteration in the final gene product. This altered protein may not have any biological activity or may have an abnormal activity.

Example: Sickle cell anemia, in which there is an amino acid substitution at the 6th position of the beta globin chain. Valine is substituted in the place of glutamine. This result in the formation of a newer type of hemoglobin called the **sickle hemoglobin (HbS)** in the red blood cells. When the red cells with HbS are subjected to hypoxia, this newer hemoglobin undergoes polymerization and coverts the biconcave shape of the red cells into a sickle cell shape which interferes with the normal oxygen delivery function of hemoglobin.

Deletion or insertion: Deletion or insertion of a base within a triplet code leads to alteration in the reading frame of the codon. This type of mutations is called the **frame shift mutations.** This may either result in total shutdown of synthesis of a particular protein or malfunctioning of a protein.

Example: Thalassemia syndromes are type of hemoglobinopathies in which there is a shutdown of synthesis of a particular globin chain. If there is shut down of alpha chain—the disease is called **alpha thalassemia** and defective beta chain synthesis leads to beta thalassemia.

Splice mutations: In this type of mutations, there is a defect in the normal splicing of the introns and exons during the formation of a mRNA. This leads to complete failure of synthesis of the particular genetic product.

GENE MAPPING

These are processes in which a particular DNA sequence is mapped in a specific chromosome. There are two types of mapping–chromosome mapping and DNA mapping. The chromosome mapping can be done by somatic cell hybridization or in situ hybridization. The DNA mapping can be done by pulsed field gel electrophoresis, chromosome jumping analysis and yeast artificial chromosome (YAC contigs).

GENE CLONING

If a gene in question is required in large amounts, the gene can be inserted into a vector and passed into the host cell. If the host cell accepts the vector and the genetic command, it will produce protein molecules according to the command of the cloned gene.

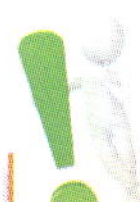

Points to Ponder

Mutation is defined as a permanent change in the structure of DNA. Mutations of the germ cells are transmitted to the progeny and give rise of inherited diseases and that of the somatic cells can induce carcinogenesis and malformations.

ASSESSMENT QUESTIONS

1. **Define mutation.**
2. **Enlist the common types of mutation.**

MULTIPLE CHOICE QUESTIONS

1. **A permanent change in DNA is known as:**
   A. Insertion
   B. Translocation
   C. Mutation
   D. Mendelian disorder
2. **Frame shift mutation includes all, *except*:**
   A. Insertion
   B. Deletion
   C. Point mutation
   D. Translocation
3. **An example of missense mutation is:**
   A. Thalassemia
   C. Down's syndrome
   B. Sickle cell anemia
   D. Cystic fibrosis
4. **What is the purpose of gene mapping?**
   A. To identify the specific sequence of nucleotides within a gene
   B. To determine the location of genes on chromosomes and their relative distances from each other
   C. To analyze the expression levels of genes in different tissues
   D. To study the biochemical pathways regulated by genes

5. What is gene cloning primarily used for?

A. Creating genetically modified organisms

B. Studying the expression patterns of genes

C. Producing large quantities of a specific DNA sequence

D. Analyzing the interactions between proteins

Answer Key for MCQs

1	2	3	4	5
C	D	B	B	C

Recombinant DNA Technology

Learning Objectives

At the end of reading this chapter, the student shall be able to:

- Describe the methodology of various recombinant DNA technology methods.

INTRODUCTION

It is one of the recent advances in the field of genetics. It involves synthesis of a new DNA molecule from the DNA sequences. The desired DNA sequence is cut with the help of a special family of enzymes called the **restriction endonucleases**, this DNA sequence is introduced into a vector to generate multiple copies of the DNA. Then the desired DNA is harvested and used for the generation of proteins.

APPLICATIONS OF RECOMBINANT DNA TECHNOLOGY

This technology can be used

- For the synthesis of various hormones for therapeutic use, e.g., insulin, growth hormone
- For synthesis of vaccines, e.g., hepatitis B virus
- For understanding the molecular basis of various diseases, such as sickle cell disease, cystic fibrosis and others
- For gene therapy in sickle cell disease, thalassemia and other diseases.

VARIOUS TECHNIQUES OF RECOMBINANT DNA TECHNOLOGY

Southern Blotting Technique (Fig. 40.1)

This method was first described by Edwin Southern (1975). It is a type of DNA-DNA hybrid. This is used to detect whether that particular DNA of interest is present in the test sample. The DNA of the test sample is separated with the help of the restriction enzymes and various fragments are separated by the agarose gel electrophoresis. Then the DNA is denatured with an alkali to form single stranded structure. To this denatured DNA, an artificial DNA probe containing the genetic sequence of interest is added and allowed to hybridize. If the test sample contains the particular DNA sequence, it will hybridize with the probe producing a visible band in the electrophoresis.

Applications

It is an extremely specific, sensitive and simple technique. Some of the applications of this technique include:

- Analysis of genes
- Important for confirming DNA cloning results
- To detect the minute quantities of DNA in Forensic science.

Northern Blotting Technique (Fig. 40.2)

This method is similar to the above. But is a RNA—DNA hybridization reaction. In this method, the mRNA is isolated and run on an electrophoretic gel. Hybridization is done with the help of a radiolabeled probe which determines the amount of mRNA.

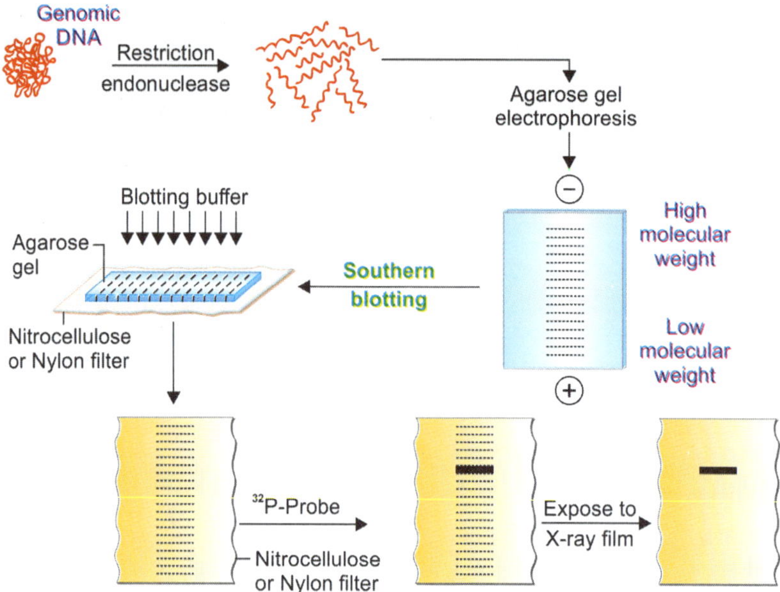

Fig. 40.1: Southern blotting.

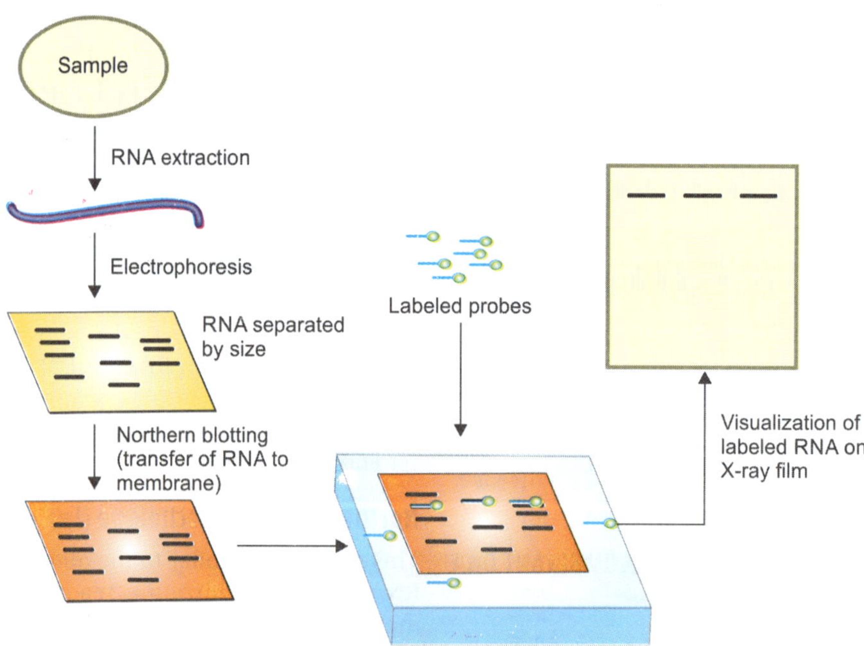

Fig. 40.2 : Northern blot technique.

Dot Blotting

It is a modification of Southern and Northern blotting techniques. Here the nucleic acid is directly spotted onto the filters and they are not subjected to electrophoresis. This is extremely useful in obtaining quantitative data for the evaluation of gene expression.

In Situ Hybridization Technique

This is more advanced than the above two procedures. The major advantage of this method is that there is no need to extract the nucleic acid from the cells and it also allows spatial resolution of the genetic material. Here the nucleic acid is exposed well with sequential steps of digestion and the sample is allowed to hybridize with the specific DNA/RNA probe of interest. The final product of hybridization can be visualized by direct fluorescence tagging or by immunohistochemical methods using various chromogens. The advantage of this procedure is that it can be used not only on fresh tissue samples but also on archival paraffin embedded tissue with preserved nucleic acid structures. This is regularly used in the detection of genomes of human *papillomavirus* in warty lesions and Epstein-Barr virus in lymphomas.

Florescence In Situ Hybridization

Fluorescence in situ hybridization (FISH) is a method used to identify specific parts of a chromosome (**Fig. 40.3**). For example, if you know the sequence of a certain gene, but you do not know on which chromosome the gene is located, you can use FISH to identify the chromosome in question and the exact location of the gene. Or, if you suspect that there has been a translocation in a chromosome, you can use a probe that spans the site of breakage/translocation. If there has been no translocation at that point, you will see one signal, since the probe hybridizes to one place on the chromosome.

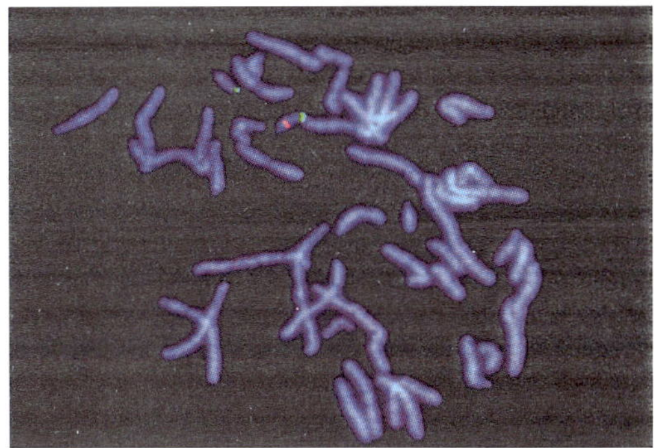

Fig. 40.3: Detection of parts of chromosome using FISH.

If, however, there has been a translocation, you will see two signals, since the probe can hybridize to both ends of the translocation point.

Polymerase Chain Reaction (PCR)

This technique was first described by Kary Mullis. It is now a powerful tool in molecular genetics.

It is an in vitro method of synthesis of nucleic acids.

Principle: There are three important steps in PCR. They include denaturation, renaturation and synthesis.

The double stranded DNA of interest is denatured (denaturation) to separate two individual strands. Each strand is then allowed to hybridize with a primer (renaturation). The primer template duplex is used for DNA synthesis (synthesis). The specific DNA sequence is rapidly amplified with the help of templates and primer. These three steps are repeated again and again to generate multiple copies of the DNA.

So within a very short time, a large number of copies of the desired DNA sequence are obtained. It is a very rapid and sensitive tool for analysis of DNA. It needs the presence of a very small quantity of genetic material. A wide range of samples, such as peripheral blood, bone marrow, sperm, hair follicle or even paraffin embedded tissues can be used.

Applications

- In prenatal diagnosis of inherited diseases by chorion villous biopsy samples
- Diagnosis of retroviral infections
- Diagnosis of bacterial infections—tuberculosis
- Diagnosis of malignancy—viral induced malignancies
- For identification of the suspects in forensic medicine.

DNA Finger Printing Technology

This was promoted by Dr Alec Jeffrey, a pioneer British genetic scientist. It is now used as a routing methodology in crime investigations for the identification of the criminals. The DNA is extracted from the material obtained in the crime scene and matched with the DNA of the suspected individual.

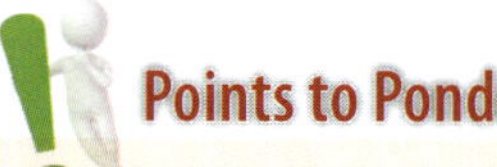

Points to Ponder

Recombinant DNA Technology is one of the recent advances in the field of genetics. It involves synthesis of a new DNA molecule from the DNA sequences. The desired DNA sequence is cut with the help of a special family of enzymes called the restriction endonucleases, this DNA sequence is introduced into a vector to generate multiple copies of the DNA. Then the desired DNA is harvested and used for the generation of proteins.

ASSESSMENT QUESTIONS

1. **What is recombinant DNA technology? Describe in detail the various methods. Add a note on the practical application of this technology.**
2. **Polymerase chain reaction.**
3. **Florescence in situ hybridization technique.**

MULTIPLE CHOICE QUESTIONS

1. **The florescence in situ hybridization technique (FISH) technique is:**
   A. A banding technique
   B. For studying karyotype
   C. An interphase cytogenetic technique
   D. All of the above
2. **What is the main purpose of the polymerase chain reaction (PCR)?**
   A. To amplify and replicate specific DNA sequences
   B. To create recombinant DNA molecules
   C. To analyze gene expression patterns
   D. To determine the genetic code of an individual

Answer Key for MCQs

1	2
C	A

CHAPTER 41

Chromosomal Aberrations

Learning Objectives

At the end of reading this chapter, the student shall be able to:

- Describe in detail the mechanism of chromosomal aberrations.

INTRODUCTION

Errors can occur either in the number or structure of the chromosomes. They are referred to as the numerical and structural chromosomal aberrations.

NUMERICAL CHROMOSOMAL ABERRATIONS

The normal number of chromosomes in human beings is 46. Any deviation from this number of chromosomes is called as **numerical chromosomal aberrations**. The normal chromosomal number is referred to as **Diploid [2n = 46]**. This pattern is seen in all somatic cells. **Haploid** refers to half the number of chromosomes [23 chromosomes]. This pattern is seen in gametes.

Polyploidy refers to increase in the number of chromosomes in multiples of n.

Triploidy means 69 chromosomes [3n] and **tetraploidy** means 92 chromosomes [4n]. When the total number of chromosomes is not an exact multiple of n it is called as **aneuploidy**. It may either increase in the total number or decrease in the total number of chromosomes [2n - 1 or 2 n + 1].

Common Causes for Aneuploidy

Aneuploidy occurs mostly due to failure of separation of chromosomes during cell division. This is called as **non-dysjunction**. Nondisjunction can occur during first meiotic division, second meiotic division or during mitosis. This results in unequal distribution of chromosomes in the daughter cells.

COMMON TYPES OF STRUCTURAL ANOMALIES OF CHROMOSOMES

They include:

- Balanced structural alterations—referred to as translocations
    - Reciprocal translocations
    - Robertsonian translocations
- Deletions—loss of genetic material from a chromosome
- Inversion—form of rearrangement of chromosome—pericentric or paracentric
- Ring chromosome—due to break at the two telomeric ends and an end to end fusion.
- Isochromosome—transverse division of the centromere—produces two short arms and two long arms.

Translocations

These are balanced structural alterations between two chromosomes in which the genetic material of one gets detached and gets itself attached to another chromosome. There are two types of translocations:

1. Balanced reciprocal translocations
2. Robertsonian translocation

Balanced Reciprocal Translocations (Fig. 41.1)

In this, there is exchange of genetic material distal to the break. It occurs mostly in nonhomologous chromosomes. There is perfect balance of transfer of genetic material. No chromosomal material is lost.

G-banded karyotypes of chromosomes: There is a balanced translocation. Chromosomes 1 and 22 have exchanged segments (arrows). The translocation is described as 46, XX, t (1:22) (q25; q13).

Robertsonian Translocation

This type occurs in acrocentric chromosomes (groups D and G). The short arm of one fuse with the short arm of another. The new fragment formed by their fusion is lost. This process is also called as **centric fusion** **(Fig. 41.2)**.

Insertion (Fig. 41.3)

It is a rare form of non-reciprocal translocation in which a fragment of chromosome is transferred to a nonhomologous chromosome. Two breaks occur in one chromosome which releases a fragment and one break occurs in the other to admit this fragment.

Inversion

This is a form of chromosomal aberration in which the genetic material is transferred within the same chromosome. They are of two types—pericentric and paracentric.

In pericentric inversion break occurs on both the p and q arms and the genetic material is transferred whereas in paracentric form, it involves either the short arm or the long arm. This does not produce any abnormal phenotype.

Isochromosome

In this, there is an abnormal split along the centromere leading to separation of the arms.

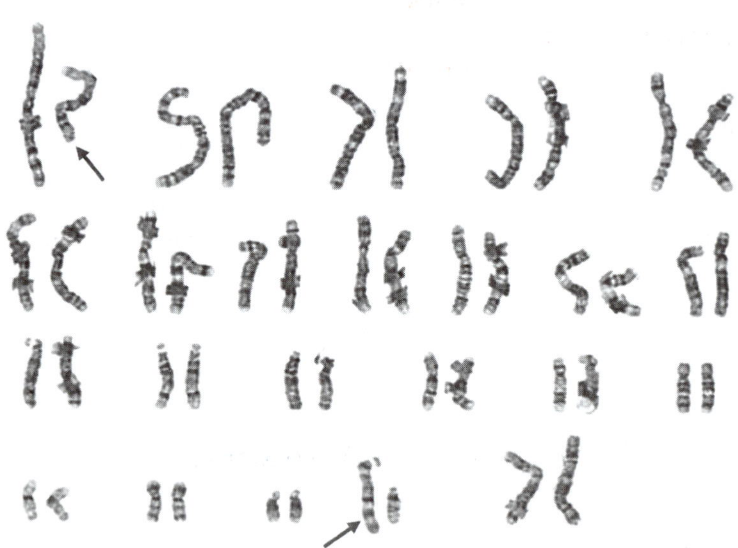

Fig. 41.1: Balanced reciprocal translocation.

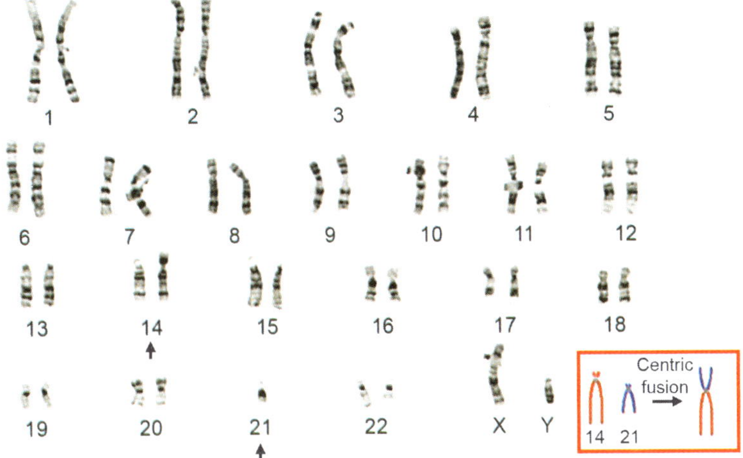

Fig. 41.2: Karyogram showing fusion.

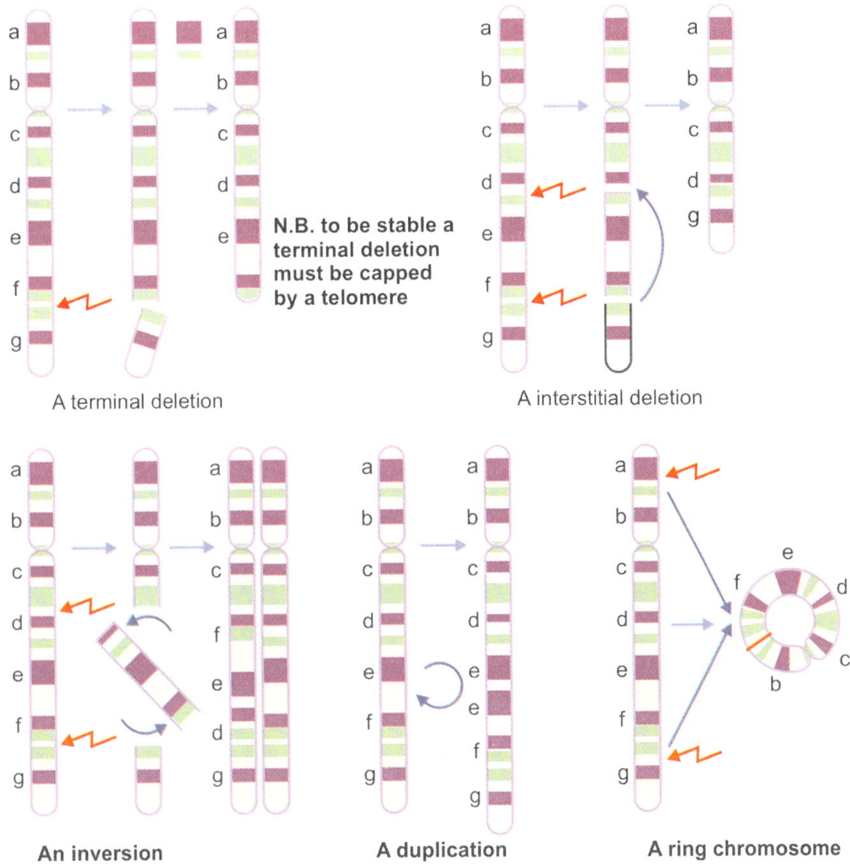

Fig. 41.3: Various types of structural alterations in a chromosome.

Ring Chromosome

It involves break at the terminal portions of the chromosomes followed by fusion of the cut ends. This is seen in cases of Turner's syndrome.

Deletion (Fig. 41.3)

This involves loss of a part of chromosome. It can be of two types terminal and interstitial.

Terminal Deletion

It is characterized by the deletion of a terminal part of the chromosome following a single break. Example Cri-du-chat syndrome (5p–).

Interstitial Deletion

It is characterized by two breaks and loss of the intervening portion. Example, WAGR syndrome, Prader-Willi syndrome and others.

CLINICAL PROFILE OF COMMON CHROMOSOMAL ABERRATIONS

Clinical profiles of some of the common chromosomal aberrations involving the autosomal chromosomes.

Down's Syndrome (Fig. 41.4)

This occurs due to trisomy 21. It was first identified by Langdon Down (1866). These individuals have 47 chromosomes. The extra chromosome is found in the 21 chromosome.

Trisomy 21 (47, XY, +21) is an extra chromosome 21 is the classic chromosomal constitution of individuals with Down syndrome. Partial trisomy's of chromosome 21 and mosaicism has also been observed associated with Down syndrome. The major clinical features include the following:

- Mental retardation
- Low IQ levels
- Hypotonia of muscles
- Low set malformed ears
- Prominent epicanthic folds
- Mongoloid slant
- Flat nose with low nasal bridge
- Wide opened mouth with protruding tongue
- High arched palate with delayed dentition
- Incurving of the little finger (clinodactyly)
- Presence of Simian crease
- Congenital heart defects

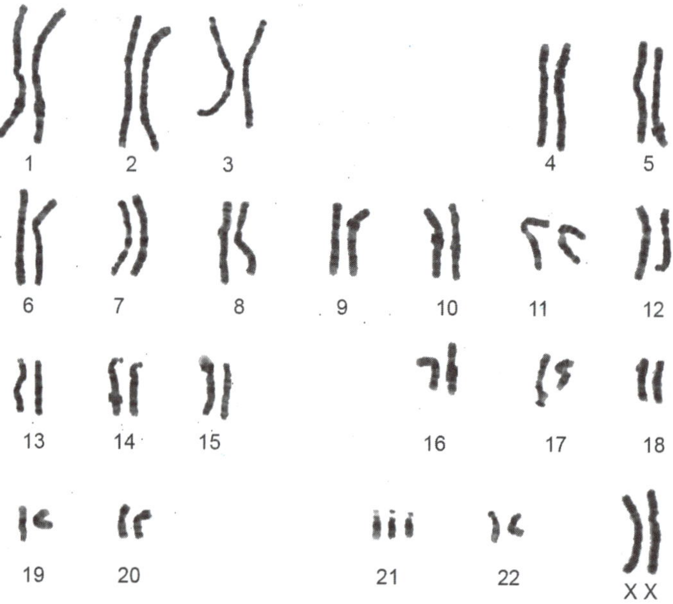

Fig. 41.4: Karyotype showing trisomy 21.

Edward's Syndrome

Edward's syndrome is due to trisomy of chromosome 18 and is characterized by:

- Mental retardation
- Prominent occiput
- Micrognathia
- Low set ears
- Short neck
- Overlapping fingers
- Congenital heart defects
- Renal malformations
- Limited hip abduction
- Rocker bottom feet

Patau Syndrome

Patau syndrome is due to Trisomy of chromosome 13. It is characterized by:

- Microcephaly and mental retardation
- Microphthalmia
- Cardiac defects
- Umbilical hernia
- Cleft lip/palate
- Renal defects
- Rocker bottom feet

CHROMOSOMAL ABERRATIONS INVOLVING SEX CHROMOSOMES

Clinical profiles of some of the common chromosomal aberrations involving the sex chromosomes.

Klinefelter's Syndrome (Fig. 41.5)

This was first described by Harry Klinefelter in 1942.

It is an important example for sex chromosome trisomy. About 80–90% of the affected individuals have a 47, XXY karyotype.

In this, the patients have testicular dysgenesis, gynecomastia, osteoporosis, lack of secondary male sexual characters, low mean IQ, tall, thin, eunuchoid features.

Turner's Syndrome

This disorder was first described by Turner in 1938.

It is an example for monosomy (45, XO). The clinical features include:

- Webbed neck
- Short stature

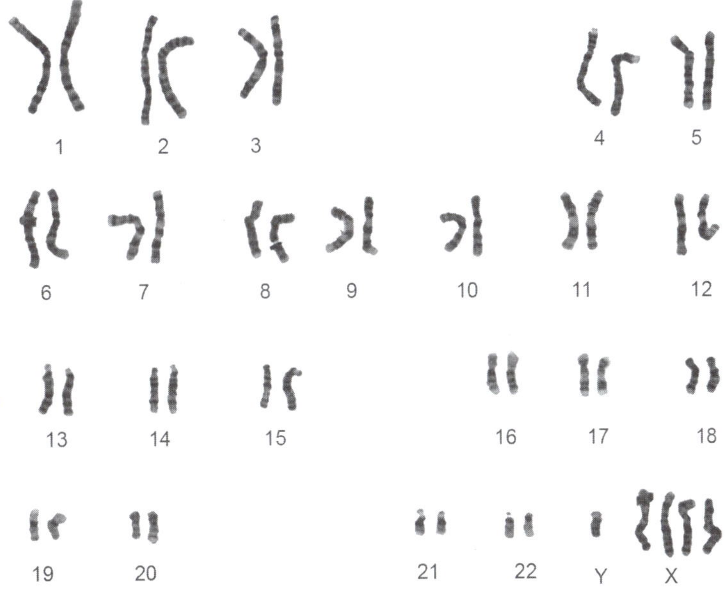

Fig. 41.5: Klinefelter's syndrome.

- Low posterior hairline
- High arched palate
- Swelling of the dorsum of hand and feet
- Congenital heart diseases, such as coarctation of aorta and bicuspid aortic valve
- Failure of development of secondary sexual characters
- Infantile genitalia
- Inadequate breast development
- Primary amenorrhea
- Horseshoe kidney, renal hypoplasia

OTHER SEX DEVELOPMENT DISORDERS

There are various criteria to assign a gender to an individual. They include:

1. *Genetic sex*—based on the presence or absence of Y chromosome
2. *Gonadal sex*—based on the histology of the gonads
3. *Ductal sex*—presence of derivatives from mullerian/wolffian ducts
4. *Phenotypic sex*—appearance of external genitalia.

Various abnormalities can occur in assigning the gender. The most common types are the following:

- *True hermaphrodite*: It is a term which implies the presence of both testicular and ovarian tissue in a same individual.
- *Pseudohermaphrodite*: This term is used to indicate a disagreement between the phenotypic and gonadal sex. This can be seen in both male and females. The most common cause for a female pseudohermaphroditism is congenital adrenal hyperplasia. Hyperplastic adrenals release increased amount of androgens which lead to masculinization. The common causes for male pseudohermaphroditism are gonadal dysgenesis during embryogenesis, abnormalities in the secretion of gonadotrophins, inborn biosynthetic defects in the metabolism of testosterone and androgen.

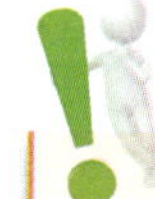

Points to Ponder

Errors can occur either in the number or structure of the chromosomes. They are referred to as the numerical and structural chromosomal aberrations.

ASSESSMENT QUESTIONS

1. **Describe the various types of chromosomal translocations.**
2. **Describe the clinical features of the following:**
   A. Down's syndrome
   B. Klinefelter's syndrome
   C. Turne's syndrome

MULTIPLE CHOICE QUESTIONS

1. **Gene deletion can affect:**
   A. Insertion B. Translation
   C. Transcription D. Deletion
2. **The most common cause of aneuploidy is:**
   A. Nondisjunction B. Isochrome formation
   C. Deletion D. Ring chromosome formation

3. **Robertsonian translocation is between:**
   A. One metacentric acid and one submedian chromosome
   B. Two submetacentric chromosomes
   C. Two median chromosomes
   D. Two acrocentric chromosomes
4. **Which of the following chromosomal abnormalities is associated with Klinefelter syndrome?**
   A. Trisomy 21
   B. Turner syndrome
   C. XYY syndrome
   D. 47, XXY
5. **Which of the following chromosomal abnormalities is associated with Edward's syndrome?**
   A. Trisomy 21
   B. Trisomy 18
   C. Turner syndrome
   D. Klinefelter syndrome

Answer Key for MCQs

1	2	3	4	5
C	A	D	D	B

CHAPTER 42

Modes of Inheritance

Learning Objectives

At the end of reading this chapter, the student shall be able to:

- Describe in detail the various modes of inheritance.

INTRODUCTION

The genetic disorders can be generally grouped as:

- *Chromosomal disorders*: Due to errors in the number and structure of the chromosomes (discussed in the earlier chapter).
- *Single gene disorders*: Due to mutation in a single gene. These are also called as **Mendelian disorders**. The defect can be in the autosomes or the sex chromosomes. These diseases are inherited in any one of the following patterns:
  - Autosomal dominant
  - Autosomal recessive
  - X-linked dominant
  - X-linked recessive
- *Diseases with multifactorial inheritance*: These are disorders which occur as a result of interaction of genetic factors in association with environment factors, infectious agents, radiation, drugs and chemicals and others.

Autosomal Dominant Pattern of Inheritance

The following are the important characters of an autosomal dominant disorder:

- The affected person will have an affected parent.
- The affected person will have normal and abnormal offsprings (50% chance).
- Both men and women are equally affected
- The disease appears in every generation without skipping.
- Normal children of the affected person do not transmit the disease.
- The mutations occur mostly in genes coding for regulatory proteins (e.g., membrane receptors) or structural proteins (e.g., collagen, hemoglobin).
- The diseases have a delayed onset of presentation.
- The persons will have variable clinical expression.

Table 42.1 gives few clinical examples of disorders inherited in an autosomal dominant pattern.

TABLE 42.1: Examples of autosomal dominant disorders.

Category	*Name of the disorder*
Hemopoietic	♦ Hereditary spherocytosis ♦ Von Willebrand disease
Nervous	♦ Huntington's disease ♦ Neurofibromatosis ♦ Myotonic dystrophy ♦ Tuberous sclerosis
Skeletal	♦ Marfan's syndrome ♦ Osteogenesis imperfecta ♦ Achondroplasia
Metabolic	♦ Familial hypercholesterolemia ♦ Acute intermittent porphyria
GIT	Familial polyposis coli
Renal	Polycystic kidney disease

Autosomal Recessive Pattern of Inheritance

The following are the important characters of an autosomal recessive disorder:

- The expression of the defect is uniform.
- Complete penetrance is common.
- Onset is frequently early in life.
- Both men and women have an equal chance of getting affected.
- Consanguinity is very common predisposing factor.
- **An heterozygote of an autosomal recessive trait is called a carrier.**
- If both the parents are affected, then all their children will be affected.
- Many in born errors of metabolism follows this pattern of inheritance.

Table 42.2 gives few clinical examples of disorders inherited in an autosomal recessive pattern.

TABLE 42.2: Examples of autosomal recessive disorders.

Category	*Name of the disorder*
Hemopoietic	♦ Sickle cell anemia ♦ Thalassemia
Endocrine	Congenital adrenal hyperplasia
Skeletal	♦ Ehler–Danlos syndrome ♦ Alkaptonuria
Metabolic	♦ Cystic fibrosis ♦ Phenylketonuria ♦ Galactosemia ♦ Lysosomal storage disorders ♦ Wilson's disease ♦ Alpha 1 antitrypsin deficiency ♦ Hemochromatosis ♦ Glycogen storage disorders
Nervous system	♦ Neuromuscular atrophy ♦ Friedreich ataxia ♦ Spinal muscular atrophy

X-linked Pattern of Inheritance

The sex chromosomes in male are XY and in female it is XX. These group of disorders are transmitted to future generations through the sex chromosomes. Genes on the Y chromosome shows a holandric pattern of inheritance and they are very uncommon. So almost all cases under this category are inherited through the X chromosomes. The X-linked disorders can be dominant or recessive. Practically, the dominant disorders are very rare. The well-known example for an X-linked dominant disorder is vitamin D resistant rickets.

The following are few general characters of an X-linked recessive disorders.

- The disease is usually symptomatic in men
- Women act as carriers of the disease.
- The women will manifest the disease very rarely, when there is aberrant lionization or mutations in the germ line.

Table 42.3 gives some of the examples of the X-linked recessive disorders.

TABLE 42.3: Examples of X-linked recessive disorders.

Category	*Name of the disorder*
Hemopoietic	♦ Hemophilia A and B ♦ Chronic granulomatous disease of childhood ♦ Glucose 6 phosphate dehydrogenase deficiency
Immune	♦ Agammaglobulinemia ♦ Wiskott-Aldrich syndrome
Metabolic	♦ Diabetes insipidus ♦ Lesch-Nyhan syndrome
Nervous system	Fragile X syndrome
Musculoskeletal	Duchenne muscular dystrophy

The following are few general characters of X-linked dominant disorders:

a. This trait is more frequent in women than in men.
b. Men have generally a milder expression of the disease.
c. Affected male transmits the trait to all his daughters not to his sons.

Example: Vitamin D resistant rickets.

There are certain terminologies used in the mode of inheritance.

Gene expression: It refers to the degree of expression of a particular gene and clinically it can be mild, moderate or severe.

Gene penetrance: It is term used to determine the fact whether a particular gene will be expressed or not.

Gene pleiotropy: Normally every gene will have a direct primary effect. When a gene produces multiple phenotypic effects it is called a **genetic pleiotropism**.

Genetic heterogeneity: It is a reverse of genetic pleiotropy, where several group of genes produce a single phenotypic defect.

For example congenital deafness can occur due to various autosomal dominant, autosomal recessive and X-linked disorders.

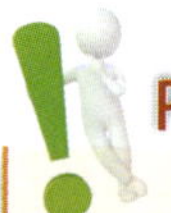

Points to Ponder

There are various modes of inheritance which includes:

- Autosomal dominant
- Autosomal recessive
- X-linked recessive
- Each will have unique patter of clinical significance.

ASSESSMENT QUESTION

1. **X-linked recessive disorders.**

MULTIPLE CHOICE QUESTIONS

1. **When both alleles are fully expressed in a heterozygote it is called:**
   A. Codominance B. Variable expressivity
   C. Polymorphism D. Pleiotropism
2. **An example of co-dominance is:**
   A. Sickle cell anemia B. Hemolytic anemia
   C. Blood group antigens D. Spermatic antigens
3. **Mutation in single genes produces:**
   A. Deletions and insertions B. Chromosomal disorders
   C. Mendelian disorders D. All of the above
4. **All are autosomal recessive disorders, *except*:**
   A. Homocystinuria B. Huntington's disease
   C. Wilson's disease D. Friedreich's ataxia
5. **Most common mendelian disorder is:**
   A. Cystic fibrosis B. Colonic polyposis
   C. Retinoblastoma D. Familial hypercholesterolemia
6. **All are autosomal dominant disorders, *except*:**
   A. Huntington's chorea B. Hereditary spherocytosis
   C. Adult polycystic kidney D. Phenylketonuria

Answer Key for MCQs

1	2	3	4	5	6
A	C	C	B	D	D

43

CHAPTER

Prenatal Diagnosis

Learning Objectives

At the end of reading this chapter, the student shall be able to:

- Enlist the common indications for prenatal diagnosis.
- Enumerate the common methods of prenatal diagnosis.

INTRODUCTION

With the advances in the field of medical genetics, it is now possible to diagnose many of the genetic disorders in utero. This forms an integral step in genetic counseling.

INDICATIONS

Prenatal diagnosis has to done in the following situations:

- It is very much essential for a genetic disorder for which there is unsatisfactory treatment.
- When the risk of pregnancy is very high.
- Disorder in which an accurate prenatal test is possible.
- If the maternal age is more than 35 to 40 years of age.
- If one of the parent is a known carrier.
- When the couple already have a child with genetic defects.

METHODOLOGIES OF PRENATAL DIAGNOSIS

There are various methods available for diagnosis of genetic disorders prenatally. They include:

- Amniocentesis
- Chorion villous biopsy
- Ultrasonography
- Fetoscopy
- Fetal blood sampling
- Cord blood sampling
- Maternal blood sampling
- Preimplantation diagnosis
- Techniques using recombinant DNA technology

Amniocentesis (Fig. 43.1)

This is one of the best known prenatal diagnostic techniques for certain congenital disorders. It is usually performed between the 13th and 15th weeks of pregnancy. In this procedure, a careful evaluation of the location of the placenta and fetus is done with an ultrasound.

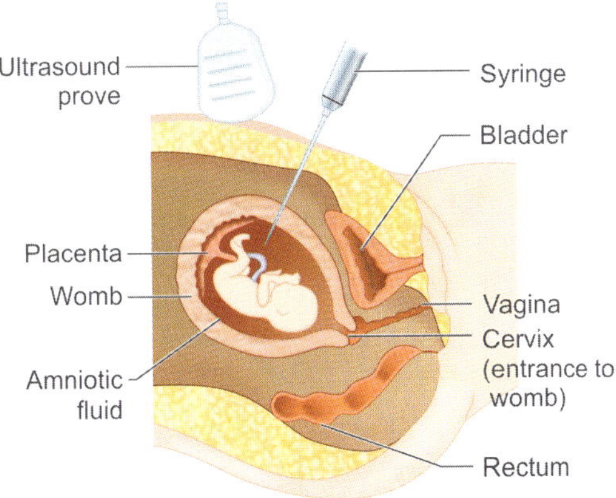

Fig. 43.1: Procedure of amniocentesis.

A thin, hollow needle is inserted into woman's uterus through the abdomen under local anesthesia, guided by ultrasound avoiding damage to placenta and the fetus. Around 10 to 20 mL of the amniotic fluid is aspirated. The fluid is subjected to centrifugation to separate the cells. The cells are then cultured for further karyotyping studies and the fluid is subjected to various biochemical tests for the detection of substances, such as the alpha fetoprotein, carcinoma embryonic antigen and others. Fetal cells floating in the fluid can be analyzed to detect chromosomal abnormalities, more than 100 metabolic disorders and some anatomic defects.

There is low-risk of miscarriage or infection following the procedure. Results of the test are ready in one to three weeks.

Chorionic Villous Biopsy [Chorion Villous Sampling (CVS)] (Fig. 43.2)

CVS is generally performed about the 8th or 11th week of pregnancy. CVS requires taking a small piece of the chorionic villi. Either a needle is inserted through the abdomen or a slim tube is inserted through the vagina to take a tiny tissue sample from outside the sac where the baby develops. The tissue is analyzed for chromosome disorders or various genetic conditions. Results are usually ready in one to two weeks. CVS is not routinely offered to all pregnant women because the test carries a risk of miscarriage, and possibly other complications. The merits of this procedure are the following:

- It can be done much earlier of gestation than the amniocentesis and is easily acceptable.
- The cellular yield is better than amniocentesis which allows rapid results.
- Termination of pregnancy is safer following chorionic villous biopsy as it is done in early weeks of gestation.

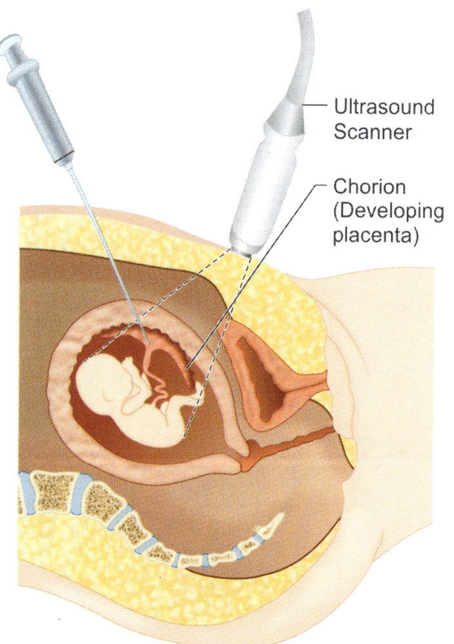

Fig. 43.2: Chorion villous sampling.

Alpha-fetoprotein Screening

This blood test is most often done between 16 and 18 weeks. The test identifies pregnancies at higher-than-average risk of certain serious birth defects, such as spina bifida and down syndrome. In most cases, an abnormal test result does not indicate a problem with the fetus.

Alpha-fetoprotein (AFP) is a substance produced by the liver of the fetus. A small amount of AFP passes into the mother's bloodstream. AFP levels can be measured during pregnancy by taking a sample of either the mother's blood or the amniotic fluid. This test cannot diagnose a birth defect, it can only indicate an increased risk. Neural tube defects are among the most common and severe problems associated with high test levels. Low test level results are sometimes associated with chromosomal abnormalities, such as Down syndrome.

Cordocentesis

Umbilical vein sampling (cordocentesis): In this procedure, a fine needle is passed through the mother's abdomen into the fetal vein in the umbilical cord. The technique allows fetal blood to be tested, facilitates intrauterine blood transfusions, and enables drugs to be injected directly into the baby if necessary.

Role of Ultrasound in Prenatal Diagnosis

The ultrasound is very much useful in most of the prenatal diagnostic procedures. The most important functions include the following:

- Localization of the fetus and the placenta
- Ascertaining the gestational age
- Recognizing congenital defects, such as anencephaly, spina bifida, microcephaly, hydrocephalus, meningocele, myelomeningocele and others.

Fetoscopy

This is a fiberoptic self-illuminated instrument used for visualizing the fetus in utero. It is inserted in the amniotic cavity under local anesthesia best between 18 and 22 weeks of gestation.

Preimplantation Diagnosis

This is mostly done in conceptus produced as a result of in vitro fertilization. The fertilized oocyte is allowed to develop up to 8 cell blastocyst stage. A single blastomere is removed and the DNA is extracted from the cell. This DNA is amplified to several copies with the help of polymerase chain reaction (PCR) and a through genetic analysis is made. If the conceptus is free of any genetic errors, it is implanted into the mother.

Recombinant DNA Technology

Recombinant DNA technology also helps in the prenatal diagnosis of a variety of disorders. A variety of DNA probes are now available for this purpose. It is now mostly followed for the prenatal diagnosis of hemoglobinopathies.

Points to Ponder

- Prenatal diagnosis has to done in the following situations:
  - It is very much essential for a genetic disorder for which there is unsatisfactory treatment.
  - When the risk of pregnancy is very high. Disorder in which an accurate prenatal test is possible.
  - If the maternal age is more than 35 to 40 years of age.
  - If one of the parent is a known carrier.
  - When the couple already have a child with genetic defects.

ASSESSMENT QUESTION

1. **Methods of prenatal diagnosis.**

MULTIPLE CHOICE QUESTION

1. **Which can make the earliest prenatal diagnosis of congenital disorders?**
   A. Amniocentesis
   B. Maternal urine examination
   C. Umbilical venous blood analysis
   D. Chorionic villi biopsy

Answer Key for MCQs

1
D

CHAPTER 44

Genetic Counseling

Learning Objectives

At the end of reading this chapter, the student shall be able to:

- Discuss in detail the role of nurses in prenatal diagnosis and genetic counseling.

INTRODUCTION

Genetic counseling is usually done by qualified genetic counselors, who will conduct genetic tests, evaluate the family history and medical records to identify the possibility of passing any genetic disorders to the baby. Some of the genetic disorders that could be identified are Down's syndrome, cystic fibrosis, sickle cell disease, Tay-Sachs disease and spina bifida. Some reputed hospitals offer genetic counseling as part of their maternity care program.

Genetic counseling also involves:

- Educating the affected couple to understand the nature of the genetic disorder.
- Giving counseling and psychological support.
- Providing the necessary information on support groups and services to manage the genetic condition.

Ideally, it is best to seek genetic counseling before becoming pregnant. It will be especially beneficial if the baby is at risk of inheriting genetic disorders.

DEFINITION

Genetic counseling is the process by which patients or relatives, at risk of an inherited disorder, are advised of the consequences and nature of the disorder, the probability of developing or transmitting it, and the options open to them in management and family planning in order to prevent, avoid or ameliorate it.

COMMON INDICATIONS FOR GENETIC COUNSELING

- If a standard prenatal screening test yields an abnormal result.
- Either parent or a close relative has an inherited disease or birth defect.
- Either parent already has children with birth defects or genetic disorders.
- If the age is over 35.
- History of miscarriages before.

GENETIC COUNSELOR

A genetic counselor is a medical genetics expert with a master of science degree. Most enter the field from a variety of disciplines, including biology, genetics, nursing, psychology, public health and social work. They work as members of a healthcare team and act as a patient advocate as well as a genetic resource to physicians. Genetic counselors provide information and support to families who have members with birth defects or genetic disorders, and to families who may be at risk for a variety of inherited conditions.

They identify families at risk, investigate the problems present in the family, interpret information about the disorder, analyze inheritance patterns and risks of recurrence and review available testing options with the family.

Genetic counselors are present at high risk or specialty prenatal clinics that offer prenatal diagnosis, pediatric care centers, and adult genetic centers. Genetic counseling can occur before conception (i.e., when one or two of the parents are carriers of a certain trait) through to adulthood (for adult onset genetic conditions, such as Huntington's disease or hereditary cancer syndromes).

FUNCTIONS OF A GENETIC COUNSELOR

- Any person may seek out genetic counseling for a condition they may have inherited from their biological parents. A woman may be referred for genetic counseling if pregnant and undergoing prenatal testing or screening. Genetic counselors educate the patient about their testing options and inform them of their results.
- If a prenatal screening or test is abnormal, the genetic counselor evaluates the risk of an affected pregnancy, educates the patient about these risks and informs the patient of their options.
- A person may also undergo genetic counseling after the birth of a child with a genetic condition. In these instances, the genetic counselor explains the condition to the patient along with recurrence risks in future children. In all cases of a positive family history for a condition, the genetic Counselor can evaluate risks, recurrence and explain the condition itself.

OTHER FUNCTIONS OF THE COUNSELOR

- Genetic counselors provide supportive counseling to families, serve as patient advocates and refer individuals and families to community or state support services.
- They serve as educators and resource people for other healthcare professionals and for the general public.
- Some counselors also work in administrative capacities. Many engage in research activities related to the field of medical genetics and genetic counseling.
- The field of genetic counseling is rapidly expanding and many counselors are taking on "non-traditional roles" which includes working for genetic companies and laboratories.
- Genetic counseling is a communication process which deals with human problems associated with the occurrence, or the risk of occurrence of a genetic disorder in a family. This process involves an attempt by one or more appropriately trained persons (genetic counselors) to help the individual or family to:
    - Comprehend the medical facts, including the diagnosis, the probable course of the disorder, and the available management
    - Appreciate the way heredity contributes to disorder, and the risk of recurrence in specified relatives
    - Understand the options for dealing with the risk of recurrence
    - Choose the course of action which seems appropriate to them in view of their risk and the family goals and in accordance with the decision and make the best possible adjustment to the disorder in the affected family member and/or the risk of recurrence of that disorder.

Presently, genetic counseling goes beyond mere presentations of risk facts and figures to the prevention and cure of disease, the relief of pain and the maintenance of health. For many disorders, it is only possible to give precise recurrence risk conditions and also the order of risk.

Moral, ethical and philosophical aspects involved in genetic counseling are now emerging as major issues with the development of the application of various diagnostic techniques as amniocentesis and fetoscopy during pregnancy.

NURSES AS GENETIC COUNSELORS

Knowledge of genetics will help nurses to:

- Development of nonjudgmental attitudes about genetics and related disorders.
- Knowledge of information needs to be collected before providing genetic counseling.
- Application of traditional nursing skills, such as patient education, confidentiality, and counseling about genetic information.
- In developing countries, there is less awareness about genetic disorders and healthcare facilities offering services for testing and management of genetic disorders. Nurses are the primary healthcare providers who can direct them to right place for their diagnosis and management. So that, genetic information will equip nurses to provide effective referral services to their genetic clients.

ETHICS IN PRENATAL DIAGNOSIS AND THE SUBSEQUENT ABORTIONS

Moral problems arise constantly in social life with the need to resolve conflicts between moral rules and principles to help, regulate and modify desires. For example, when genetic risks are high, the desire to have a healthy child and to avoid danger to oneself, family and society are frequently in conflict. Although 96% of the counseling sessions end well with no or very little chances for the occurrence of the disease, the remaining 4% people in the high-risk category are left with three options:

i. Prenatal diagnosis and abortion if required
ii. Artificial insemination
iii. Gene therapy

In a broader view, the problems of moral choices can be, in decreasing order of frequency and difficulty as: (i) abortion choices, (ii) problems related to access and distribution of prenatal diagnosis as a service, and (iii) problems related to research on prenatal diagnosis.

Abortion Choices

The choice to abort any pregnancy is a moral problem wherever duties to protect the interests of the woman, the fetus and the society are held to be in conflict. Historically some of the earliest conflicts about prenatal diagnosis were on the question of whether abortion was its primary goal. One group argued that the destruction of certain fetuses was the morally unacceptable goal of prenatal diagnosis outweighing the possibility that it might give reassurance to some at-risk parents that their child would (likely) be unaffected. The other group contended that since prenatal diagnosis was done largely with an intent to abort an affected fetus, the practice contradicted the basic purpose of medicinal science.

Abortion choices, after prenatal diagnosis present difficulties and dilemmas for several reasons:

- The high moral status of the woman carrying the fetus at mid-trimester.
- The wide spectrum of severity in some diagnosable genetic disorders.
- The treatability of some disorders.
- The possibility of diagnosing twins where one is affected and the other healthy.
- Claims that the practice of mid-trimester abortion creates a precedence for pediatric/euthanasia, selective abortion.
- Decisions about treatment of handicapped newborns.

With the involvement of euthenics, i.e., state-of-the-art of treatment for genetic disorders by modification of the environment to allow the genetically abnormal individual to develop normally and to live a relatively normal life, abortion choices will become predictably more complicated.

Euthenics can be applied both medically and socially—examples of phenylketonuria (PKU) treatment by diet control, use of human growth hormone for growth disorders, purified factor VIII for hemophilia A, etc., illustrate medical euthenics, while special schools for deaf children, illustrate social euthenics.

Problems Related to Access to and Distribution of Prenatal Diagnosis Service

Access to and distribution of prenatal diagnosis and genetic services is the central moral problem in medical ethics. Except for Denmark where about 80% of the women who need prenatal diagnosis receive it, most of the countries do not meet the true need for services. Further, women who undergo prenatal diagnosis belong largely to higher economic groups. Lack of financial resources and adequate planning have restricted the distribution of genetic services in almost every country.

ETHICAL PROBLEMS FACED BY THE COUNSELOR

There cannot be a universal model for genetic counseling because counseling is an understanding of a set of facts according to the counselors' frame of reference, background in the science of genetics, and previous training and experience in effectively communicating with the consultee. In order to communicate effectively, the counselor must consider the educational background of the consultee, what to disclose and how to limit the ways in which he can communicate.

- It has been found that the principal obstacles to the effective use of genetic counseling are emotional conflicts, and lack of knowledge of genetics and biology
- An equally difficult assignment for the counselor is presenting his knowledge in an unbiased manner. It is difficult for a counselor to impart unbiased information because of the consultee's personal and family history, such as parental age, ethnic background, reproductive history, i.e., abortions, stillborn or dead siblings, and the age, sex and health of the living children. This may lead the counselor to adopt a directive rather than a non-directive approach to genetic counseling.
- The major difference between directive and non-directive counseling is whether or not the counselor actively participates or helps the consultees to make a decision. Directive counseling has a positive influence on the consultee's decision. The non-directive approach involves presentation of the facts in an unbiased manner, leaving the entire responsibility of decision with the consultee.
- Counselors can be and have been fooled with respect to certain inherited conditions because of improper measurements and observations and/or because of similar symptoms of many genetic diseases. However, the counselor probably cannot completely disassociate himself from his/her own values and present the information in such a way that the recipient is not completely free to make his own judgment. For example, in interpreting the probability even for a single gene disease, the counselor, depending on his level of personal emotional involvement in the particular case, may bias or slant the data. The Counselor may not change the truth but his tone, manner of speech and other facial and body gestures can influence the information transfer. For example, in a case where a counselor feels that a pregnancy might be best for a family, he could say to Mr and Mrs X, 'there is only one chance in four that your child would be affected. Your chances for a healthy birth are very high, three chances out of four or 75%'. For family Y with these same inherited defects, but a

different social history, the counselor may emphasize more on probable disorder.

- During counseling, the counselor may come across other findings, that may put him in a situation of ethical dilemma. Some of these are fetal sex, findings of questionable or potentially harmful significance, false paternity, etc.
- Occasionally, disputes arise about the significance of laboratory findings especially about the true v/s pseudomosaicism or by possibility of contamination by maternal cells. Another example is when sonography suggests an irregularity of the fetal head but the amniotic fluid is normal for alpha-fetoprotein. The issue is whether the disclosure of a finding of probably small significance will result in severe parental anxiety leading to psychological problems. Medical geneticists learn.
- Many family secrets, such as previous abortions, previous abnormal births, and occasional false paternity. The findings can be made after prenatal diagnosis of a recessive disorder and testing the carrier parents or in the context of genetic screening after the birth of an affected infant. The putative father believes that he must be a carrier, but tests are negative. The option left is partial or total deception.

ETHICAL GUIDANCE IN GENETIC COUNSELING

A proposal for guidelines for prenatal diagnosis, genetic counseling and screening has been made. The proposal assumes that consensus exists among medical geneticists, obstetricians and parents about some key ethical principles and approaches to difficult choices:

- Parental autonomy in abortion choices
- Non-directive counseling
- Prenatal diagnosis that must be provided when parents need the information to prepare themselves for the birth of a possibly affected child.
- Practitioners need to disclose to the consultee the risks and benefits of each procedure in prenatal diagnosis.
- Information of XY females and XX males with great care that casts no ambiguity on the patient's social and phenotypic sexual identity.
- In case putative father is not the biological father of the fetus, the mother to be informed first to avoid social problems and she may be left to take final decision.
- Medical geneticists to decide which of the disorders warrants the options of prenatal diagnosis and termination of pregnancy.
- Consequences from the above to be evaluated in terms of basic ethical principles, and critical tests of what is best for the individuals, groups and society.

ANALYSIS OF GENETIC DISORDER: ROLE OF PARAMEDICAL PERSONNEL

While dealing with a case of probable genetic origin, the first step is recording the family history of the index case or proband. Proband is an affected individuality are also called as propositus if he is a male and proposita if she is a female. The common symbols used in a pedigree analysis is given in **Figure 44.1**.

The information that are usually gathered includes:

Age of onset, duration of complaints and presence of any other major illness.

The next step is to examine the first-degree relatives—parents, siblings and offspring of the proband. The information should be properly recorded in the form as given below:

- Does any relative suffer from similar illness?
- This will help to decide the pattern of inheritance and the recurrence risk of the present disorder.
- Does the relatives show any other disease which is not present in the proband?

  For example, in case of dissecting aneurysm caused by Marfan's syndrome,

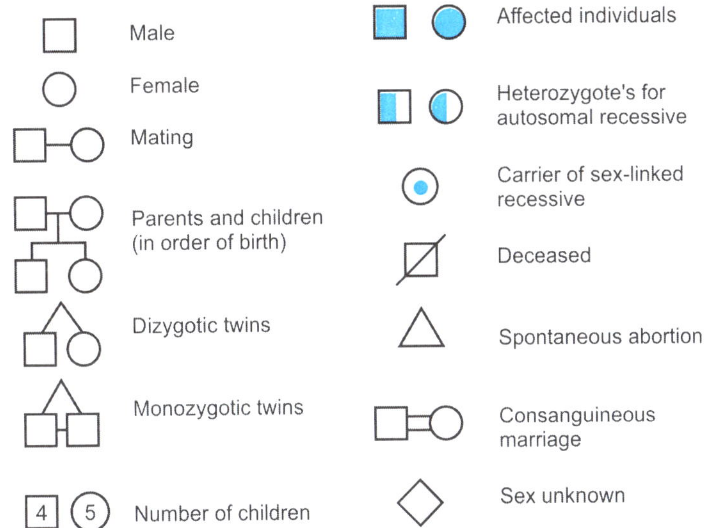

Fig. 44.1: Common symbols in pedigree analysis.

kindly ask about the presence of cardiac anomalies, ocular manifestations and skeletal manifestations.

- Is the proband an outcome of consanguineous marriage?
- This is very important because most of the outcomes of the consanguineous marriages have disorders with autosomal recessive mode of inheritance.
- What is the ethnic group of the family? This is again important because certain illness are common in certain ethnic groups.
- Any information regarding infant deaths, still births, abortions should be recorded with due importance.
- Any deformity in the fetus or the deceased infant must also be recorded.
- Illegitimacy should be borne in mind and proper enquiry with the family doctor and medical social worker should be carried out.
- The full family address of the proband and the relatives must be recorded as it will be helpful in contacting them in future.

Genetic counseling is a practical method of calculating risk figures, intended for information regarding the unborn, and we ought to use it in an efficient manner but in a direction, which our ethics and morality point to. The decision taken by the parents after the counseling session must leave them satisfied instead of placing them in a state of dilemma.

CONCLUSION

Application of science and scientific principles has two faces. To decide the correct use, man must deal with his conscious, individual and social status and the ethics underlying the applications.

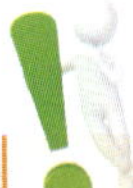

Points to Ponder

Genetic counseling is the process by which patients or relatives, at risk of an inherited disorder, are advised of the consequences and nature of the disorder, the probability of developing or transmitting it, and the options open to them in management and family planning in order to prevent, avoid or ameliorate

ASSESSMENT QUESTION

1. **Discuss in detail the role of nurses as genetic counselors.**

MULTIPLE CHOICE QUESTIONS

1. **What is the primary role of a genetic counselor?**
   A. To perform genetic testing on patients
   B. To diagnose genetic disorders in patients
   C. To provide information and support to individuals and families regarding genetic conditions, inheritance patterns, and available testing options
   D. To administer gene therapy to patients with genetic disorders
2. **Which of the following is NOT a typical responsibility of a genetic counselor?**
   A. Interpreting genetic test results for patients
   B. Performing surgical procedures to correct genetic abnormalities
   C. Providing emotional support and counseling to individuals and families affected by genetic conditions
   D. Educating healthcare professionals about genetics and genetic testing

Answer Key for MCQs

1	2
C	B

Recent Advances in Medical Genetics and Gene Therapy

Learning Objectives

At the end of reading this chapter, the student shall be able to:

- Describe the recent advances happening in field of biomedical genetics.

INTRODUCTION

There are various advancements and improvements in the field of medical genetics. The most important one is the human genome project and gene therapy.

HUMAN GENOME PROJECT

The human genome project was conceived in 1984 and the work for it officially began in 1990. The primary objective of the project was to determine the nucleotide sequence of the entire human nuclear genome. James Watson was the first director of this project.

It is a major attempt to map and sequence the entire human genome. It has been found that the human genome contains 50,000–100,000 genes with a total 3,200,000,000 base pairs. Approximately, 1.1 to 1.5% of the genome codes for the proteins. The number of protein coded genes is in the range of 30,000 to 40,000. Genes associated with many diseases, breast cancer, muscle diseases, deafness and blindness have been identified. This will help in improving our knowledge about various genetic factors and will also help in the management of various genetic disorders. Some of the benefits of the human genome project are:

- Identification of human genes and its function
- Understanding polygenic disorders, such as cancer, diabetes, hypertension
- Improvements in gene therapy
- To formulate genetic basis of psychiatry disorders
- To improve knowledge on various mutations

GENE THERAPY

This is a process of inserting genes into the cells to treat diseases. The newly introduced gene will encode the missing protein and correct the deficiency.

There are two forms of gene therapy:

1. *Gene augmentation therapy*—in which a new gene is introduced into the genome to replace the missing gene product.
2. *Gene inhibition therapy*—here an antisense gene is used to inhibit the expression of the dominant gene.

This involves replacement of a defective gene by a normal gene. The normal gene is delivered through proper vectors and it is introduced into the appropriate cell. It requires introduction of foreign DNA sequences with stable integration and gene expression.

The newly introduced gene usually replaces the missing gene. The gene is introduced into the cell by two methods:

1. The desired cells are removed from the individual, an appropriate gene is introduced into these cells and they are transplanted back to the patient.
2. In the second method, the newly synthesized gene is directly introduced into the target tissue.

   There are several methods for introducing the gene into the target tissue. They include direct physical methods, such as the:

   - Liposome mediated DNA transfer
   - Receptor mediated endocytosis or through indirect vector-based methods. The common vectors used are the retroviruses, adenoviruses and occasionally herpes virus.

The common target tissue includes the hepatocytes, bone marrow cells, cells of the central nervous system and muscular tissue.

The common diseases treated by gene therapy includes various types of cancers, peripheral vascular disease, coronary artery disease and acquired immunodeficiency syndrome.

The future of gene therapy is promising and it is likely that this technology will be applied to treat a wide range of diseases in the near future.

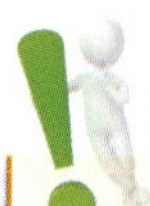

Points to Ponder

There are various advancements and improvements in the field of medical genetics. The most important one is the human genome project and gene therapy.

Answer Key for MCQs

1
B

Index

Page numbers followed by *f* refer to figure, *fc* refer to flowchart, and *t* refer to table.

A

C

F

G

N

O

P

R

S

U

V

W

X

Y

Z